Gynecologic Urology and Urodynamics

Theory and Practice

Gynecologic Urology and Urodynamics

Theory and Practice

Edited by

Donald R. Ostergard, M.D.

With contributions by   *Mogens Asmussen, M.D.*
William E. Bradley, M.D.
Philip J. DiSaia, M.D.
C. Paul Hodgkinson, M.D.
Thomas A. McCarthy, M.D.
Donald R. Ostergard, M.D.
Jack R. Robertson, M.D.
Stuart L. Stanton,
F.R.C.S., M.R.C.O.G.
Charles B. Stone, M.D.
Emil A. Tanagho, M.D.

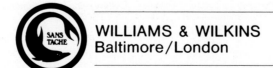

WILLIAMS & WILKINS
Baltimore/London

Copyright ©, 1980
The Williams & Wilkins Company
428 E. Preston Street
Baltimore, MD 21202, U.S.A.

Made in the United States of America

Reprinted 1981

Library of Congress Cataloging in Publication Data

Main entry under title:

Gynecologic urology and urodynamics.

   "Based upon presentations by the authors to post graduate courses ... [held] in
Los Angeles, California, June 22–23, 1978; Anaheim, California, March 14–16, 1979;
and North Hollywood, California, December 6–9, 1979."
   Includes index.
   1. Bladder—Diseases. 2. Urethra—Diseases. 3. Urinary stress incontinence.
4. Gynecology. I. Ostergard, Donald R. II. Asmussen, Mogens. [DNLM: 1. Genital
diseases, Female—Congresses. 2. Urologic diseases—Congresses. 3. Urodynamics—
Congresses. 4. Urinary incontinence—Congresses. WJ190 P857g 1978–1979]
RC484.G97   616.6   80-11894
ISBN 0-683-06645-5

Composed and printed at the
Waverly Press, Inc.
Mt. Royal and Guilford Aves.
Baltimore, MD 21202, U.S.A.

Dedication

I gratefully dedicate this book to my loving wife, Charlene, for putting up with my many hours of editing and for her help and suggestions in the writing of this text.

Preface

The multiplicity of different procedures, operations, concepts and evaluations relating to female urinary incontinence bespeaks the complexity of this problem. In spite of the "80%" surgical cure rate reported by various writers, all too often the gynecologist must care for the patient who is still incontinent after more than one operative procedure. There is genuine uneasiness by all who are confronted by the patient's question: "Will *this* operation cure my incontinence?"

The custom of performing a vaginal reparative operation on the basis of history alone continues to be the norm. When the vaginal operation fails, a retropubic procedure follows. The physician refers those patients who are still incontinent after the second operation with an air of resignation that little hope is in prospect.

From time to time questions arise about the scope of responsibility of the obstetrician-gynecologist regarding urinary tract symptoms in the female and the nature of the preoperative evaluation. All too often failures of operative treatment are due to the lack of proper assessment of the lower urinary tract before surgery.

The goal of this text is to promote a more active role of the obstetrician-gynecologist in the evaluation of the lower urinary tract regardless of how obvious the patient's symptoms of stress incontinence may seem. Office procedures are now available to adequately screen the lower urinary tract. More sophisticated techniques are now available to accurately diagnose alterations of vesicourethral physiology. The physician rapidly learns the skills necessary to perform or interpret the results of these evaluations.

The medical literature of the past few years contains information concerning the neurophysiology, maturation of micturition, new techniques for evaluation of the lower urinary tract and the fascinating new field of urodynamics. Unfortunately, most of this material is in publications which the practicing obstetrician-gynecologist does not regularly review. This text collates the relevant medical literature in a readily comprehensive format. The contributors to this text are experts in such diverse areas of medicine as neurology, urology, gynecology and psychiatry. The foundation of their collective clinical experience with a sound basis in the medical literature leads to the formulation of a logical, orderly, practical evaluation of the patient's lower urinary tract. The thoroughness of this evaluation ensures the likeliness of clinical success. The clinical evaluation and triage plans provide a clinical diagnosis and treatment programs which are unique for each individual patient.

This text brings together the known facets of lower urinary tract physiology and pathophysiology which are needed for an in-depth understanding of the basis of urinary complaints of the individual patient. The "anatomy of failure" in the past has largely been a failure to apply the correct treatment to the specific urinary malfunction and to a preoccupation with incontinence as the only symptom of the female urinary tract. The availability of modern urodynamic evaluation equipment now allows us to alter this myopic view of the lower urinary tract. A comprehensive urodynamic evaluation of the patient in a step-by-step fashion allows the establishment of a specific diagnosis. The physician then treats specific problems either medically or surgically. Surgical procedures are applied only when indicated for that patient with true anatomical stress incontinence. The education of the physician in the establishment of specific therapies based upon appropriate diagnosis is the goal of this text.

The material in this text is based upon presentations by the authors to *Postgraduate Courses in Gynecologic Urology, Theory and Practice*, in Los Angeles, California, June 22–23, 1978; Anaheim, California; March 14–16, 1979; and North Hollywood, California, December 6–9, 1979.

Contributors

Mogens Asmussen, M.D.
Research Fellow
Gynecological Oncology Department
The Norwegian Radium Hospital
Oslo, Norway

William E. Bradley, M.D.
Professor of Neurology and Obstetrics and Gynecology
Department of Obstetrics and Gynecology and Neurology
University of California at Irvine
Chief, Section of Neurology
Veteran's Administration Hospital
Long Beach, California

Philip J. DiSaia, M.D.
Professor and Chairman
Department of Obstetrics and Gynecology
University of California, Irvine

C. Paul Hodgkinson, M.D.
Consultant and Former Chairman
Department of Obstetrics and Gynecology
Henry Ford Hospital
Detroit, Michigan

Thomas A. McCarthy, M.D.
Assistant Professor of Obstetrics and Gynecology
UCLA School of Medicine
Los Angeles County Harbor/UCLA Medical Center
Torrance, California

Donald R. Ostergard, M..D.
Associate Medical Director
Women's Hospital
Memorial Hospital Medical Center
Long Beach, California
Professor of Obstetrics and Gynecology
University of California at Irvine

Jack R. Robertson, M.D.
Clinical Professor
Department of Obstetrics and Gynecology
University of California at Irvine

Stuart L. Stanton, F.R.C.S., M.R.C.O.G.
Honorary Senior Lecturer
Urodynamic Unit
Department of Obstetrics and Gynecology
St. George's Hospital
University of London
London, England

Charles B. Stone, M.D.
Associate Clinical Professor
Department of Psychiatry
UCLA School of Medicine
Los Angeles County Harbor/UCLA Medical Center
Torrance, California

Emil A. Tanagho, M.D.
Professor and Chairman
Department of Urology
University of California School of Medicine
San Francisco, California

Acknowledgments

The contributors to this text wish to gratefully acknowledge the artistic talents of Carol Beckerman and Meg Newton for preparing the majority of the illustrations used in this book.

Contents

Appendices

Introduction and Historical Perspectives:

THE TIME HAS COME

Philip J. DiSaia, M.D.

"There is no more distressing lesion than urinary incontinence—a constant dribbling of the repulsive urine soaking the clothes which cling wet and cold to the thighs, making the patient offensive to herself and her family and ostracizing her from society."

Howard A. Kelly, M.D., 1928

It is somewhat paradoxical that the field of gynecological urology which gave birth to the greater discipline of gynecology has been so long in becoming a science of its own. In his book *Genitourinary Problems in Women*, Robertson discusses the ancient writing of the Kahun papyrus written approximately 2000 years B.C., devoted to diseases of women and including a discussion of diseases of the urinary bladder. Indeed, the Ebers papyrus in 1550 B.C. classified diseases by systems and organs. Robertson states that in Section 6, of this latter papyrus, there was a description for the cure of a woman who suffers from a disease of her urine, as well as her womb. Henhenit was one of six women attached to the court of Menuhotep II, of the 11th dynasty, who reigned in Egypt about 2050 B.C. Her mummified body was found in 1955; radiographs of this mummy revealed that she had an extensive urinary fistula.

It was one of our own, Marion Simms, who is credited with the birth of modern gynecology through his pioneer work in the treatment of obstetrical urinary fistulas. Robertson writes that Marion Simms chose to study medicine, much to his father's disgust, as the elder had only contempt for the medical profession. Simm's father felt that there was no science in medicine and there was no longer honor to be achieved by going from house to house with a box of pills in one hand and a squirt in the other. However, Marion

Simms did enter the field of medicine and started his practice in Lancaster, South Carolina. His first two patients were infants who died from cholera. He was so disturbed that he moved to Mount Meigs, Alabama, where he earned the reputation of a great surgeon and he married his childhood sweetheart, Eliza Theresa Jones, in December, 1836. His practice had flourished at that point and his income was a wholesome $3000 per year.

Robertson tells us of the birth of gynecology with a specific case. Evidently, Simms' settled life was changed by an event which eventually led to his great medical achievement. A Mrs. Merril was thrown from a horse and this resulted in an impacted retroverted uterus. She was brought to Simms after many other physicians had failed to help her. Although Simms did not like to examine women, he did recall the advice of one of his professors from medical school. He placed her in a knee-chest position and reluctantly applied pressure to the vagina. The impacted uterus suddenly yielded and Mrs. Merril had immediate relief. His success with this particular patient led him to consider examining several slave women with vesicovaginal fistulas, utilizing the same rather advantageous knee-chest position. He found that this position allowed careful examination of the vagina which had hitherto been very difficult. When examining patients with a fistula he was able to clearly see the opening, and he began thinking of methods for repair. As is well known, his first attempts at fistula repair utilized silk sutures, but these attempts failed. His first success was with a slave girl named Anarcha, where the fistula repair was accomplished with silver wire sutures. Her fistula had first occurred at the age of 17 following childbirth and she seemed doomed forever to be a disgusting object to herself as well as to everyone who came near her. It was this that led to the motivation which allowed her to submit to so many surgeries. Simms had convinced his jeweler to make the wire out of unalloyed silver drawn out as thin as a horse hair. It was in May of 1849 when he prepared Anarcha for her 13th operation. He brought the edges of the fistula close together with four of his five flexible new silver wires, passing them through little strips of lead to keep them from cutting into the tissue and fastening them tightly by using, once again, his perforated lead shot. Then he introduced the essential catheter into the bladder and readied himself for the tedious week of waiting. On a score or more of earlier occasions, he had been sure that when the week was over, he would witness a successful cure; this time he was filled with anxieties. It seemed to him that he had played his last trump; if he had failed to win now, the game was really lost; even with his fanatical devotion he could not keep on forever. At the week's end, almost four years to the day from the time when he had first seen those gaping, mocking holes which were Anarcha's souvenirs of child-birth labor, he had Anarcha placed again on the operating table. With pounding heart and fearful mind, he introduced the speculum. There lay the suture apparatus just as he had fixed it, quite undisturbed by swelling and inflammation. There was no longer any fistula. Its edges had joined close in a perfect union. Anarcha's recovery with the silver sutures in place was uncomplicated and she remained dry for the rest of her life. This was a great relief for this particular patient because her fistula not only opened into the bladder but into the rectum as well.

In 1852, Simms reported the cure of 252 fistulas out of 320 attempts. It was apparently the use of silver wire sutures that turned repeated failures into predictable successes. Shortly thereafter, Simms left Alabama for New York where he became one of the founders of the Women's Hospital in that city. He toured Europe and operated successfully on patients throughout the continent.

His success did not end with his accomplishments in fistula surgery. The Internal Medical Congress in London in 1881 was perhaps the most satisfactory medical meeting in the life of Marion Simms. Simms' thesis and his valedictory address was "Progress in Peritoneal Surgery." Dr. Simms prefaced his remarks by saying, "that he was prompted to discuss the subject as a result of what he had seen and heard in the surgical and obstetric sections at the International Medical Congress." His object was to lay before the Academy a synopsis of the progress of peritoneal surgery in his own pioneer practice. In his address, the physically afflicted 68-year-old pioneer surgeon was ardent in his plea for surgeons to adopt the new methods—aseptic technique in particular—in dealing with any wound that invaded the peritoneal cavity. He pleaded for the adoption of Lister's principle for preventing infection in all wounds, particularly with the abdomen. "Ovariotomy is the parent of peritoneal surgery," said Simms, and he gave credit to Ephraim McDowell and Washington Atlee, whom he called the "great ovariodomists."

Marion Simms died quietly in 1883 while working on his autobiography entitled "The Story of My Life," a book that was to be released by his son, Harry Marion Simms, a year after his father's death.

The spirit of Marion Simms was to be assumed by Howard A. Kelly who was appointed the first professor of gynecology at the Johns Hopkins Medical School. Like Simms, Kelly believed that gynecology and urology were so closely related that they could not be separated. It is interesting that this conference and the new society of gynecologic urology, which embryonically lingers in the wings of this conference, is the fulfillment of the beliefs of Marion Simms and Howard Kelly.

In 1893, Kelly invented the cystoscope. According to Robertson, he utilized the so-called air cystoscope with the patient in knee-chest position. Robertson relates that the cystoscope originally was a hollow tube with a handle and a glass partition which prevented water from running out of the bladder. The bladder had been distended with the installation of water prior to the insertion of the cystoscope and light was reflected from a head mirror. One day, an assistant to Dr. Kelly dropped the scope and the glass shattered. Kelly had noticed that the vagina ballooned with air when the patient was in the knee-chest position. He concluded that the bladder might be distended with air in a similar manner. He inserted the broken cystoscope and when he removed the obturator, the bladder ballooned with air and he was able to satisfactorily inspect the bladder mucosa. Kelly's interest in urologic problems of the female intensified, and in 1949, he and Burnham co-authored a text entitled *Diseases of the Kidney, Ureters and Bladder*.

Kelly wrote, "The commonest form of incontinence is the result of childbirth, entailing an injury to the neck of the bladder; it is occasionally seen in elderly nullipara and is most common after the age of forty. It is usually progressive, beginning with an occasional dribble, later becoming more frequent and occurring on slight provocation. In its incipiency, a strain, cough, sneeze or stepping up to get on a tram car starts a little spurt of urine which, in the course of time, initiates the act which empties the bladder. The list of operations devised to overcome the incontinence is legion; most unsuccessful, but occasionally, temporarily at least, affording some control. The best plan, often successful, is to set free the thickened musculature (sphincter) at the neck of the bladder (Bell's muscle) and to suture it so as to overlap its ends, forming a good internal sphincter." This was to be the forerunner of the Kelly plication as a component of the anterior colporrhaphy. The individuals at the Johns Hopkins Medical School that followed Kelly were similarly interested in female urology. Guy Hunner described the Hunner's ulcer, which today is called intestinal cystitis. Houston Everett succeeded Hunner; his important contribution was the relationship of the urinary tract to cervical cancer. His concepts are fundamental in modern concepts of gynecological oncology. He is the author of *Gynecologic and Obstetrical Urology* and co-author of *Female Urology*.

In 1914, Latzko described a new operation for closure of the posthysterectomy vesicovaginal fistula. His simple method consisted of an upper vaginectomy and was easily applicable to a large number of patients in the United States who have a small fistula posthysterectomy. Many modifications of this technique have been proposed during the last several decades, but the fundamental methodology remains unchanged.

As stated above, a surgical approach to stress incontinence was begun by Howard A. Kelly who reported on 20 cases of incontinence treated by plication of the vesical neck with success in sixteen cases. In 1949, Marshall, Marchetti and Krantz reported a new operation in which they had treated 50 patients with stress incontinence; 25 of these patients had previous unsuccessful surgical procedures for incontinence. Their overall success rate was 82%. This retropubic suspension of the bladder neck has been modified by many individuals over the last three decades. The procedure described by Burch in 1968 has received great popularity. This procedure accomplishes the retropubic suspension by suturing the periurethral tissue to Cooper's ligament.

Most recently, the evaluation of bladder dynamics has been more carefully and scientifically approached. This began with the report by Robertson of the use of the culdoscope which had been modified to accommodate the physician in his inspection of the bladder and urethra. The standard culdoscope, used for many years in gynecology, could not be used to visualize the vesical neck or the urethra because of the right angle of the lens and the heat from the bulb. Robertson modified the Kelly air cystoscope to overcome these obstacles. The new urethroscope had optical glass fibers enclosed between double walls of a stainless steel barrel. An electric source in the handle transmitted cold light around the circumference at the distal end. This allowed magnification at the proximal end. An air vent allowed a closed system by placing a fingertip over the vent. The development of fiberoptic telescopes revolutionized endoscopy and has made many changes in the practice of gynecology. Robertson developed a new female urethroscope with a direct view telescope which looks into an open barrel tube. The fiberoptic cord and the gas tubing are attached to the head. Carbon dioxide is used for distention of the urethra and bladder. This flexible system allows both thorough inspection of the urinary tract mucosa and the beginnings of analysis of bladder and urethral function. Recently, utilizing this instrument and modifications thereof, a more sophisticated system for dynamic assessment of bladder and urethral function has been pioneered with a more thorough understanding of the entire process of micturition.

It would appear that the discipline which gave birth to the

larger specialty of gynecology has finally come of age. Many of us have been frustrated by the paucity of concrete knowledge in the area of stress incontinence and related problems. The number of surgical procedures which have been devised over the last century to accommodate and improve these afflicted patients is legion. Undoubtedly, the fundamental problem was a serious lack of understanding of the etiology. Developments in the last few years would suggest that our understanding of the mechanisms involved in the proper function of the healthy and diseased bladder and urethra are at hand, and appropriate procedures are forthcoming to improve the well being of this large group of afflicted patients.

References

1. **Kelly, H. A., Dumm, W. M.** Urinary Incontinence in Women Without Manifest Injury to the Bladder. *Surg. Gynecol. Obstet.* 18: 444, 1914.
2. **Robertson, J. R.** *Genitourinary Problems in Women.* Charles C Thomas, Springfield, Ill., 1978.
3. **Robertson, J. R.** Gynecological Urethroscopy. *Am. J. Obstet. Gynecol.* 115: 986, 1973.

THE NORMAL LOWER URINARY TRACT

1 Embryology and Anatomy of the Female Bladder and Urethra

Donald R. Ostergard, M.D.

Information concerning the embryological development and the anatomy of the bladder and urethra continues to be the subject of research. Although agreement exists in most of the major areas relating to this topic, common consensus is not apparent in many of the details. This chapter presents a compilation of opinion as currently stated in the medical literature.

EMBRYOLOGY OF THE BLADDER AND URETHRA

The cloaca appears during the fourth fetal week in the embryo of 4 mm length (Figure 1.1). This endodermal structure consists of the expanded blind end of the hind gut and receives the hind gut, the tail gut, the allantois and the urinary excretory ducts. The primitive kidney (pronephros) becomes visible in the third fetal week and its pronephric duct extends to the cloaca. During the fourth fetal week the mesonephros appears as the second primitive kidney and replaces the non-functional pronephros which subsequently degenerates. The mesonephros begins to function in the sixth fetal week and utilizes the pronephric duct, which becomes the mesonephric duct. The mesonephros begins to degenerate during the third and fourth months of development. More caudally in the embryo during the fourth fetal week the metanephric duct buds off the mesonephric duct near the point where the mesonephric duct empties into the cloaca. This duct induces the surrounding metanephrogenic mesenchyme to form the metanephros, which

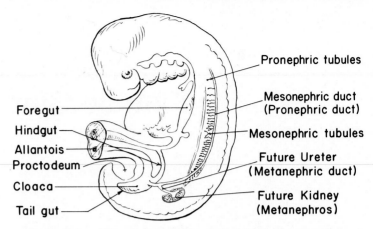

Foregut
Hindgut
Allantois
Proctodeum
Cloaca
Tail gut

Pronephric tubules
Mesonephric duct
(Pronephric duct)
Mesonephric tubules
Future Ureter
(Metanephric duct)
Future Kidney
(Metanephros)

Figure 1.1.   The embryo of 4 mm length in the fourth fetal week. (Redrawn with permission from *The Ciba Collection of Medical Illustrations*, Vol. 6, Copyright 1973.)

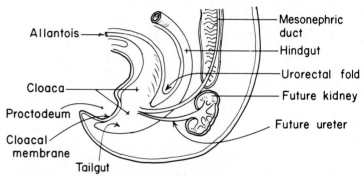

Allantois

Cloaca

Proctodeum

Cloacal
membrane

Tailgut

Mesonephric
duct
Hindgut
Urorectal fold
Future kidney
Future ureter

Figure 1.2.   Further development and differential growth causes the future ureter to enter into the cloaca. (Redrawn with permission from *The Ciba Collection of Medical Illustrations*, Vol. 6, Copyright 1973.)

becomes the permanent kidney. Beginning shortly thereafter, a differential growth process causes the metanephric duct to enter into the future bladder. This same process absorbs the mesonephric duct, which now enters into the future urethra (Figures 1.2 and 1.3).

Also during the fourth fetal week an ectodermal depression forms which contacts the cloacal wall to form the cloacal membrane (Figure 1.2). This ectodermal depression is the proctodeum and has endodermal cells forming its mucous membrane. The urorectal fold divides the cloaca during the fourth fetal week (Figure 1.2). A lateral ingrowth of mesenchyme in the lower portion of the cloaca may also contribute to this cloacal division. The caudal migration of the urorectal fold causes a division of the cloaca into the posterior portion which becomes the rectum and the ante-

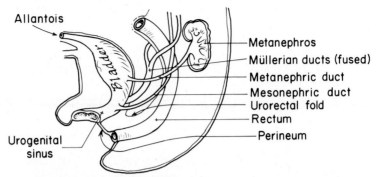

Figure 1.3.   Continued differential growth now places the ureter into the bladder. (Redrawn with permission from *The Ciba Collection of Medical Illustrations*, Vol. 6, Copyright 1973.)

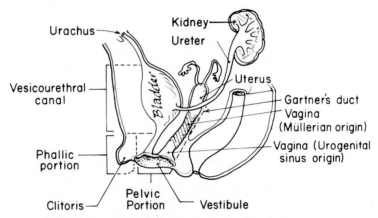

Figure 1.4.   The embryo at the end of the fourth month. (Redrawn with permission from *The Ciba Collection of Medical Illustrations*, Vol. 6, Copyright 1973.)

rior portion which becomes the urogenital sinus (Figure 1.3). The latter is primarily of endodermal origin.

The urogenital sinus differentiates into two parts (Figure 1.4). The first part is the vesicourethral canal which forms the bladder and the upper urethra. The bladder itself gradually enlarges to incorporate the lower portion of the allantois. In the adult the upper portion of the allantois becomes the urachus. The second definitive portion of the urogenital sinus differentiates into pelvic and phallic components (Figure 1.4). The pelvic portion develops into the main part of the urethra, including the urethral and periurethral glands, a part of the vestibule and approximately one-fifth of the lower vagina. The phallic portion becomes a part of the female vestibule. Most of this differentiation concludes by the fourth month when the definitive muscular structure of the bladder and urethra appears. The posterior urethral and

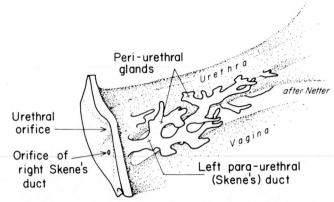

Figure 1.5. The urethra and periurethral glands. (Redrawn with permission from *The Ciba Collection of Medical Illustrations*, Vol. 2, Copyright 1954 and 1965.)

trigonal musculature are of the same embryological origin with a recognizable direct muscular continuation between the trigone and posterior urethral musculature. The anterior urethral musculature is continuous with bladder musculature and is formed by vaginal canal derivatives.

In the female the mesonephric duct largely degenerates and remains as the paravaginal duct of Gartner (Figure 1.4). Occasionally this duct persists and explains the ectopic location of a ureter in the urethra, vagina, cervix or uterus.

The major urethral glands eventually become known as Skene's ducts which have their orifices at the junction of the lower and middle thirds of the external urethral meatus (Figure 1.5). Additional glands empty directly into the posterior portion of the urethra and constitute the homologue of the male prostate. These glands have considerable importance in the pathophysiology of the urethral syndrome.

ANATOMY OF THE BLADDER AND URETHRA

The classical description of the bladder musculature includes three layers. These layers are the outer longitudinal, a middle circular and an inner longitudinal (Figure 1.6). The outer longitudinal layer is continuous with the outer circular layer of the urethra. The middle circular layer ends at the internal meatus and connects to the deep trigonal musculature. The inner longitudinal layer continues down the anterior portion of the urethra. Embryologically the bladder musculature develops separately from the trigonal musculature. Its development also precedes the formation of the trigone. Although the classic description of the bladder musculature includes these three layers, each individual muscle bundle in the bladder interconnects with all other muscle bundles (Figure 1.7). Therefore, the detrusor musculature forms a meshwork of broad-to-narrow muscle fascicles which run in many different directions and change

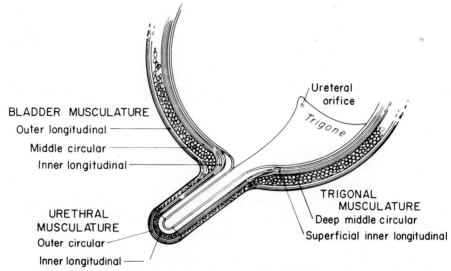

Figure 1.6.   The muscular layers of the bladder, trigone and urethra.

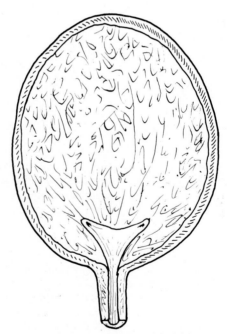

Figure 1.7   The interdecussation of bladder muscular fibers.

planes and orientation in various parts of the bladder. This elaborate interconnection of muscle fibers is important in the propagation of a coordinated detrusor contraction.

ANATOMY OF THE TRIGONE

The trigone develops separately and distinctly from the bladder and has two layers of musculature. These two layers are derivatives of mesenchyme and are a direct continuation of the lower ureteral musculature without interruption or

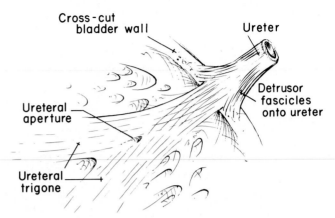

Figure 1.8.   The ureter and the trigone.

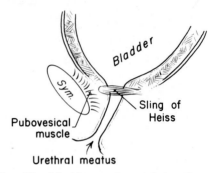

Figure 1.9.   The bladder outlet and the sling of Heiss.

loss of any muscle tissue. Essentially, the ureter changes from a tubular structure to a sheet-like structure in the formation of the trigone (Figure 1.8). The two muscular layers are the inner longitudinal layer and the outer circular layer. The inner longitudinal layer forms the superficial trigone and extends down into the urethra and also between detrusor muscle fibers. Therefore, it is continuous with both vesical and urethral musculature. The outer longitudinal or deep trigonal musculature terminates at the internal meatus. The deep trigonal musculature passes laterally into the detrusor muscle and forms a direct connection between these two organs. This connection between the trigone and the detrusor musculature introduces a mechanism whereby trigonal activity influences detrusor function. The deep trigonal musculature and the detrusor middle circular layers surround the bladder outlet.

URETHRAL ANATOMY

The urethral musculature contains two layers, the inner longitudinal and the outer circular (Figure 1.6). The fibers of the outer circular layer are continuous with the outer longitudinal layer of the bladder and have an oblique course as they surround the urethra. The inner longitudinal layer is continuous with the inner longitudinal layer of the bladder and also the superficial trigonal musculature. At the level of the bladder outlet there is a smooth muscular structure in the shape of a horseshoe which surrounds the anterior urethra and inserts into the trigonal musculature posteriorly. This is the sling of Heiss (Figure 1.9).

The urethral musculature also has a striated muscular component. This is a circular arrangement of striated muscular fibers which extends from the bulbocavernosus muscle in the lower portion of the urethra to the lower edge of the detrusor muscle. It is most abundant inferiorly in the middle third of the urethra and gradually diminishes in size near the detrusor.

An additional urethral muscular component which serves to support the bladder and urethra anteriorly is the pubovesical muscle, which is a derivative of the outer circular layers of the bladder and urethra (Figure 1.9). It terminates in the retropubic connective tissue.

References

1. **Brockis, J.G.** The Development of the Trigone of the Bladder with a Report of a Case of Ectopic Ureter. *Br. J. Urol.* 24: 192–200, 1952.
2. **Campbell, M.F.** Developmental Anatomy of the Urinary System. In *Gynecological Urology*, edited by A. F. Youssef. Charles C Thomas, Springfield, Ill., 1960, p. 16–28.
3. **Crelin, E.S.** Normal and Abnormal Development of the Ureter. *Urology* 12:51–56, 1978.
4. **Donker P.J.** Anatomy of the Bladder, the Urethra and the Pelvic Floor. Proceedings of the Annual Meeting, International Continence Society, Antwerp, Belgium, 1976.
5. **Droes, J.T.** Observations on the Musculature of the Urinary Bladder and the Urethra in the Human Foetus. *Br. J. Urol.* 46:179–185, 1974.
6. **Hartl, H.** Anatomy of the Bladder and Urethra, Their Sphincter Mechanism and Their Supports. In *Gynecological Urology*, edited by A. F. Youssef. Charles C Thomas, Springfield, Ill., 1960.
7. **Huffman, J.W.** The Development of the Periurethral Glands in the Human Female. *Am. J. Obstet. Gynecol.* 45:773–785, 1943.
8. **Hutch, J.A.** *Anatomy and Physiology of the Bladder, Trigone and Urethra*. Appleton-Century-Crofts, New York, 1972.
9. **Okonkwo, J.E.N., Crocker, K.M.** Cloacal Dysgenesis. *Obstet. Gynecol.* 50:97–101, 1977.
10. **Parrott, T.S.** Urologic Implications of Imperforate Anus. *Urology* 10:407–413, 1977.
11. **Tanagho, E.A., Meyers, F.H., Smith, D.R.** The Trigone: Anatomical and Physiological Considerations. 1. In Relation to the Ureterovesical Junction. *J. Urol.* 100:623–632, 1968.
12. **Tanagho, E.A., Smith, D.R., Meyers, F.H.** The Trigone: Anatomical and Physiological Considerations. 2. In Relation to the Bladder Neck. *J. Urol.* 100:633–639, 1968.
13. **Tanagho, E.A., Smith, D.R.** Mechanism of Urinary Conti-

nence. 1. Embryologic, Anatomic and Pathologic Considerations. *J. Urol.* 100:640–646, 1968.
14. **Wendelken, J.R., Sethney, H.T., Halverstadt, D.B.** Urologic Abnormalities Associated with Imperforate Anus. *Urology* 10: 239–242, 1977.
15. **Woodburne, R.T.** Anatomy of the Bladder and Bladder Outlet. *J. Urol.* 100:474–487, 1968.
16. **Zornow, D.H.** Embryology of Urinary Incontinence. *Urology* 10: 293–300, 1977.

2 The Neurology of Micturition

William E. Bradley, M.D.

The neurological control of the voluntary micturition reflex is both a central and peripheral nervous system function which includes a variety of reflex arcs extending anatomically from the cerebrum to the bladder itself. It is the maturation of these central nervous system pathways which provides for the attainment of continence in early childhood. Thus, the human establishes the volitional control of the detrusor reflex which allows the important social function of suppressing the micturition reflex when it occurs spontaneously, so that its activation may occur subsequently at a more appropriate occasion.

CEREBRAL CORTEX

The micturition center of the cerebral cortex receives sensory pathways from the periphery, including the bladder muscle, the periurethral striated muscle and also the brain stem nuclei (Figure 2.1). In turn it sends signals back to the brain stem (Loop I).

Table 2.1 lists the diagnostic neurological entities associated with urinary bladder dysfunction. In the brain, occlusive cerebrovascular disease affects approximately 2 million individuals in this country with about 200,000 to 300,000 patients added to this group each year. The incidence of urinary incontinence in these patients is unknown, but probably is quite high. Cerebrovascular disease is of two types, either ischemic or occlusive. The latter is quite common and occurs with atherosclerosis due to aging, diabetes

11

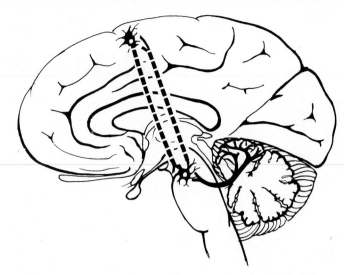

Figure 2.1. Cerebral neurological connections of reflexes involved in micturition control (Loop I) including cerebellum.

Table 2.1. Diagnostic Entities Related to Urinary Bladder Dysfunction

BRAIN
  Cerebrovascular disease
  Trauma
  Parkinson's disease
  Multiple sclerosis
  Dementia
  Tumors
SPINAL CORD
  Injury
  Vascular disease
  Dysraphia
    Meningomyelocele
  Spinal stenosis
  Myelopathies
  Tumors
  Spondylosis of lumbar or cervical spine
  Multiple sclerosis
  Cauda equina lesions
  Conus medullaris lesions
  Sacral agenesis
  Spinal arachnoiditis
PERIPHERAL INNERVATION
  Autonomic neuropathy
  Diabetes mellitus
  Hypothyroidism
  Uremia
  Extensive pelvic surgery

mellitus and hypertension. Infarction secondary to occlusion of these vessels affects the cranial end of Loops I and IV in the detrusor motor area and causes detrusor hyperreflexia through a release of the detrusor muscle from volitional control. The cells of the cerebral cortex atrophy in a cumulative fashion as the brain ages. This process begins at birth and eventually accounts for one type of incontinence found in the aging population.

Dementia is an increasing problem, particularly when associated with urinary incontinence. Social dissolution begins when incontinence occurs and the family places the patient in a nursing home.

Figure 2.2 shows the central nervous system representation of various parts of the body in the cerebrum. Note that specific parts of the brain represent corresponding areas of the body, both somatic and visceral. As with other structures the periurethral striated muscle and the detrusor muscle have a one-to-one representation in the brain.

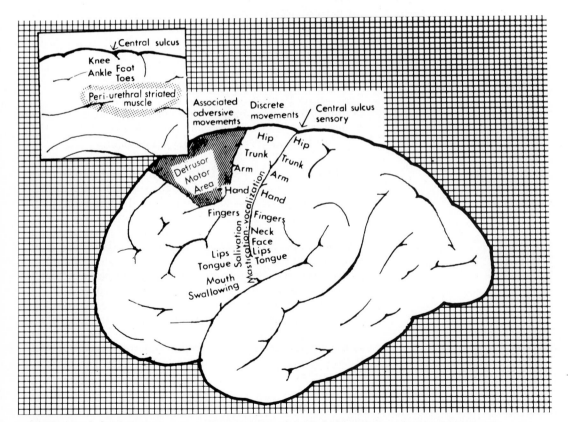

Figure 2.2. Central nervous system representation of peripheral structures in the cerebrum.

INTERNAL CAPSULE

All nervous pathways from the cerebral cortex pass through the internal capsule en route to the brain stem (Figure 2.1). Its strategic location, and the concentration of central nervous system pathways contained within it, places all of these neurons in an extremely vulnerable position and only minor insults produce severe functional derangements. Unfortunately, this is a favored site for occlusive cerebral vascular disease which occurs with interruption of the blood supply to that particular part of the brain. The resulting weakness on the opposite side of the body, hemiplegia or partial hemiplegia, frequently brings about urinary incontinence as a result of interruption of the reflex arcs involved in voluntary control of the bladder.

LIMBIC SYSTEM

A further influence on this central circuit is the limbic system, which controls all autonomic functions. The importance of the limbic system in relation to urinary incontinence and bladder control relates to its association with the affective reactions of the individual to her personal life. It mediates such reactions as how one feels, how depressed or how angry one is. Through feelings such as these the limbic system influences the control of the detrusor muscle. A further importance lies in the realization that it is a favorite site for development of epileptiform activity. In these patients seizure activity in this area may be responsible for urinary bladder dysfunction.

BASAL GANGLIA

The basal ganglia also influence voiding (Figure 2.1). In this country Parkinson's disease affects this anatomical area in approximately 1 million individuals who have slowness of movement, gait instability and tremor. Forty-five to 75% manifest various forms of urinary incontinence.

Until recently, knowledge of the neuropathology of Parkinson's disease consisted only of the recognition of the degenerative changes occurring in the cells of the brain and parts in the basal ganglia. Recent biochemical and pharmacological studies indicate that the substantia nigra manufactures dopamine and transports it to the basal ganglia. The basal ganglia controls all somatic motor movements related to posture and the neutrotransmitter agent, dopamine, determine how these cells function. In terms of control of the detrusor muscle, the basal ganglia suppress its contractile activity. Exhaustion of the transmitter occurs in Parkinson's disease, producing bladder instability in the same age group as those patients with the symptom of stress incontinence. It usually occurs after 40 and certainly after the 50s and 60s.

Patients with Parkinson's disease demonstrate detrusor hyperreflexia and urge incontinence which may masquerade as genuine stress incontinence. Therapeutic benefit results from replacement of the neutrotransmitter with L-dopa therapy and from concomitant sedation with anticholinergics.

CEREBELLUM

The cerebellum is the main sensory afferent pathway from the detrusor and the periurethral striated muscles and coordinates all micturition related activities of the brain stem (Figure 2.1). Since the cerebellum coordinates all other motor activities, it is not surprising that it is also a coordinating center for muscular activity involving these structures. The whole purpose of the cerebellum is to say "no." It says no to all other motor systems by means of an electrophysiologic or neurophysiologic code. The clinical analog is that when cerebellar function decreases through any of the diseases which also affect the cerebrum, uninhibited bladder contractions result. That is, abnormal detrusor reflex contractions occur which the patient cannot suppress on command; the detrusor muscle is no longer subject to cerebellar inhibition. Clinically, cerebellar disease characteristically produces spontaneous, high amplitude detrusor reflex contractions.

Multiple sclerosis is a disease of the young affecting approximately a half million individuals, most of whom are in the most productive periods of their lives. The incidence of urinary incontinence from central nervous system involvement is in excess of 90%.

BRAIN STEM MICTURITION CENTER

In the experimental animal the concept of a sacral micturition center is now in doubt. Microelectrode stimulation and signal tracing techniques place the detrusor motor nucleus in a discrete portion of the pons in the brain stem (Figure 2.1). Stimulation of this area produces a smooth contractile response in the detrusor muscle with a smooth rise in intravesical pressure. This technique demonstrates that the pons contains the final common pathway for detrusor motor neurons and casts doubt upon the existence of a sacral micturition center. This places the brain stem center in an important functional position. Any subsequent modulation of the micturition reflex in the sacral cord becomes of secondary importance. Therefore, the brain stem has the capacity to develop detrusor reflex contractions rather than or in addition to the sacral autonomic neurons.

SPINAL CORD

The next major area for central nervous system organization of the micturition reflex resides in the spinal cord (Figure 2.3). The efferents from the brain stem pass all the way to the sacral gray matter (Loop II). En route they pass through recognizable anatomic areas. The bony spinal column protects the soft tissue of the spinal cord and has definite numbering and locations consisting of cervical, thoracic and lumbar vertebrae. A similar numbering system exists

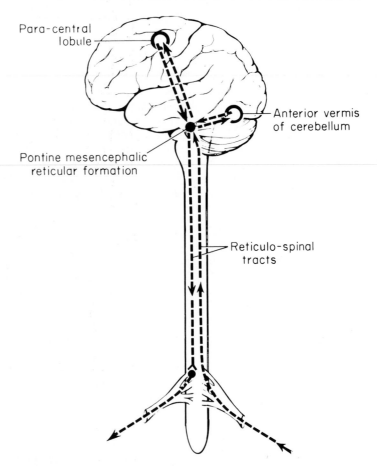

Figure 2.3.   The spinal cord showing anatomy, long routing and sacral nuclei (Loop II).

in the spinal cord itself. However, as the organism progresses from fetal life to infancy and subsequently to adolescence, the spinal cord shortens in relative length and eventually terminates somewhere around the first lumbar bony vertebral body. This results in a consistent disparity between the spinal cord origin of motor neurons and the actual bony vertebral level. The site of termination of the spinal cord is the conus medullaris which contains the autonomic neurons concerned with the peripheral innervation of the detrusor muscle. The conus medullaris is quite short and contains the entire first to fifth sacral spinal segmental innervation. In addition to detrusor innervation it also contains fibers concerned with rectal and sexual functions derived from their respective brain stem centers.

The pelvic and pudendal nerves contain the sensory afferent input from the detrusor and periurethral striated musculature (Figure 2.4). Most of these fibers long route to the brain stem with little segmental crossing after entering the sacral spinal cord. Long routing allows these fibers to bypass any neuronal connection in the sacral cord with the first synapse in the brain stem (Figure 2.3). One of the principal characteristics of this long routing approach to the brain stem is to provide for temporal gain or increase in duration of the detrusor reflex. This is the second most important characteristic of the detrusor reflex. The individual must not only be able to volitionally control micturition but must also generate a detrusor contraction which is long enough to achieve the desired end result: total evacuation of intravesical contents. Neuroanatomically, the long routing of bladder sensory fibers to the brain stem amplification system increases the duration of the reflex response.

In the sacral gray matter are two pairs of nuclei: the detrusor motor nuclei and the pudendal motor nuclei. The former provides motor impulses to the detrusor and the latter to the periurethral striated musculature. These nuclei reside in separate anatomical locations in the sacral cord. Therefore, disease states or injury to the lower spine can selectively damage one of these structures to the exclusion of the others with resultant neurological effects localized to a particular peripheral anatomical site.

These nuclei in the sacral gray matter have separate and distinct inputs from different structures in the periphery. Neuroanatomically, each nucleus interacts with all other nuclei. Stimulation of any of the peripheral inputs produces an evoked response in any of the other projecting pathways. The neurologist uses this information to analyze disease of

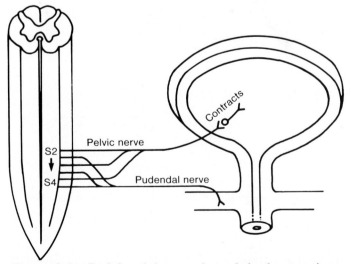

Figure 2.4. Peripheral innervation of the lower urinary tract. Pelvic and motor nerves to the bladder, urethra and striated sphincter.

the conus medullaris which is frequently asymptomatic. He also uses this technique to evaluate the presence of peripheral or central neuropathies. Neuropathy is a disease of peripheral neurons originating in the sacral gray matter. Frequently, the only abnormality associated with clinical complaints is a delay in the time required from stimulation of the end organ to the evoked response in another organ. This manifests a delay in transit time. The response will not appear at all if there is a disease of the intrinsic gray matter of the sacral spinal cord. Clinically, in some patients with the symptom of stress incontinence, using this technique it is possible to find evidence of neuropathic involvement of the urethra. This neuropathic incontinence does not respond to surgical therapy!

Disease of the spinal cord also affects vesical function. Spinal cord injury affects approximately 250,000 individuals in the United States. Spinovascular disease is an increasing problem associated with atherosclerosis and diabetes mellitus. Incomplete fusion of the spinal cord, dysrhaphia, includes meningomyelocele, a spinal cord malformation which is fairly common. Spinal stenosis occurs in patients with long histories of back pain, a common complaint of patients with the symptom of stress incontinence.

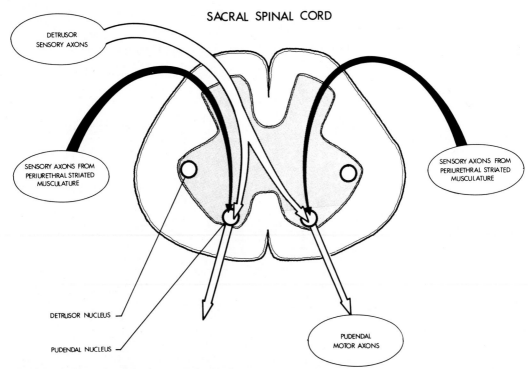

Figure 2.5.   Diagram of detrusor sphincteric relaxing reflex (Loop III).

Myelopathies are spinal cord diseases of unknown etiology. Spinal cord tumors also occur. The demyelinating plaques of multiple sclerosis characteristically affect vesical function, particularly in the younger female with the symptom of stress incontinence. Since this disease causes incontinence, detrusor hyperreflexia and urge incontinence, its diagnosis is important. Documentary evidence, however, on either neurologic exam or special investigations frequently is unobtainable.

Diseases of the bony spine, such as lumbar or cervical spondylosis, produce active reflexes in the knees and coexist with an extensor plantar response. The physician elicits this response by stroking the outer and lateral aspect of the foot to stimulate the upgoing toe. This indicates the involvement of the pyramidal tract (Loop IV in Figure 2.6).

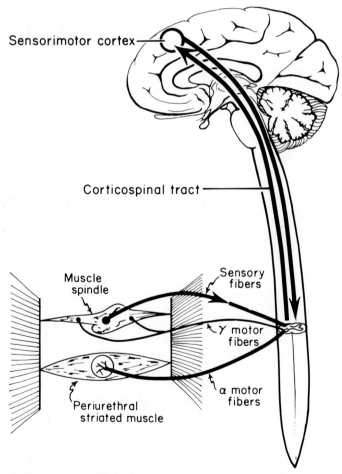

Figure 2.6. Diagram of the peripheral and central innervation of the periurethral striated muscle (Loop IV).

REFLEXES INVOLVED IN MICTURITION SYNERGISM

An important reflex pathway facilitates reciprocal relaxation of the periurethral striated muscle when the detrusor muscle contracts (Figure 2.5). This reflex originates in detrusor sensory afferent impulses generated in the bladder musculature which pass to the pudendal nucleus in the sacral cord, resulting in inhibition of this tonically active nucleus. In the normal patient the pudendal nucleus tonically generates motor impulses to the periurethral striated muscle in the waking and sleeping states; the only interruption to this constant flow of impulses is the voluntary cerebral inhibition of the pudendal nucleus which facilitates perineal relaxation during a willed detrusor muscle contraction. In some patients this reciprocal relationship between detrusor muscle contraction and the activity of periurethral striated muscle is abnormal. Instead of reciprocal relaxation there is dyssynergia with an actual contraction of the periurethral striated muscle. Sometimes this prevents the patient from voiding properly by developing a relative increase in urethral resistance. Increased residual urine volume and a prolonged intermittent voiding pattern results.

NEUROLOGY OF THE PERIURETHRAL STRIATED MUSCLE

The innervation of the periurethral striated muscle (Loop IV) consists of two reflex arcs, a segmental peripheral one and a central one which originates in the motor cortex (Figure 2.6). The periurethral striated muscle has its own sensing elements in the muscle spindles which are the same as in other striated muscles. When the periurethral striated muscle stretches in response to a detrusor contraction, sensory fibers carry signals back to the spinal cord. If voluntary micturition is not appropriate, motor impulses cause the periurethral striated muscle to contract and to prevent urine flow. If voluntary micturition is appropriate, reciprocal relaxation occurs.

An additional influence is the gamma motor system which controls the sensitivity of these sensing elements (Figure 2.7). The gamma motor system has its own diseases which may produce a supersensitivity of these spindles. Under these conditions, instead of responding in a normal way to stretch, they may respond abnormally and maintain a long sustained contraction of the periurethral striated muscle.

The end result of neurophysiologic activity of these loops and pathways under normal circumstances is to provide a smooth rise in intravesical pressure secondary to a gradual increase in pelvic motor nerve discharge. Concurrently, a reciprocal relaxation of the periurethral striated muscle occurs which is due to inhibition of the tonic pudendal motor nerve discharge.

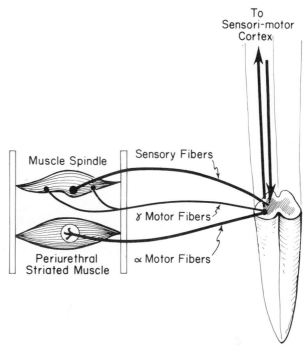

Figure 2.7. The sensing elements in the muscle spindles and the gamma motor spindles.

PELVIC GANGLIA AND MOTOR END PLATES

When the pelvic nerve motor impulses emerge from the sacral spinal roots, they pass through another transformation station: the autonomic ganglion (Figure 2.8). Most of these parasympathetic pelvic ganglia lie in the substance of the detrusor muscle where they are inaccessible to any kind of anatomic dissection. Unfortunately, this also makes them vulnerable to any type of end organ disease, such as overstretch or infection. Additional problems accrue from the use of tranquilizing agents such as the phenothiazines which inadvertently block the release of the neurotransmitter acetylcholine. The result is an interference with neurotransmission in the ganglia with subsequent urinary retention or improper voiding.

When the motor end plate releases its neurotransmitter, depolarization or excitation of the adjoining muscle cell generates motor impulses resulting in a detrusor muscle contraction (Figure 2.8). The synaptic endings have little vesicles which contain acetylcholine. Motor impulses stimulate these vesicles to move to the periphery and release acetylcholine. This neurotransmitter then migrates across the synaptic space to cause depolarization on the postsynaptic side. Alterations in the function of the neurotransmitter release mechanism cause clinically recognizable abnor-

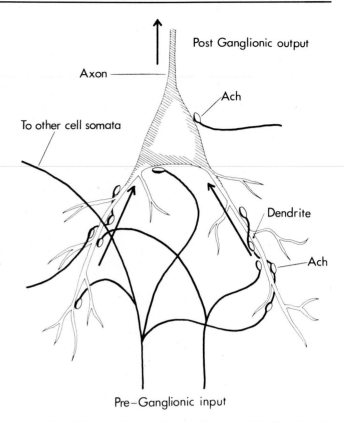

Post Ganglionic output

Axon

Ach

To other cell somata

Dendrite

Ach

Pre-Ganglionic input

Figure 2.8. The pelvic ganglion with acetylcholine (Ach) vesicles.

malities. An example is the symptom of stress incontinence from the use of phenothiazines. This is also the site where propantheline and methantheline exert their anticholinergic effects. These drugs interfere with neurotransmitter release.

In sites other than ganglia there is another type of innervation of the detrusor muscle. The postganglionic motor axon has varicosities which contain the transmitter agents for the detrusor muscle. Unfortunately, the exact transmitter agent for the detrusor muscle is unknown at this time. Acetylcholine or some other type of transmitter agent may fulfill this role. This arrangement of vesicles provides for a sustained effect of transmitter release by necessitating diffusion across the synapse to reach the individual smooth muscle cell (Figure 2.9). The diffusion process results in a long sustained contraction. Initially, the transmitter agent causes depolarization of the key or pacemaker cell. Since cells in the detrusor muscle do not have direct innervation by axons, a structure called the tight junction fuses the muscle cells to a pacemaker cell. Clinically, the tight junction is vulnerable to overdistention of the bladder. If over-

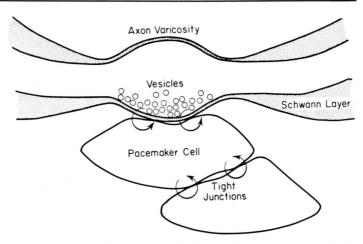

Figure 2.9. The motor end plate with pacemaker cells in the bladder.

distention of the bladder ruptures these tight junctions, collagen deposition results which interferes with effective detrusor contraction. The lack of fusion of the smooth muscle cell to the pacemaker cell interferes with the transmission of postganglionic motor impulses. Residual urine is the inevitable result of this process.

A detrusor muscle bundle consists of 12 to 15 individual muscle fibers. A collagen tendon surrounds each muscle bundle with its mucopolysaccharide lubricant. Collagen in the normal human detrusor accounts for approximately 25% of the muscle bulk. This collagen transmits all the tension generated during activity of the muscle. It is of equal importance with the muscle itself in producing the actual opening of the bladder neck during a detrusor contraction. The detrusor muscle bundles interconnect with other bundles by means of individual muscle fibers to produce a coordinated propagation of excitation and subsequent vesical contraction (see Chapter 1).

MOTOR END PLATES OF SKELETAL MUSCLE

The innervation of the periurethral striated muscle is different than the pattern of innervation of the smooth muscle bundle (Figure 2.10). The characteristic pattern of innervation of skeletal muscle is via myelinated motor axons. Blockade of the periurethral striated muscle with succinylcholine is difficult due to its tonically active nature and the organization of its neuromuscular junctions.

DISEASES OF PERIPHERAL INNERVATION

Diseases of the peripheral innervation represent one of the most common neurological causes of bladder dysfunction. The prototype of these diseases is the autonomic neuropathy which affects the peripheral innervation of the detrusor muscle. The commonest cause is diabetes mellitus with

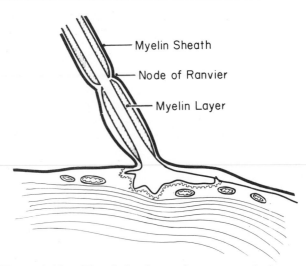

Figure 2.10. The skeletal muscle motor end plates.

approximately 10 million individuals affected. Almost all patients with juvenile onset diabetes or with insulin dependent diabetes have evidence of autonomic neuropathy. It also occurs with a variety of other metabolic diseases, including uremia and hypothyroidism, and may occur secondary to any central reflex dysfunction where there is a long history of recurrent vesical overdistention or infection.

Sacral agenesis is another disease of the peripheral innervation which may occur in the younger patient and causes bladder dysfunction which mimics genuine stress incontinence. Sacral x-rays reveal the diagnosis. Tumors or injury of the conus medullaris or cauda equina produce evidence of impairment of the bulbocavernosus or anal sphincter reflexes or cause loss of perineal sensation. Similar impairments occur in the patient with multiple laminectomies for back pain. These patients frequently have myelography and develop spinal arachnoiditis.

Extensive pelvic surgery, such as a Wertheim hysterectomy or abdominal perineal resection of the rectum for cancer, produces similar findings.

SENSORY INNERVATION

Sensory innervation of the bladder consists of nerve endings in the collagen capsules which surround individual muscle bundles. Stimulation of these sensory fibers occurs with any degree of stretch or reflex contraction. Other nerve endings associated with pain, temperature and touch lie free in the mucosa and submucosa. These additional fibers in the individual muscle fascicles drive the motor nucleus and constitute the peripheral arm of Loop II. Disease states either at the periphery or in the spinal cord interfere with these nerve endings and produce impairment of reflex excitation with resultant detrusor areflexia. Proprioceptive fibers have a long route to travel. They may contribute to the functioning of Loop II or long route to the CNS. The fibers concerned with pain, temperature and touch project across the spinothalamic tracts and then all the way to the cerebrum. An understanding of bladder neuroanatomy emphasizes that disease of the bladder itself results in the sensory disturbance symptoms of frequency and urgency associated with the symptom of stress incontinence.

MICTURITION EVENT

The anatomy of the detrusor muscle is such that the individual coalescing muscle bundles at the bladder neck produce a smooth coordinated opening of the vesicle neck (see Chapter 1). The presence of periurethral striated muscle at the distal third of the urethra and the variable and interindividual reflection of the striated muscle to the bladder neck complicates this process. The initiation of voiding probably requires contraction of the anterior reflection of the periurethral striated muscle originating from the urogenital diaphragm. The muscular arrangement at the bladder neck consists of intersecting loops of detrusor muscle and a trigonal loop which normally maintain continence. When a normal smooth coordinated micturition begins, the cranially inserted muscle fibers pull these two groups of muscles apart. This results in the opening of the bladder neck, expulsion of intravesical contents into the proximal urethra, urethral shortening and a lowering of intraurethral resistance to urine flow.

SUMMARY

In summary, there are four reflex loops concerned with innervation of the detrusor. The cortical loop provides the volitional control of the reflex and the spinal one provides for sufficient temporal duration of the reflex to completely evacuate intravesical contents. The gain provided by the spinal loop is important because its interruption by spinal cord injury, by spinal vascular disease associated with diabetes or atherosclerosis or by various lumbar spondylytic processes produces a reflex which does not last long enough to completely empty the bladder. This reflex may become hyperreflexic and mimic genuine stress incontinence. The patient may or may not demonstrate increased residual urine volume.

In a clinical situation it is important to emphasize that both motor and sensory phenomena in the micturition reflex exist. For example, patients with genuine stress incontinence whose reflex functions are normal seem to have an abnormality of sensory innervation of the urethra or bladder.

Similar symptoms occur when the patient translates disease of central nervous system structures as disease of the end organ and appears clinically as referred pain. The sensory abnormalities of voiding which are due to disease of central nervous system structures are extremely difficult to treat.

References

1. **Andrew, J., Nathan, P.W.** The Cerebral Control of Micturition. *Proc. R. Soc. Med.* 58:553–555, 1965.
2. **Andrew, J., Nathan, P.W., Spanos, N.C.** Disturbances of Micturition and Defecation due to Aneurysms of Cerebral Arteries. *J. Neurosurg.* 24:1, 1966.
3. **Barrington, F.J.F.** The Component Reflexes of Micturition in the Cat, Part III. *Brain* 64:239–243, 1941.
4. **Barrington, F.J.F.** The Localization of the Paths Subserving Micturition in the Spinal Cord of the Cat. *Brain* 56:126–148, 1933.
5. **Barrington, F.J.F.** The Relation of the Hindbrain to Micturition. *Brain* 44:23–53, 1921.
6. **Barrington, F.J.F.** The Effect of Lesions on the Hind and Midbrain on Micturition in the Cat. *Q.J. Exp. Physiol.* 15: 181–202, 1915.
7. **Barrington, F.J.F.** The Nervous Mechanism of Micturition. *Q. J. Exp. Physiol.* 8:33–71, 1915.
8. **Bowen, J.M., Timm, G.W., Bradley, W.E.** Some Contractile and Electrophysiological Properties of the Periurethral Striated Muscles of the Cat. *Invest. Urol.* 13:327–330, 1976.
9. **Bradley, W.E.** Micturition Reflex Amplification. *J. Urol.* 101: 403–407, 1969.
10. **Bradley, W.E.** Regulation of the Micturition Reflex by Negative Feedback. *J. Urol.* 101:400–402, 1969.
11. **Bradley, W.E., Conway, C.J.** Bladder Representation in the Pontine-mesencephalic Reticular Formation. *Exp. Neurol.* 16: 237–249, 1966.
12. **Bradley, W.E., Teague, C.T.** Cerebellar Regulation of the Micturition Reflex. *Exp. Neurol.* 23:399–411, 1969.
13. **Bradley, W.E., Teague, C.T.** Innervation of the Vesical Detrusor Muscle by the Ganglia of the Pelvic Plexus. *Invest. Urol.* 6:251–266, 1968.
14. **Bradley, W.E., Teague, C.T.** Spinal Cord Organization of Micturition Reflex Afferents. *Exp. Neurol.* 22:504–516, 1968.
15. **Bradley, W.E., Scott, F.B., Timm, G.W.** Innervation of the Detrusor Muscle and Urethra. *Urol. Clin. North Am.* 1(1):69–80, 1974.
16. **Bradley, W.E., Timm, G.W., Scott, F.B.** Cystometry IV: Neuromuscular Transmission in the Urinary Bladder. *Urology* 6: 520–524, 1975.
17. **Bradley, W.E., Timm, G.W., Scott, F.B.** Cystometry V: Sensation. *Urology* 6:654–658, 1975.
18. **Bradley, W.E., Griffin, D., Teague, C.T., Timm, G.W.** Sensory Innervation of the Mammalian Urethra. *Invest. Urol.* 10:287–289, 1973.
19. **Edvardsen, P.** Nervous Control of Urinary Bladder in Cats. I: The Collecting Phase. *Acta Physiol. Scand.* 72:157, 1968.
20. **Edvardsen, P.** Nervous Control of Urinary Bladder in Cats. II: The Expulsion Phase. *Acta Physiol. Scand.* 72:172, 1968.
21. **Garry, R.C., Roberts, T.D.M., Todd J.K.** Reflexes Involving the External Urethral Sphincter in the Cat. *J. Physiol.* 149: 653–665, 1959.

22. **Gjone, R., Seteklew, J.** Excitatory and Inhibitory Responses to Stimulation of the Cerebral Cortex in the Cat. *Acta Physiol. Scand.* 59:337, 1963.

23. **Heimburger, R.F., Freeman, L.W., Wilde, N.J.** Sacral nerve innervation of the human bladder. *J. Neurosurg.* 5:154, 1948.

24. **Kock, N.G., Pompeius, R.** Inhibition of Vesical Motor Activity Induced by Anal Stimulation. *Acta Chir. Scand.* 216:244–250, 1963.

25. **Kuru, M.** Nervous Control of Micturition. *Physiol. Rev.* 45: 426, 1965.

26. **Lewin, R.J., Dillard, G.V., Porter, R.W.** Extrapyramidal Inhibition of the Urinary Bladder. *Brain Res.* 4:301, 1967.

27. **Martner, J.** Influences on the Defecation and Micturition Reflexes by the Cerebellar Fastigial Nucleus. *Acta Physiol. Scand.* 94:95–104, 1975.

28. **Mathews, P.B.C.** Muscle Spindles and Their Motor Control. *Physiol. Rev.* 44:219, 1964.

29. **McLeod, J.G.** The Representation of the Splanchnic Afferent Pathways in the Thalamus of the Cat. *J. Physiol.* 140:462, 1958.

30. **Murnaghan, G.F.** Neurogenic Disorders of the Bladder in Parkinsonism. *Br. J. Urol.* 33:403, 1961.

31. **Nathan, P.W., Smith, M.C.** The Centrifugal Pathway for Micturition within the Spinal Cord. *J. Neurol. Neurosurg. Psychiatry* 21:117, 1958.

32. **Nathan, P.W., Smith, M.C.** The Contripetal Pathway from the Bladder and Urethra within the Spinal Cord. *J. Neurol. Neurosurg. Psychiatry* 14:262,1951.

33. **Oliver, J.E., Bradley, W.E., Fletcher, T.F.** Spinal Cord Representation of the Micturition Reflex. *J. Comp. Neurol.* 137: 329, 1969.

34. **Rockswold, G.L., Bradley, W.E., Chou, S.N.** Effect of Sacral Nerve Blocks on the Function of the Human Urinary Bladder. *J. Neurosurg.* 40:83, 1974.

35. **Tang, P.C.** Levels of Brain Stem and Diencephalon Controlling the Micturition Reflex. *J. Neurophysiol.* 18:583, 1955.

3 The Neurological Control of Micturition and Integral Voiding Reflexes

Donald R. Ostergard, M.D.

An understanding of the neurology of micturition is important to every practicing gynecologist or urologist. Until recently, mystique, vagary and uncertainty shrouded this subject to the point that most practicing physicians found it to be of no clinical significance. This is unfortunate since a basic comprehension of the neurology of micturition by the practicing physician enables him to more thoughtfully prescribe medications for the treatment of various urogynecological disorders. Similarly, he is better able to understand the effect of a variety of non-urologic medications upon the lower urinary tract. The purpose of this chapter is to assemble the contemporary knowledge of the neurological mechanisms involved with the control of micturition.

CENTRAL NERVOUS SYSTEM LOOPS AND CIRCUITS

The current conceptualization of the neurological control of the lower urinary tract permits the identification of four loops and circuits as described by Bradley (4–5). Although this is a convenient categorization for discussion purposes, interrelationships exist between all four loops such that successful function of one loop depends upon the integrity of the remaining loops. Most importantly, the successful integration of the micturition reflex requires a balanced contribution by all four loops. Although specific tests may suggest malfunction of a specific loop or circuit, the exact localization of the central nervous system abnormality requires a thorough neurological evaluation.

The following paragraphs describe each of these loops and circuits according to anatomical origin and termination, function, clinical abnormalities associated with malfunction, clinical indications of malfunction, and tests for integrity of the intact reflex.

Loop I: The Cerebral-Brain Stem Circuit

Origin and Termination. Loop I originates in the frontal lobes of the cerebral cortex and terminates in the pontine-mesencephalic reticular formation of the brain stem. The cerebellum and basal ganglia provide additional input (Figure 3.1).

Function. This loop coordinates volitional control of the micturition reflex.

Associated Abnormalities. Various disease entities may interrupt or alter this circuit. Examples of such abnormalities are: Parkinson's disease, brain tumors, trauma, cerebral vascular disease, multiple sclerosis and local lower urinary tract disease.

Clinical Indications of Malfunction. Interruption of this circuit severs the micturition reflex from volitional control.

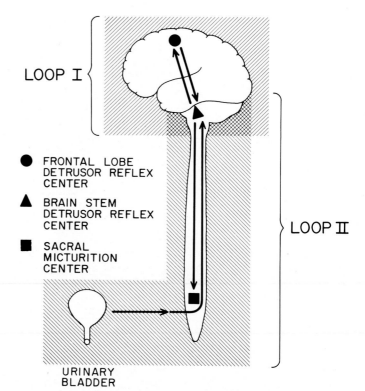

Figure 3.1. The origins and terminations of Loop I (the cerebral-brain stem loop) and Loop II (the brain-stem-sacral loop).

Therefore, the bladder functions autonomously without the benefit of volitional control.

Tests for Integrity. The cystometrogram tests the integrity of Loop I. This test determines the ability of the patient to voluntarily suppress detrusor contractions.

Loop II: The Brain Stem Sacral Loop

Origin and Termination. Loop II originates in the pontine-mesencephalic reticular formation of the brain stem and terminates in the sacral micturition center. Additionally, sensory afferents originate in the bladder musculature and travel directly from the bladder to this brain stem center without synapsing. These afferents bypass the sacral micturition center (Figure 3.1).

Function. This loop provides for a detrusor muscle contraction which is of sufficient temporal duration to allow total evacuation of intravesical contents.

Associated Abnormalities. Abnormalities which alter the function of Loop II are spinal cord trauma, multiple sclerosis and spinal cord tumors.

Clinical Indications of Malfunction. Total interruption of this circuit produces an absence of vesical contractions.

Tests for Integrity. The cystometrogram is the primary means of testing the integrity of Loop II. Loop II is intact if a terminal detrusor contraction appears in the cystometrogram as the physician instructs the patient to urinate.

Loop III: The Vesical-Sacral-Sphincter Loop

Origin and Termination. Loop III originates with sensory afferents in the detrusor muscle which travel to the detrusor nucleus in the sacral micturition center. From there, interneurons influence the closely located pudendal motor nucleus. Pudendal motor neurons terminate in the striated muscular component of the urethral sphincter (Figure 3.2).

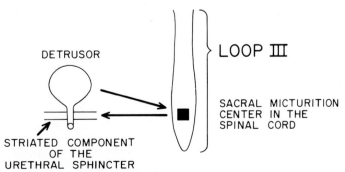

Figure 3.2. The origin and termination of Loop III (the vesical-sacral-sphincter loop).

Function. Loop III provides the circuitry for coordination of detrusor and the urethral muscular activity during voiding. That is, the integrity of this loop allows the tonically contracted external striated muscular sphincter of the urethra to relax in synchrony with contraction of the detrusor muscle. Loop IV may override this effect (see below).

Associated Abnormalities. These include multiple sclerosis, spinal cord trauma, spinal cord tumors, the peripheral neuropathy of diabetes mellitus and local urinary tract disease.

Clinical Indications of Malfunction. Absence of urethral sphincter relaxation during micturition produces symptoms of obstruction such as hesitancy and prolongation of the total time required to void.

Tests for Integrity. Tests for the integrity of Loop III require the application of sophisticated neurophysiologic techniques designed to trace signals and measure the transit time from one area of the peripheral nervous system to another. That is, this technique traces and times a signal applied to the urethra as it travels to the rectal sphincter via the spinal cord (see Chapters 8 and 24).

Loop IV: The Cerebral Sacral Loop

Origin and Termination. Loop IV originates in the frontal lobe of the cerebral cortex and terminates in the pudendal nucleus located in the sacral micturition center (Figure 3.3).

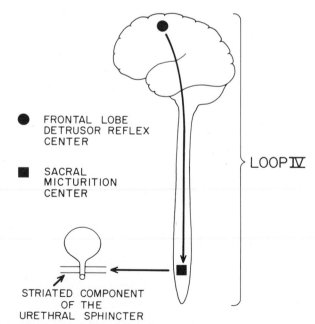

Figure 3.3. The origin and termination of Loop IV (the cerebral-sacral loop).

Function. This loop provides for volitional control of the striated external urethral sphincter.

Associated Abnormalities. These include multiple sclerosis, cerebral or spinal cord trauma or tumors, cerebral vascular disease, and local lower urinary tract disease.

Clinical Indications of Malfunction. Interruption of this loop abolishes voluntary contraction of the external striated urethral sphincter on command.

Test for Integrity. Electromyographic evidence of voluntary contraction of the external striated urethral sphincter demonstrates an intact Loop IV.

AUTONOMIC CONTROL OF THE LOWER URINARY TRACT

The lower urinary tract is under the control of the autonomic nervous system. Both the sympathetic and parasympathetic components influence the lower urinary tract (2, 4, 8).

Parasympathetic Nervous System

Origin and Termination. The parasympathetic nervous system originates in the sacral spinal cord segments S2 through S4. Its long preganglionic fibers terminate in ganglia located within the wall of the innervated end organ. Both the long preganglionic fibers and the short postganglionic fibers release the neurotransmitter acetylcholine. Anatomically, the pelvic nerve contains parasympathetic nerve fibers.

Function. The parasympathetic nervous system stimulates the detrusor muscle contraction and inhibits urethral smooth muscle contraction.

Sympathetic Nervous System

Origin and Termination. The sympathetic nervous system originates from thoracic spinal cord segments 10 to 12 to the second lumbar segment. Preganglionic sympathetic fibers are short and terminate in ganglia generally located at some distance from the end organ. These fibers also release the neurotransmitter acetylcholine. The long postganglionic sympathetic fibers terminate in parasympathetic ganglia and in the innervated end organ. The sympathetic postganglionic fiber releases the neurotransmitter norepinephrine. The sympathetic nervous system has alpha and beta adrenergic components. Although both the bladder and the urethra receive alpha and beta fibers, the beta fibers terminate primarily in the detrusor muscle with only minimal beta adrenergic innervation of the urethra. The converse is true for the alpha component which terminates primarily in the urethra. Anatomically, the hypogastric nerve contains sympathetic nerve fibers.

Function. The alpha adrenergic component stimulates contraction of the bladder neck and urethra and produces relaxation of the detrusor muscle. The beta adrenergic component relaxes the urethra and the detrusor muscle. The sympathetic nervous system also depresses transmission within parasympathetic ganglia. This modulation of the parasympathetic nervous system by sympathetic neurons provides the basis for a complex interaction between the two major components of the autonomic nervous system at the end organ level.

INTEGRAL REFLEXES CONCERNED WITH VOIDING

An alternative and complementary method of comprehending the neurology of micturition involves an understanding of the 12 reflexes which are important for coordinated micturition. These reflexes subserve the functions of continence, storage, initiation, continuation and cessation of micturition. Mahoney and associates recently described these reflexes (15).

Continence Favoring Reflexes

Four reflexes subserve the function of favoring continence and storage.

Sympathetic Detrusor Inhibiting Reflex (7)

Origin and Termination. This reflex originates in the detrusor musculature and travels to the sacral spinal cord. From the cord it returns to the detrusor musculature (Figure 3.4).

Function. This reflex inhibits the contractility of the detrusor muscle in response to increasing tension of its own muscular walls.

Sympathetic Sphincter Constrictor Reflex (7, 10, 14)

Origin and Termination. The reflex originates in the detrusor muscle and travels to the sacral spinal cord. It terminates in the internal (smooth muscle component) urethral sphincter (Figure 3.4).

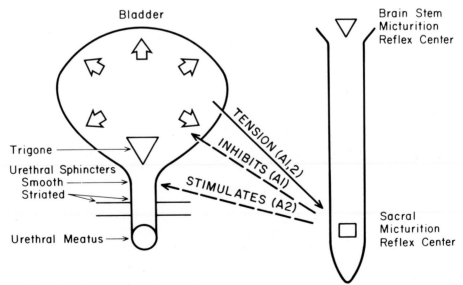

Figure 3.4. Continence favoring reflexes: Increasing detrusor mural tension leads to inhibition of detrusor contractility (Reflex A1) and contraction of the smooth muscle component of the urethral sphincter (Reflex A2).

Function. This reflex stimulates the contractility of the smooth sphincter in response to increasing tension of the detrusor muscle.

The Perineodetrusor Inhibitory Reflex (3, 6)

Origin and Termination. This reflex originates from the perineal and pelvic floor muscles and travels to the sacral micturition reflex center. It terminates in the detrusor muscle (Figure 3.5).

Function. The function of this reflex is to inhibit detrusor contractility in respone to increasing voluntary tension in the perineal and pelvic floor muscles.

Urethrosphincteric Guarding Reflex (10, 14)

Origin and Termination. This reflex originates in the bladder trigone and the proximal urethra and travels to the sacral cord. It terminates in the external striated sphincter of the urethra (Figure 3.6).

Function. This reflex stimulates contraction of the external striated portion of the urethral sphincteric mechanism in response to increasing tension in the bladder trigone or the presence of urine in the proximal urethra.

Initiation of Micturition Reflexes

Two reflexes contribute to the initiation of micturition.

Perineobulbar Detrusor Facilitative Reflex (14)

Origin and Termination. This reflex originates in the pelvic floor and perineal musculature. It travels from these muscles to the detrusor constrictor center in the brain stem and in turn to the detrusor relaxor center. It then proceeds to the sacral micturition center and subsequently terminates in the detrusor muscle (Figure 3.7).

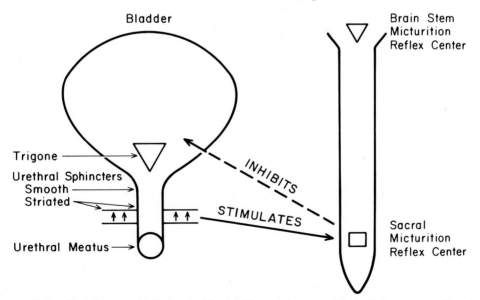

Figure 3.5. Continence favoring reflexes: Increasing tension of the external striated sphincter leads to inhibition of detrusor contractility (Reflex A3).

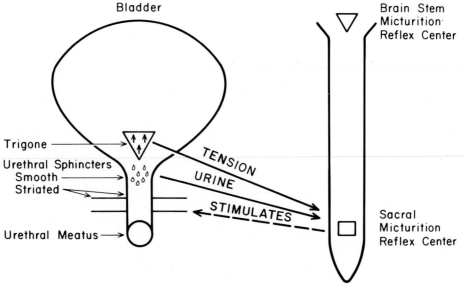

Figure 3.6. Continence favoring reflexes: Increasing tension in the trigone or the presence of urine in the proximal urethra leads to contraction of the external striated urethral sphincter (Reflex A4).

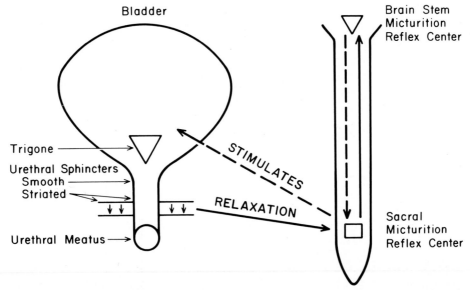

Figure 3.7. Initiation of micturition reflexes: Voluntary contraction of the diaphragmatic and abdominal musculature with simultaneous relaxation of the perineal and pelvic floor musculature leads to vesical contraction (Reflex B1).

Function. This reflex assists with the initiation of detrusor contraction at the beginning of micturition in response to abdominal and diaphragmatic muscular contraction and perineal and pelvic floor muscular relaxation.

Detrusodetrusor Facilitative Reflex (1, 9, 13, 14)

Origin and Termination. This reflex originates in the detrusor musculature and travels to the spinal cord and hence to the brain stem reflex center. It then proceeds to the sacral micturition center and terminates in the detrusor musculature (Figure 3.8).

Function. This reflex stimulates detrusor contraction at the beginning of the actual act of micturition in response to increasing detrusor mural tension.

Intramicturition Reflexes

Five reflexes are operative during the actual act of micturition.

Detrusourethral Inhibitory Reflex (1)

Origin and Termination. This reflex originates in the detrusor musculature and travels to the sacral reflex center. It terminates in the bladder neck and the proximal urethra (Figure 3.9).

Function. This reflex inhibits contraction of the bladder neck and the proximal urethra (smooth muscle component) in response to increasing detrusor mural tension prior to micturition.

Detrusosphincteric Inhibitory Reflex (1, 14)

Origin and Termination. This second reflex of the same name also originates in the detrusor musculature and travels to the sacral reflex center. It terminates in the external striated component of the urethral sphincter (Figure 3.9).

Function. This reflex inhibits the external striated component of the urethral sphincter.

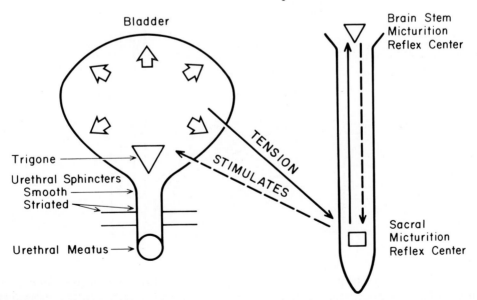

Figure 3.8. Initiation of micturition reflexes: Increasing detrusor mural tension facilitates detrusor contraction (Reflex B2).

Urethrodetrusor Facilitative Reflex (1, 10, 14, 16)

Origin and Termination. This reflex originates in the proximal urethra and travels to the brainstem reflex center and subsequently to the sacral micturition reflex center. It terminates in the detrusor muscle (Figure 3.10).

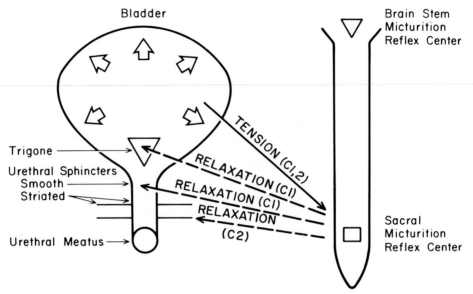

Figure 3.9. Intramicturition reflexes: Increasing detrusor mural tension leads to relaxation of the trigone and smooth muscle of the proximal urethra (Reflex C1) and to relaxation of the external striated component also (Reflex C2).

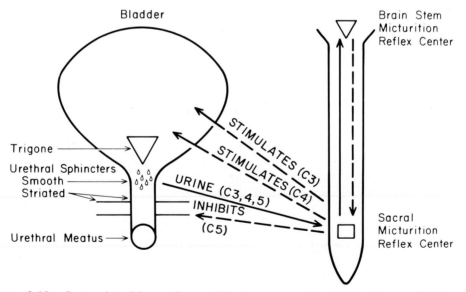

Figure 3.10. Intramicturition reflexes: The presence of urine in the proximal urethra causes an increase in detrusor muscle contractility (Reflex C3 incorporates the brain stem reflex center which is not included in Reflex C4) and inhibits the external striated urethral sphincter.

Function. This reflex stimulates detrusor muscle contraction in response to the presence of urine in the proximal urethra.

Urethrodetrusor Facilitative Reflex (1, 10, 14)

Origin and Termination. The second reflex by the same name originates in the urethra and travels to the sacral micturition reflex center. It terminates in the detrusor musculature (Figure 3.10). This reflex does not have a brain stem component.

Function. This reflex stimulates detrusor contraction in response to the presence of urine in the urethra.

Urethrosphincteric Inhibitory Reflex (1)

Origin and Termination. This reflex originates in the proximal urethra and travels to the sacral reflex center. It terminates in the external striated portion of the urethral sphincter (Figure 3.10).

Function. This reflex inhibits the voluntary (striated portion) of the external urethral sphincter during micturition.

Micturition Cessation Reflex

A single reflex aids the cessation of micturition and the resumption of the storage phase.

Perineobulbar Detrusor Inhibitory Reflex (11, 12, 14)

Origin and Termination. This reflex originates in the perineal and pelvic musculature and travels to the sacral reflex center and subsequently to the brainstem center. It returns to the sacral micturition reflex center and terminates in the detrusor musculature (Figure 3.11).

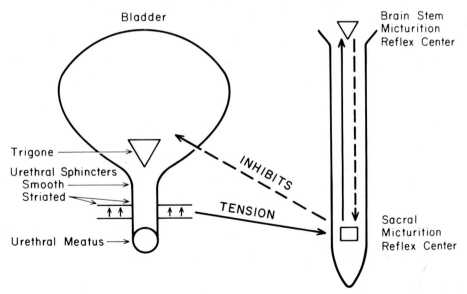

Figure 3.11. Micturition cessation reflex: Increasing tension in the perineal and pelvic floor musculature at the termination of micturition inhibits contraction of the detrusor muscle (Reflex D1).

Function. This reflex inhibits contraction of the detrusor muscle at the termination of micturition in response to voluntary contraction of the perineal and pelvic floor musculature. This facilitates the cessation of micturition and initiates the storage phase.

SUMMARY OF REFLEXES

Reflexes which originate from increased detrusor mural tension subserve several functions (Table 3.1). Some favor continence and retention while others assist in the initiation and maintenance of micturition. The seemingly contradictory nature of these reflexes emphasizes the delicate balance between stimulatory and inhibitory influences which exist in the micturition process.

An additional reflex originates from increasing trigonal mural tension with or without the presence of urine in the proximal urethra, and others originate solely from the

Table 3.1 Summary of Micturition Reflexes

Reflex	Function	Effect
I. Reflexes Originating from Increased Detrusor Mural Tension		
A1	Favor retention and	Inhibits detrusor contractility
A2	continence	Stimulates smooth muscle component of urethral sphincter
B2	Initiation of micturition	Facilitates detrusor contraction
C1	Maintenance of micturition	Relax smooth muscle of trigone and proximal urethra
C2	Maintenance of micturition	Relax striated muscle of the urethra
II. Reflex Originating from Increased Trigonal Mural Tension and/or the Presence of Urine in the Proximal Urethra		
A4	Favors continence and retention	Stimulates contraction of external striated urethral sphincters
III. Reflexes Originating from the Presence of Urine in the Proximal Urethra		
C3	Maintenance of micturition	Stimulates detrusor contractility
C4	Maintenance of micturition	Stimulates detrusor contractility
C5	Maintenance of micturition	Inhibits external striated urethral sphincter
IV. Reflexes Originating from Increased Tension in the Perineal or Pelvic Floor Muscles		
A3	Favors continence	Inhibits detrusor contractility
D1	Terminates micturition	Inhibits detrusor contractility
V. Reflex Originating from Decreased Tension in Perineal and Pelvic Floor Muscles		
B1	Initiation of micturition	Stimulates contractility of detrusor

presence of urine in this location (Table 3.1). Again, checks and balances are evident from opposing forces.

Other reflexes originate from increased tension in the perineal or pelvic floor muscles as well as decreased tension in these same muscles. Similar opposing influences are evident.

COMMENT

From the foregoing discussion of the reflexes and reflex arcs involved in the neurology of micturition, it is evident that a variety of loops, circuits and integral voiding reflexes are important in the voluntary act of voiding. All of these circuits must be intact in order for normal voiding to occur. Although lack of complexity is not a virtue inherent in the reflex arcs of normal micturition, the practicing gynecologist benefits from an understanding of the contemporary knowledge of this complex mechanism. An example is the patient with vesical neck funnelling associated with stress incontinence who demonstrates uninhibited bladder contractions in addition to anatomical stress incontinence. An understanding of the effect of urine in the funnelled proximal urethra (Reflexes C3 and C4) provides an explanation of this phenomenon and suggests a rationale for surgical therapy. These reflexes may be operative when opposing influences are absent.

In the clinical practice of gynecologic urology, it is very common to encounter a variety of abnormalities which affect the ability of the patient to maintain continence and to initiate or terminate voiding at will. An understanding of these reflexes, loops and circuits helps to place these problems in perspective.

Finally, an understanding of the neurology of micturition also allows a better comprehension of the effect of various pharmacologic agents on the lower urinary tract. Knowledge of the effects of these pharmacologic agents upon the lower urinary tract allows an understanding of clinical malfunctions resulting from medical therapy of unrelated disease. Similarly, urogynecologic disorders may be effectively treated by definitive pharmacologic therapy. In many instances this alleviates the need to subject the patient to an unnecessary surgical procedure.

References

1. **Barrington, F.J.F.** The Component Reflexes of Micturition in the Cat. *Brain* 54:177–188, 1931.
2. **Bissada, N.K., Finkbeiner, A.E., Welch, L.T.** Lower Urinary Tract Pharmacology, II. Review of Neurology. *Urology* 9:113–118, 1977.
3. **Bors, E.** Segmental and Peripheral Innervation of the Urinary Bladder. *J. Neurol. Mental Disorders* 116:572–578, 1952.
4. **Bradley, W.E., Timm, G. W., Scott, F.B.** Innervation of the

Detrusor Muscle and Urethra. *Urol. Clin. North Am.* 1:3–27, 1974.

5. **Bradley, W.E., Rockswold, G. L., Timm, G. W., Scott, F.B.** Neurology of Micturition. *J. Urol.* 115:481–486, 1976.

6. **Denny-Brown, D., Robertson, E.** On the Physiology of Micturition. *Brain* 56:149–191, 1933.

7. **Edvardsen, P.** Neurophysiological aspects of Enuresis. *Acta. Neurol. Scand.* 48:220, 1972.

8. **Gosling, J.A., Dixon, J.S., Lendon, R.G.** The Autonomic Innervation of the Human Male and Female Bladder Neck and Proximal Urethra. *J. Urol.* 118:302–305, 1977.

9. **Kamikawa, K., Matsuo, S., Koshino, K., Kuru, M.** Analysis of Lateral Column Units Related to Vesical Reflexes. *Exp. Neurol.* 6:271–284, 1962.

10. **Karlson, S.** Experimental Studies on the Functioning of the Female Urinary Bladder and Urethra. *Acta Obstet. Gynecol. Scand.* 32:285–307, 1953.

11. **Kuru, M., Kurati, T., Koyama, Y.** The Bulbar Vesico-Constrictor Center and the Bulbo-Sacral Connections Arising from It. *J. Comp. Neurol.* 113:365–388, 1957.

12. **Kuru, M., Koyama, Y., Kurati, T.** The Bulbar Vesico-Relaxer Center and the Bulbo-Sacral Connections Arising from It. *J. Comp. Neurol.* 115:15–25, 1960.

13. **Kuru, M., Makuya, A., Koyama, Y.** Fiber Connections between the Mesencephalic Micturition Facilitary Area and the Bulbar Vesico-Motor Centers. *J. Comp. Neurol.* 117:161–178, 1961.

14. **Kuru, M.** Nervous Control of Micturition. *Physiol. Rev.* 45: 425, 1965.

15. **Mahoney, D.T., Laberte, R.O., Blais, D.J.** Integral Storage and Voiding Reflexes: Neurophysiologic Concept of Continence and Micturition. *Urology* 10:95–106, 1977.

16. **Nathan, P.W., Smith, M.C.** The Centripetal Pathway from the Bladder and Urethra Within the Spinal Cord. *J. Neurol. Neurosurg. Psychiatry* 14:262–280, 1951.

II EVALUATION OF THE LOWER URINARY TRACT

4 Medical History and Physical Examination

Thomas A. McCarthy, M.D.

As in every area of clinical medicine, the patient's history is of primary importance. The more accurate and complete the history, the better the subsequent urologic evaluation maximizes available diagnostic resources. Equally important is the thorough physical examination which complements the history and gives initial clues to the patient's basic problem. This chapter outlines the important elements of the urological history and physical examination in the evaluation of the incontinent patient.

MEDICAL HISTORY

It is important to realize that lower urinary tract symptoms have their basis in a wide variety of structural and functional abnormalities. It is incumbent upon the physician to sort out these symptoms to reach a final diagnosis; the urologic history aids the physician in this process. However, unlike most areas of medicine, the history is not helpful in arriving at a precise diagnosis; its primary value is to direct further investigative efforts wisely. The reasons for this are twofold. First, lower urinary tract symptoms are generally overlapping and non-specific. For example, urgency and frequency of urination occur not only in patients with urinary tract infections but also in patients with uninhibited bladder contractions. Surprisingly, both infection and uninhibited bladder contractions occur in patients even without these symptoms. Secondly, in addition to the lack of specificity, urinary symptoms frequently result from a non-urologic disease process. For example, normal micturition

45

depends upon an intact and normally functioning neurologic system. A wide variety of disease processes, such as diabetes, thyroid disease and senile atrophy affect the central and peripheral nervous system and produce a symptomatic alteration of normal micturition patterns. Similarly, since the conscious level controls much of the micturition process, psychiatric disorders often include urinary complaints as well.

Although non-specific, the urologic history highlights general categories of pathology. In general, pathology in five major areas causes lower urinary tract symptoms: (1) intrinsic urinary tract pathology; (2) extrinsic local anatomic changes; (3) neurologic disorders; (4) psychiatric disorders; and (5) local effects of systemic disease or its treatment. Specific questions in the medical history suggest a categorization of the patient's problem into one of these general areas rather than trying to focus on a specific diagnosis.

A more reliable and complete history derives from written questions which the patient answers in private in a yes or no fashion. This programmed history taking avoids the majority of both patient and physician errors inherent in the history taking proces. Appendix III, Form 1A displays the historical questionnaire which the patient completes prior to interview by the physician. The questionnaire reviews topics such as previous urologic disease and family history of urologic disorders, trauma or previous surgery, medical disease, neurologic history, current medication and the specifics of the patient's current urologic problem. Allowing the patient to complete the questionnaire in the waiting room prior to interview by the physician is convenient and allows the patient as much time as she needs to accurately present her problem. The physician then reviews the positive responses with the patient. Although the questionnaire is not a substitute for an adequate history, it serves to highlight and focus on the patient's problem, allowing further definition by the physician.

PHYSICAL EXAMINATION

The physical examination is as important in patients with urological complaints as it is in every other field of medicine. In particular, when dealing with lower urinary tract complaints, the physician emphasizes the neurologic and pelvic examinations. Chapter 5 discusses the urologically oriented neurologic examination. It is of particular importance for the physician to search for neurological disease in any patient with urologic symptoms. The first manifestations of many neurologic diseases are lower urinary tract symptoms, epecially in those patients with incontinence. Appendix III, Form 2 displays the form used to record the urologically oriented physical examination.

The pelvic examination is of primary importance in the evaluation of the patient with lower urinary tract symptoms. Estrogen deprivation not only manifests itself with atrophic changes in the vulva and vagina but also produces a variety of lower urinary tract symptoms. Similarly, since both fistula and urethral diverticula produce incontinence, a thorough search may reveal their presence.

Slight variations in technique allow an easier and more productive examination. The Sims speculum helps to evaluate cystocele, diverticula and urinary fistula. Careful palpation of the suburethral tissues occasionally reveals induration or sacculation suggesting the presence of a diverticulum. Although urethral diverticula and urinary fistula are difficult to diagnose on physical examination, the physician must rule out their presence in any incontinent patient.

There are several special diagnostic maneuvers performed during the pelvic examination of the patient complaining of incontinence. These tests attempt to differentiate between genuine stress incontinence and the uninhibited bladder.

The first of these is the Q-tip test which is useful to determine the amount of vesical neck descent on straining. With the patient in the supine position, the physician inserts a lubricated Q-tip into the urethra to the level of the urethrovesical junction and measures the angle between the Q-tip and the horizontal, using an orthopedic goniometer. The patient then strains maximally which produces a new angle of the Q-tip with the horizontal. At rest, the angle in the non-parous woman is normally from 10° to 15° above the horizontal with minimal change on straining. In the patient with geniune stress incontinence, this angle usually increases by 20° or more, frequently in the range of 50° to 60°. This suggests that descent of the vesical neck is due to weakness of normal anatomical support. Unfortunately, not all patients with genuine stress incontinence have a positive Q-tip test nor do all patients with a positive Q-tip test have genuine stress incontinence. This test gives the physician information on the amount of vesical neck descent with straining and usually obviates the need for a chain cystogram.

The stress test is also a useful diagnostic aid especially when performed simultaneously with urethral closure pressure studies. The physician examines the patient with a full bladder in the standing position. While the physician closely observes the urethral meatus, the patient coughs. If short spurts of urine escape simultaneously with each cough, this suggests genuine stress incontinence. A delayed leakage or the loss of large volumes of urine suggests the diagnosis of uninhibited bladder contractions as the etiology of the patient's incontinence rather than genuine stress incontinence.

In those patients demonstrating a "stress-type" leakage of urine during the stress test, other tests purport to help determine the beneficial effects of surgical elevation of the bladder neck. The Bonney test utilizes two vaginal fingers to elevate the bladder neck toward the umbilicus, taking care not to compress the urethra. Urethroscopically, however, urethral compression almost always occurs, thereby, negating the predictive value of the Bonney test. The Marchetti test, using local anesthesia and Allis clamps, and the Read test, using rubber shod clamps, also compress the urethra. Because occlusion of the urethra or vesical neck prevents leakage regardless of the pathophysiology of the patient's incontinence, these tests are of limited value.

SUMMARY

A properly performed history and physical examination contribute substantially to the diagnosis of the basic urologic disturbance. Rarely, the history and physical examination alone reveal the precise diagnosis. Usually they only suggest which path to take for further evaluation which ultimately provides the proper diagnosis. Except for physical defects such as fistula or diverticula, it is erroneous to make a diagnosis on the basis of the history and physical examination alone. Almost always, further corroboration requires endoscopic, radiologic, urodynamic or pharmacologic testing procedures.

References

1. **Chrystle, C.D., Charmel, S., Copeland, W.E.** Q-tip Test for Stress Urinary Incontinence. *Obstet. Gynecol.* 38:313, 1971.
2. **Graber, E.A.** Stress Incontinence in Women: A Review. *Obstet. Gynecol. Surv.* 32:565, 1977.
3. **Pelosi, M., Apuzzio, J.J., Frattarola, A. et al.** Diagnostic Device for Stress Incontinence. *Obstet. Gynecol.* 45:223, 1975.
4. **Shingleton, H.M., Davis, R.O.** Stress Incontinence in Perspective. *J. Cont. Educ. Obstet. Gynecol.* December 1977, pp 15–26.
5. **Svigos, J.M., Matthews, C.D.** Assessment and Treatment of Female Urinary Incontinence by Cystometrogram and Bladder Retaining Programs. *Obstet Gynecol.* 50:9, 1977.

5 The Urologically Oriented Neurological Examination

William E. Bradley, M.D.

The neurologic examination of the incontinent patient is potentially very valuable. Although few patients show overt neurologic disease, the yield in patients with urinary incontinence is greater than in the normal population. Unfortunately, objective deduction from the neurological examination is not always possible, and the neurologist tends to overestimate abnormalities because of the subjectivity of the neurological evaluation. Pattern recognition is important in the interpretation of the potential constellation of neurologic findings. Since historical events may be the most important consideration, an extensive history of voiding difficulties and habits, along with information regarding bowel and sexual function, is essential to proper interpretation of neurological findings. In this subjective way the neurologist applies a diagnostic label to the patient and assigns a prognosis.

GENERAL SCREENING NEUROLOGICAL EXAMINATION

In order to localize neurological lesions the physician systematically examines the cranial nerves, the deep tendon reflexes, muscular function, coordination and, finally, body sensory function. The reflexes of importance are the jaw jerk, the bicep, tricep, knee, ankle and plantar responses. Evaluation of each of these allows him to localize the lesion to the cerebrum, brain stem, spinal cord or periphery or, alternatively, to recognize its diffuseness. Any asymmetry of reflexes or muscular function, symmetrical hyperreflexia, impairment of intellectual function or coordination indicates the need to refer the patient to a neurologist for a thorough examination.

The sensory examination is the most subjective part of the neurological evaluation and includes perception of light touch, pain, temperature, vibration, position and deep pain. Again, asymmetry of response indicates the need for referral.

LOWER URINARY TRACT SCREENING NEUROLOGICAL EXAMINATION

Since sacral spinal cord segments S2 to S4 contain the important neurons involved with micturition, the screening neurological examination relating to the lower urinary tract encompasses the sensory and motor functions represented in this area. It is not important that the referring physician arrive at a precise neurological diagnosis. It is important, however, that the referring physician know when to refer the patient with incontinence to a neurologist for a thorough evaluation.

MOTOR FUNCTION

Evaluation of the motor function of the sacral area involves testing the patient's ability to perform certain basic motor functions (Figure 5.1). The basic maneuvers are extension and flexion of the hip, knee and ankle and inversion or eversion of the foot. Figure 5.1 illustrates these manuevers and the segments of the spinal cord involved.

SENSATION

The dermatome chart of the lower extremities indicates the sacral and lumbar roots involved in the sensation of this area (Figure 5.2).

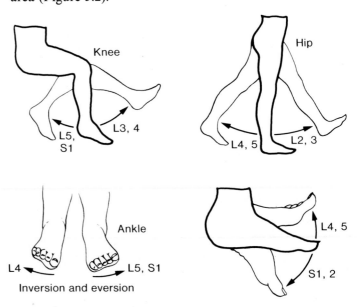

Figure 5.1.   Motor innervation of the lower extremities.

TESTS OF SACRAL CORD INTEGRITY

The external voluntary anal sphincter is representative of the pelvic floor musculature. Anal sphincter testing involves a determination of resistance to entry of the examining finger and the ability of the patient to voluntarily contract the anal sphincter. A full bladder or rectal ampulla may interfere with anal sphincter reflex activity but leaves the muscle tone unaffected.

Three reflexes help in the examination of sacral reflex activity. These are the anal sphincter, bulbocavernosus and cough reflexes. All produce a reflex contraction of the pelvic floor. Stroking the skin lateral to the anus elicits the anal reflex (Figure 5.3A). The bulbocavernosus reflex involves contraction of the bulbo- and ischiocavernosus muscles in response to tapping or squeezing the clitoris (Figure 5.3B). Pulling on a suprapubic or intraurethral Foley catheter or touching the urethral or vesical mucosa also stimulates this reflex. Since the external anal sphincter is part of this same pelvic floor musculature, it also responds in most patients. Intactness of these reflexes indicates functional normality of the fifth lumbar to the fifth sacral segments.

The cough reflex involves the same cord efferents but also the volitional innervation of the abdominal muscles (T6 to L1). Both coughing and deep inspiration causes a contraction of the periurethral striated sphincter (Figure 5.4).

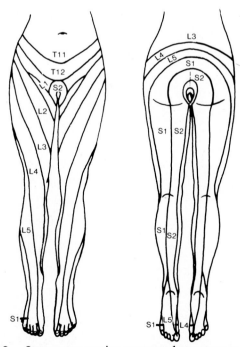

Figure 5.2.   Lower extremity sensory dermatomes.

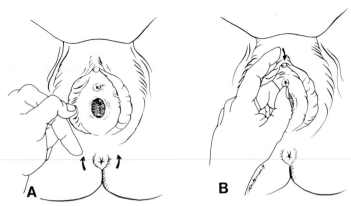

Figure 5.3. The anal and clitoral reflexes. Gentle stroking lateral to the anus causes anal sphincter contraction **(A)**. Gental tapping or pressure on the clitoris causes pelvic floor contraction **(B)**.

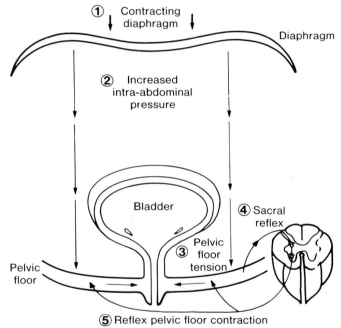

Figure 5.4. The cough reflex. The stretch spindles in the levator ani and external striated urethral sphincter are activated by increased intra-abdominal pressure and cause reflex contraction of the periurethral skeletal musculature.

Unfortunately, these reflexes are sometimes difficult to evaluate clinically due to the rapidity of response. It is possible to definitively detect the responses of all three reflexes by placing a pressure sensitive catheter in either the urethra or the anal sphincter and recording pressure changes (Figure 5.5).

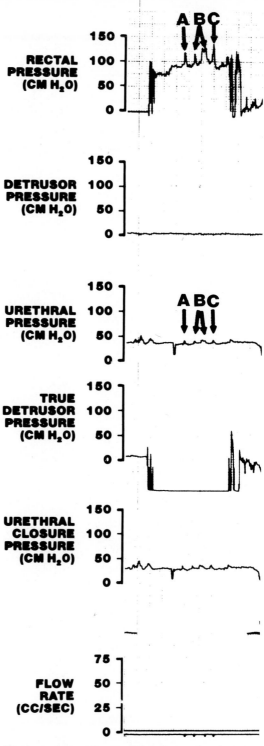

Figure 5.5. The urodynamic confirmation of voluntary, anal and clitoral reflex activity of the pelvic floor. The urethral transducer is at maximal pressure and the other transducer is in the area of peak anal pressure. The labeled arrows indicate the voluntary (**A**), anal (**B**) and clitoral (**C**) responses of intra-anal and intraurethral pressures.

SUMMARY

A variety of diseases cause urethral and bladder distur-bances and associated clinical symptoms. The primary care physician has the responsibility to perform a general screen-ing neurological examination. An abnormality discovered during this evaluation indicates the need to consult a neu-rologist. Specifically, abnormalities of the bulbocavernosus reflex, anal reflex or volitional control of the anal sphincter indicate altered sacral reflex activity and are highly sugges-tive of a central or peripheral nervous system lesion. The referring physician has a major role in performing the majority of these screening neurological examinations. However, the neurologist has the ultimate task of assigning a specific diagnosis to the abnormality.

References

1. **Adams, R., Victor, M.** *Textbook of Neurology*, W.B. Saunders, Philadelphia, 1978.
2. **Baker, A.B., Baker, L.H.,** Eds. *Textbook of Neurology*. Harper and Row, New York, 1978.

6 Introduction to the Preoperative Evaluation of the Incontinent Patient

Stuart L. Stanton, F.R.C.S., M.R.C.O.G.

INTRODUCTION

There is much controversy about the methods of evaluation of female patients with functional disorders of the lower urinary tract. Part of this stems from our knowledge and understanding of the anatomy and physiology of micturition. Despite studies by several authors (1,2,8), older concepts of the etiology of incontinence, such as the importance of the posterior urethrovesical angle, still remain. Frequently, clinicians encounter the incontinent patient who has a satisfactory posterior urethrovesical angle and, conversely, the continent patient who lacks this angle. Finally, no amount of measuring of the angle will enable a diagnosis of detrusor instability to be made.

Because of the invasive nature of these investigations, there is a low risk of urinary tract infection and they are also uncomfortable. For these reasons, the physician only performs those tests which are necessary.

Certain questions remain to be answered:
1. What is the patient's main complaint?
2. What is the etiology of her disorder?
3. Does her condition warrant major surgery?
4. If so, what kind of surgery?

To see the problem of incontinence in perspective, it is necessary to know its incidence. The medical literature contains many surveys involving varying age groups using postal questionnaires, direct interviews and other techniques (Table 6.1).

Table 6.1. The Frequency of Urinary Incontinence In Various Age Groups

Author	Age (years)	% of Population
Nemir and Middleton (4)	17–21	5
Osborne (5)	35–60	26
Thomas et al. (9)	15–64	21
Hood (3)	62–90	42

Incontinence occurs in the young nulliparous patient and the incidence of incontinence increases towards old age. The latter probably results from a combination of the following factors: cerebral atherosclerosis leading to decreased bladder inhibition and reduction of social awareness, decreased physical mobility, the effects of menopause and previous childbearing on bladder and urethral anatomical supports, constipation and urinary tract infection.

One difficulty confronting any epidemiologist is to find an acceptable definition of incontinence which takes both the severity and frequency of incontinence into account. These are subjective symptoms and some attempt to objectively measure them is important. In the absence of objective data we are unable to compare surveys like those in Table 6.1 and, more importantly, we are unable to measure the effects of surgical procedures and decide which are satisfactory and which are not.

Before investigating a patient it is important to classify the causes of incontinence (Table 6.2, see Chapter 21). The most common cause is urethral sphincter incompetence in which the sphincter mechanism is no longer able to prevent urine leaking from the normal bladder during moments of physical effort or stress. Synonyms for this include "stress urinary incontinence," "anatomic stress incontinence," "genuine stress incontinence" and "pressure equalization incontinence." The term "stress incontinence" on its own only designates the symptom and the sign but is *not* the diagnosis. This is important since "stress incontinence" occurs in many types of incontinence.

Table 6.2. Causes of Urinary Incontinence

Urethral sphincter incompetence
Detrusor instability
Urinary retention and overflow
Congenital
Urinary fistula
Functional

SYMPTOMS	MSU FOR CULTURE	URINALYSIS	URETHROCYSTOSCOPY	UROFLOWMETRY	URETHRAL PRESSURE	SUBTRACTED CYSTOMETRY	VCU / MCG	URILOS	INTRAVENOUS UROGRAM	URINE OSMOLARITY	BLOOD UREA AND CREATININE	LUMBO - SACRAL SPINE X - RAY	FLUID BALANCE CHART	URINARY DIARY	URETHRAL EMG
STRESS INCONTINENCE (NO PAST SURGERY)	●			●		●									
RECURRENT STRESS INCONTINENCE	●		●	●	●		●	●							
STRESS & URGE INCONTINENCE, NOCTURIA	●		●	●	●		●	●							
URGE & FREQUENCY (NO INCONTINENCE)	●	●	●	●		●			●	●	●		●	●	
FREQUENCY (DOMINANT)	●	●	●	●		●			●	●	●		●	●	
UROLOGICAL & NEUROLOGICAL SYMPTOMS (UMN)	●		●	●		●			●		●	●			●
VOIDING DIFFICULTIES	●		●	●	●	●			●		●	●	●		●
ENURESIS	●		●			●								●	
ELDERLY OR DISABLED WITH INCONTINENCE	●			●					●		●			●	
CONTINUOUS INCONTINENCE	●		●	●	●		●		●		●				

Figure 6.1.   A guide to appropriate investigations for urological complaints. MSU: Midstream urine; VCU/MCG: videocystourethrogram/micturating cystogram; Urilos: an electronic diaper used to record urine loss; UMN: upper motor neuron. The physician chooses the appropriate investigations dependent upon the patient's symptoms.

SELECTION OF EVALUATION PROCEDURES

The orientation of the evaluation process is towards achieving a diagnosis and includes a medical history, physical examination and urodynamic investigations. It is important to be aware that disorders outside the pelvis produce incontinence, such as the effects of multiple sclerosis, diabetes mellitus and autonomic neuropathy, and that voiding disorders sometimes remain undetected in the presence of incontinence. A simple guide illustrates the author's approach to the choice of investigations in relation to symptoms (Figure 6.1; see Chapter 25).

Medical History

The recording of the medical history is either by conventional written means or assumes the form of a yes/no questionnaire which varies in complexity according to how much information the clinician requires. The advantage of the latter is that it allows for ready computerization (Figure 6.2). Either the patient herself, the nurse or the doctor administers it. While the first two methods of administration save the physician time, direct questioning by the doctor ultimately provides more valuable and accurate data. The history includes general health, urological, gynecological, neurological and psychiatric symptoms. Also important are an account of current and past drugs, obstetric and surgical

Medical Questionnaire

URODYNAMIC DATA 1

Surname

Hosp. No. _____

Card No. | 1

Unit No. .... (2 5)

2 5

Ref. Consultant...

First Names

(10 15) Date of Birth

6 9

Date of Consultation....................................... (6 9)

Sex

PRESENT CONDITION   (9 = No Data)

Age:................................

10 15

Main Complaints   **Duration**

16 18

1)...

19 21

2)...

22 24

3)...

Duration: $0 = < \frac{1}{12}$, $1 = \frac{1 \cdot 6}{12}$, $2 = \frac{7 \cdot 12}{12}$, $3 = \frac{13}{12}$ 2yrs, 4 = 3 5yrs, 5 = 5 10yrs, 6 = >10yrs.

Frequency Day: $<$ Hourly · No. of times · 0=No, 1= $\frac{\frac{1}{2} \cdot 1}{10^+}$, 2= $\frac{2}{7 \cdot 9}$, 3= $\frac{3}{5 \cdot 6}$, 4= $\frac{4}{4}$, 5= $\frac{5}{3 \cdot 4}$ 6= $\frac{6}{3}$ 7= $\frac{7}{2 \cdot 3}$, 8= $\frac{8}{2}$

25

26

Night: No. of times · 0 = None, 1   2   3   4   5   6   7   8+   9 = No Data

Other Symptoms   0=No   1=Yes occasionally 2=Yes frequently   3=Not applicable

Stress Incontinence (27) .... Urgency (28)..............

27 | 28

Urgency Incontinence (29).............................. Wet at rest (30)..............

29 | 30

Wet on standing up (31).............................. Wet at night (32)..............

31 | 32

Ability to interrupt flow (33)..............................Complete emptying (34)..............

33 | 34

Post micturition dribble (35).............................. Good stream (36)..............

35 | 36

Straining to void (37).............................. Retention of urine (38)..............

37 | 38

Dysuria (39).............................. Aware of full bladder (40)..............

39 | 40

Aware of being wet (41).............................. Aware of prolapse/dragging (42)..............

41 | 42

Protective underwear (43).............................. Dyspareunia (44)..............

43 | 44

Rectal soiling (45).............................. Weakness of legs (46)..............

45 | 46

Cough (47).............................. Constipation (48)..............

47 | 48

Other symptoms   1)..............................

49 50

2)..............................

51 52

Periods   1 = Premen., 2 = Menopausal, 3 = Postmen., 4 = Hysterectomy +/-BSO

53

O.C.Pill.............................. Cycle.............................LMP..............

Effect of a period on a main symptom   ·   0 = No Effect   2 = Aggravated   3 = Better

54

9 = No Data or No periods

Diabetes Mellitus   0 = No   1 = Yes 9 = No Data

55

Neurological disorder   ·   0 = None 1 = UMN lesion 2 = LMN lesion 3 = Mixed 4 = Unspecified

56

5 = MS 9 = No Data

Psychological disorder   ·   0 = None 1 = Schizophrenia 2 = Other Psychosis 3 = Neurosis

57

Other Disorders   1) ....

58 59

2) ....

60 61

Present Medication   **Name**   **Success**   **Duration**

1)..............................

62 66

2)..............................

67 71

3)..............................

72 76

Success: 0 = No success   1 = Improved 2 = Cured 3 = Irrelevant 9 = No Data

Other   1)..............................

77 78

2)..............................

79 80

Figure 6.2.   St. George's Hospital Current Medical History Questionnaire. The column on the right is for computerization of questionnaire data.

history, particularly previous incontinence surgery (Figure 6.3).

Physical Examination

The physical examination comprises a general examination, and specific evaluation of the urological, gynecological and neurological systems, including the back. The physician notes the position, mobility and tenderness of the urethra, bladder neck and bladder base, together with the capacity and mobility of the vagina (Figure 6.2).

Any abnormal neurological symptoms and signs or significant psychiatric symptoms require further investigation in collaboration with the other especially knowledgeable physicians.

Investigations

Culture and sensitivity of a midstream or catheterized specimen of urine precedes any investigation. Invasive urodynamic evaluation procedure in the presence of a urinary tract infection not only aggravates the infection, but commonly invalidates the results of the investigations. The basic procedures include: urethrocystoscopy, cystometry, radiology, uroflowmetry and simultaneous urethral and bladder pressure measurements. Since subsequent chapters explain these procedures in detail, this discussion amplifies only certain points.

Urethrocystoscopy

The physician performs urethrocystoscopy under general anesthesia or with the patient awake (see Chapter 11). If cystometry reveals a reduced bladder capacity, filling the bladder under general anesthesia determines if this is a true or artefactual capacity. The interpretation of the function of the bladder neck when visualized at urethrocystoscopy necessitates an element of caution. Failure of closure of the bladder neck requires confirmation by a combination of urethrovesical pressure recordings and radiological screening during voiding.

Cystometry

The most useful urodynamic investigation is cystometry, which provides information on the filling phase of bladder function (see Chapter 7). There is still a controversial debate over whether gas or water is the best filling medium. This author prefers water due to more familiarity with it. Carbon dioxide has the disadvantages of gas leakage, compressibility and interaction of carbon dioxide with bladder mucosa. Subtracted cystometry is the technique of choice, as this allows measurement of the detrusor pressure by subtracting rectal (abdominal) pressure from the intravesical (total bladder) pressure. Regardless of the position of the patient during cystometry, the pressure transducers are always at the level of the symphysis pubis. The rate of filling is controversial. This author prefers a non-physiological rate of 100 ml per minute because this discloses detrusor instability in those patients where it is obvious or latent. The

Past Medical History & Physical Examination

URODYNAMIC DATA 2

Unit No...(2.5)

Ref. Consultant...

Date of Consultation...............................(6.9)

Surname _____   Hosp. No. _____

First Names   Date of Birth

Sex

Card No. | 2

2 5

6 9

Past History   (9 = No Data)

	Operation	Date	Success	Duration
1)				
2)				
3)				
4)				
5)				

00000 = No operation. Success · 0 = No Success 1 = Improved 2 = Cured 3 = Irrelevant
9 = No Data

Duration: $0 = <\frac{1}{12}$, $1 = \frac{1\cdot6}{12}$, $2 = \frac{7\cdot12}{12}$, $3 = \frac{13}{12}$· 2yrs, $4 = 3\cdot5$yrs, $5 = 5\cdot10$yrs, $6 = >10$yrs.

	Drug Name	Success	Duration of Therapy
1)			
2)			
3)			

Parity   0   1   2   3   4   5   6   7   8+   9 = No Data

Birth weight of heaviest infant (kg)   00 = None/No Data

Enuresis   0 = No 1 = Yes 9 = No Data   Until....................years.

Retention   0 - No 1 = Yes 9 = No Data

Urinary Tract infection   (attacks in last 2 years) 0 - None   1   2   3   4   5   6   7+
                               8 = chronic infection 9 = No Data

Examination   (9 = No Data)

Breasts....................................Height (cms.).................................(56.58)

Abdo.......................................Weight (kg.).................................(59.61)

Neuropathy   0 = None 1=mild / 2=severe > UMN   3=mild / 4=severe > LMN   5=mild / 6=severe > Mixed

Congenital lesions · 0 = None 1 = Ectopic ureter   2 = Epispadias 3 = Spina Bifida (overt)
                        4 = Spina Bifida (occult) 5 = other

Anterior Wall prolapse · 0 = None 1=slight / 2=marked > Cystourethrocoele   3=slight / 4=marked > Cystocoele

Rectocoele   · 0 = None   1 = slight   2 = marked

Enterocoele   · 0 = None   1 = slight   2 = marked

Uterine/Vault Descent · 0=None 1=1° 2=2° 3=3° 4=slight vault descent 5=marked vault descent

Uterine Size   · 0=Normal, $1 - <\frac{12}{52}$ $2 = \frac{12+}{52}$ 8= No uterus

Stress incontinence · 0= No   1 = Yes

Other pelvic pathology · 0= No   1 = Yes

Anal Sphincter tone · 0= Normal I = Decreased 2 = No tone

$S_{2, 3, 4}$ **Outflow**   0 = Normal 1=Dec. / 2=Inc. > Motor   3=Dec. / 4=Inc. > Sensory   5=Dec. / 6=Inc. > Both

Other 1)...
          2)...

(grid labels right margin): 10 14, 15 19, 20-24, 25 29, 30 34, 35 39, 40 44, 45 49, 50, 51 52, 53, 54, 55, 56 58, 59 61, 62, 63, 64, 65, 66, 67, 68, 69, 70, 71, 72, 73 74, 75 76

Figure 6.3. St. George's Hospital Past Medical History Questionnaire and Physical Examination Record Form.

physician notes the following during cystometry: residual urine, first sensation of filling, final capacity, the pressure rise on filling, the pressure rise on changing from a sitting to a standing position, and any detrusor contractions which occur during bladder filling.

If uroflowmetry is available, the patient voids with the pressure catheters still present in the urethra and bladder, in order to record to maximum voiding pressure simultaneously with the peak urine flow rate.

Radiology

Radiologic techniques allow evaluation of the voiding phase of bladder function, principally to detect the presence of stress incontinence, the position of the bladder neck and base of the bladder and to exclude ureteric reflux (see Chapter 13). This is a useful and informative procedure and with an image intensifier, the amount of irradiation during radiological screening of the voiding phase is less than that of a standard intravenous pyelogram. By combining it with cystometry it is possible to study both the filling and voiding phases of bladder and urethral function together. This enhances the value of this procedure.

A television camera displays the detrusor pressure, intravesical pressure and flow rate from the recorder and combines this with the radiological image (Figure 6.4). The resultant combined picture enters the videotape recorder, together with a verbal commentary of the patient's history and the radiologist's comments made to the patient during screening. This is a dynamic and permanent record of voiding and allows later replay and case discussion (Figure 6.5). From the videotape, the physician notes the presence of stress incontinence, the position and mobility of the bladder neck and bladder base at rest and during coughing and voiding, the ability of the extrinsic urethral sphincter to voluntarily interrupt the urinary stream and the subsequent ability of the bladder neck to close, residual urine, and ureteric reflux.

Uroflowmetry

This is a relatively unknown investigation for gynecologists but is, of course familiar to urologists (see Chapter 9). Uroflowmetry provides a method to study urine flow characteristics and is a measure of the function of the detrusor contraction and the outflow resistance. It is a non-invasive investigation. For accurate interpretation the patient must void at least 200 ml of urine during several independent and private flow measurements. As well as obtaining the maximum flow rate, the uroflowmetry also records the volume voided. A pelvic examination or urethral catheterization after voiding confirms the completeness of bladder emptying. Flow rate values below 20 ml per second during a time period of greater than 20 seconds indicate voiding disorders.

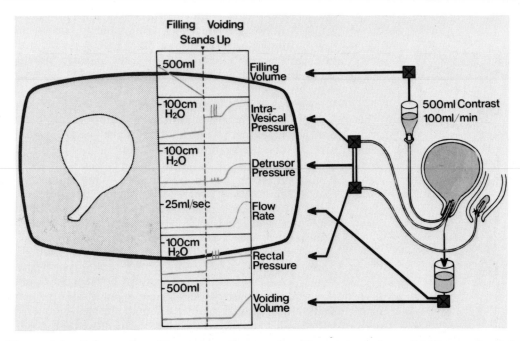

Figure 6.4. Schema for videocystourethrography. The rectangular solid line on the left outlines the events recorded on the videotape. The display includes the radiological appearance of the bladder and the urethra on the left and the urodynamic events on the right. The urodynamic tracing includes three events evaluated during the cystometrogram: the filling phase (left); the effect of standing (center); and the voiding phase (right). The left hand side of the polygraph tracing shows the simultaneous recording of bladder and rectal pressure changes during supine cystometry, combined with a display of bladder filling volume. On voiding, the bladder and rectal pressures with the voiding rate and volume are recorded on the right of the tracing. A television camera projects three parameters (intravesical pressure, detrusor pressure and voiding rate) in addition to the radiographic image of the bladder (shown on the extreme left of the schema). A sound commentary on the videotape completes the recording.

The role of this investigation is to confirm a suspected voiding disorder and to exclude voiding disorders in a patient about to undergo incontinence surgery (6–7).

Simultaneous Urethral and Bladder Pressure Measurements

The work of Enhorning on the relationship between simultaneous urethral and bladder pressure measurements before and during micturition provide the cornerstone for our understanding of the mechanism of urinary control (see Chapters 7, 9 and 10). To remain continent, the pressure in the urethra must exceed the intravesical pressure so that a *positive* urethral closure pressure exists. Stress incontinence due to urethral sphincter incompetence occurs when this is absent in the presence of pressure equalization or negative urethral closure pressures. The existence of many different techniques for these measurements makes comparison of results difficult. These include twin microtipped catheter transducers, CO_2 and water perfusion catheters and the membrane catheter. Chapters 7, 9, and 10 discuss the

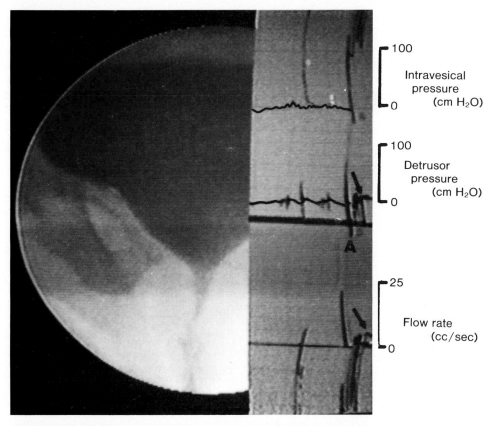

Figure 6.5. A videocystourethrogram. On the left is the radiologic image of the bladder and on the right the intravesical and detrusor pressures and urine flow rate data from a typical patient during micturition. At Point A the patient stands. Note increase of true detrusor pressure (arrow) and urine flow (arrow).

advantages and disadvantages of these various techniques. Both methods require careful attention to calibration and record in order to avoid artefacts.

CONCLUSION

The final decision as to which methods of investigation prevail depends upon the clinician's view of the factors governing the control of continence and the finances, equipment and manpower available to perform the investigations. This chapter serves as an introduction to the available methods which are detailed in succeeding chapters. A simple guide (Figure 6.1) indicates one approach to the choice of investigations in relation to the patient's symptoms (see Chapter 25).

References

1. **Enhorning, G.** Simultaneous Recording of Intravesical and Intraurethral Pressure. A Study on Urethral Closure in Normal and Stress Incontinent Women. *Acta. Chir. Scand.* 276:1–68, 1961.

2. **Gosling, J., Dixon, J., Lendon, R.** The Autonomic Innervation of the Human Male and Female Bladder Neck and Urethra. *J. Urol.* 118:302, 1977.
3. **Hood, N.** Incontinence in the Elderly. Conference at Scottish Health Service Centre, 1976.
4. **Nemir, A., Middleton, R.** Stress Incontinence in Young Nulliparous Women. *Am. J. Obstet. Gynecol.* 68:1166–1168, 1954.
5. **Osborne, J.** Post-menopausal Changes in Micturition Habits and in Urine Flow in Urethral Pressure Studies. In *Management of the Menopause and Post-menopausal Years*, edited by S. Campbell. Medical and Technical Publishing Co. Ltd., Lancaster, England, 1976, pp. 291–198.
6. **Stanton, S.L.** Pre-operative Investigation and Diagnosis. *Clin. Obstet. Gynecol.* 21:705–724, 1978.
7. **Stanton, S.L., Cardozo, L., Chandbury, N.** Spontaneous Voiding after Surgery for Urinary Incontinence. *Br. J. Obstet. Gynecol.* 85:149–152, 1978.
8. **Tanagho, E.** Anatomy and Physiology of Micturition. In *Gynecological Urology*, edited by S. L. Stanton. *Clin. Obstet. Gynecol.* W. B. Saunders, London, 1978, p. 3–26.
9. **Thomas, T., Plymat, K., Blannin, J., Meade, T.** Prevalence of Incontinence in the Community. Proceedings of the VIIIth International Continence Society Meeting, Manchester, England, p. 3–15, 1978.

7 Urodynamics: Cystometry and the Urethral Closure Pressure Profile

Emil A. Tanagho, M.D.

When evaluating a patient with serious clinical disturbance of the lower urinary tract, it is important to understand that one single test cannot reveal everything about the entirety of function of this area. This makes it necessary to use the combined results of a variety of urodynamic testing procedures in order to understand the effect of various pathological entities on the bladder and the urethra. Urodynamic studies of the lower urinary tract evaluate the dynamic functional activities of the bladder, the sphincter and the interrelation of these two organs during the voiding act itself. This dynamic functional integration of activities determines the normalcy or abnormalcy of the lower urinary tract.

BLADDER

Urodynamic or radiologic studies alone or in combination provide useful information in the study of detrusor function. Radiographic studies comprise simple cystography or the more complex combination of fluoroscopy and cinefluoroscopy. A thorough study of bladder function necessitates obtaining information about its capacity, its ability to perceive sensation, its ability to accommodate various volumes of fluids and its contractility. Specifically, analysis of bladder function provides practical knowledge regarding its unique feature of being an involuntary organ, yet under voluntary control. In defined testing situations, its responses to various drugs, both stimulants and depressants, supply an appreciation of anticipated clinical responses to these medications. Pressure recordings under specific conditions provide much of this information.

SPHINCTER

The vesical sphincter consists of two muscular sphincteric mechanisms: a smooth sphincter (involuntary) and a skeletal (voluntary) sphincter. An adequate evaluation of sphincteric function requires an understanding of the functional capabilities of each unit separately by either pressure measurements or by electromyography. Electromyography is only applicable to the skeletal sphincter, whereas pressure studies provide information regarding the activity of the voluntary as well as the involuntary sphincter.

VOIDING ACT

An evaluation of the voiding act itself comprises a simultaneous study of the functional combination of the detrusor and both components of the sphincter. The outcome of the interaction between these two organs determines the actual urinary flow rate and the efficiency of bladder emptying.

CYSTOMETRY

Bladder capacity of the average woman is normally within the range of 400 to 500 ml of water. A variety of neuropathic dysfunctions as well as diseases either reduce or increase this capacity. Table 7.1 contains a partial listing of conditions associated with reduced bladder capacity.

Increased bladder capacity also occurs from a variety of causes (Table 7.2). For example, many women train themselves to hold more urine, probably resulting from various social factors.

Actual capacity by itself has little meaning without simultaneous measurement of pressures. A decreased capacity bladder with normal pressures has little significance. How-

Table 7.1. Conditions Associated with Reduced Bladder Capacity

Enuresis
Infection
Contracted bladder
Upper motor neuron lesion
Postsurgical defunctionalization
Incontinence

Table 7.2. Conditions Associated with Increased Bladder Capacity

Social inhibitions
Sensory neuropathy
Lower motor neuron lesion
Outflow obstruction
Megalocystis

ever, a reduced capacity associated with increased pressure becomes very significant. Similarly, increased vesical capacity associated with normal pressure is of minor significance, particularly in teenagers. However, large capacity becomes very significant when associated with diminished intravesical pressure. The combination of large volume and low pressure usually signifies a definable underlying pathologic entity.

Intravesical pressure recordings (cystometrogram or CMG) provide information about the cumulative result of intra-abdominal pressure plus the true detrusor pressure (Figure 7.1). The true detrusor pressure is the total detrusor pressure minus the simultaneously measured intra-abdominal (intra-

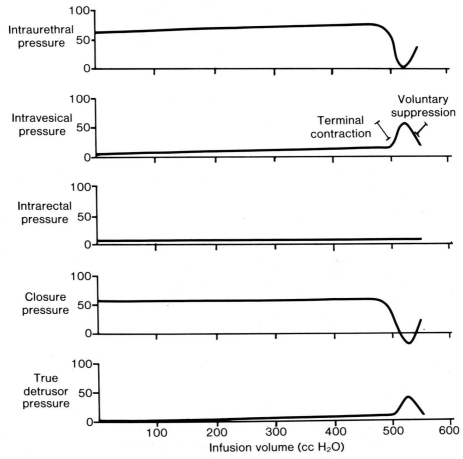

Figure 7.1.   The normal cystometrogram with an inhibitable terminal contraction. This diagrammatic representation of a urodynamic tracing shows the simultaneous measurement of intraurethral, intravesical and intrarectal pressures. The intrarectal pressure, when subtracted from the intravesical pressure, gives the true detrusor pressure. The closure pressure results from subtracting the intravesical pressure from the intraurethral pressure. All measurements of pressure are in cm of H_2O.

rectal) pressure. Total detrusor pressure alone is meaningless, since it may result from factors other than actual activity of the detrusor muscle itself. True detrusor pressure recordings are necessary to make deductions regarding the authentic muscle activity of the detrusor muscle itself. Although some pressure results from spontaneous rectal peristalsis, its contribution to total intrarectal pressure is usually insignificant.

It is possible to have either a low pressure system or a high pressure system within the normal intravesical pressure range. Low pressures with normal capacities are distinctly normal (Figure 7.1). However, low pressures with a large capacity potentially indicate either sensory neuropathic dysfunction, a flaccid bladder or the large, chronically obstructed atonic bladder (Figure 7.2).

Several subdivisions exist in the high pressure group. One

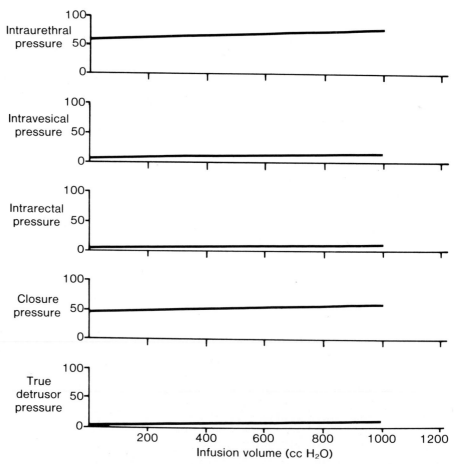

Figure 7.2. The CMG of a hypotonic bladder. Minimal intravesical pressure increase occurs despite a large intravesical volume. No terminal contraction occurs.

of these is a rapidly rising pressure demonstrable during bladder filling (Figure 7.3). The pattern occurs with reduced bladder capacity, with inflammatory changes and also with enuresis. The high pressure spikes or waves associated with a series of uninhibited bladder contractions constitute another subdivision (Figure 7.4). The intravesical pressure does not go back to baseline and gives a progressively climbing, stepladder type of bladder pressure rise which is quite common with uninhibited vesical contractions.

The third aspect of cystometric evaluation of the bladder is its power of accommodation. This very important feature reflects the resiliency of the bladder in response to stretch as indicated by its pressure response to distension. This represents the relationship of volume to pressure during actual detrusor filling (Figure 7.1).

One of the most important features of bladder function is

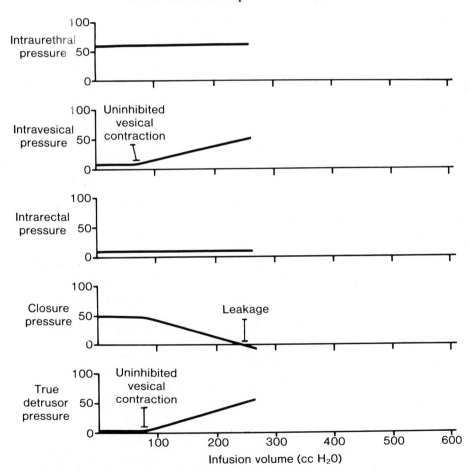

Figure 7.3.   The CMG of a hypertonic bladder. Characteristically, a gradual increase of uninhibitable bladder pressure occurs at low bladder volumes.

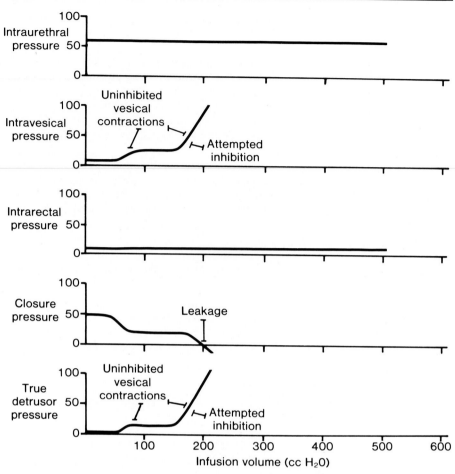

Figure 7.4. The CMG of a hypertonic bladder. A series of uninhibitable vesical contractions occur with a stairstep increase in intravesical pressure.

its ability to contract. The bladder is unique since it is an involuntary organ with voluntary control. It is also unique since, once it contracts on its own, it normally sustains a contraction until it is completely empty.

There are two aspects to contractility of the bladder. The first is whether or not detrusor contractions occur (Figure 7.1). Secondly, and more importantly, is whether the detrusor contractions are of sufficient duration to completely evacuate intravesical contents. Absent or very weak contractions result from sensory neuropathic or lower motor neuron lesions or from conscious inhibition. The latter is important since conscious inhibition of detrusor function is an unmistakable sign of normalcy but could readily be mistaken for lack of vesical contractile ability.

Uninhibited detrusor contractions signify a lack of accommodation on the part of the bladder during filling. In order to recognize these abnormal contractions during cystometry, one evaluates the voluntary control of this involuntary organ (Figure 7.4). Voluntary control has two phases, ability to initiate a contraction as well as ability to inhibit the contraction. The neurologically normal individual has sufficient voluntary control to both inhibit or initiate contractions in spite of the fact that it is a smooth muscular organ (Figure 7.1).

The final point regarding cystometry is the effect of stimulatory and inhibitory drugs on the bladder. It is important to know the range of drug effects and to decide whether this bladder is inherently overactive, overresponsive, or whether it reacts in an opposite fashion.

SPHINCTER: PRESSURE RECORDINGS VERSUS ELECTROMYOGRAPHY

There are two basic means to evaluate the sphincter, either by recording pressures or by electromyography. Electromyography utilizes either surface electrodes or needle electrodes. Needle electrodes are most precise; surface electrodes are very inaccurate. Electromyography of individual motor unit potentials is not an easy technique to master due to many artifacts from voluntary activity or injury from the needle producing a myriad of overlapping patterns. Only the expert electromyographer can separate true electromyographic motor unit action potentials from other artifacts.

URETHRAL CLOSURE PRESSURE PROFILES

The urethral closure pressure profile (UCPP) provides information regarding several aspects of urethral function (Figure 7.5). These are the total or maximum urethral pressure, the closure pressure (the difference between the

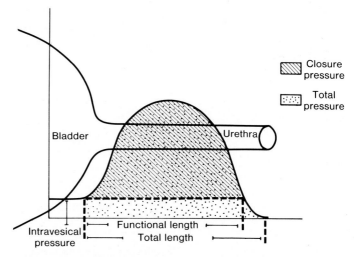

Figure 7.5. The urethral closure pressure profile of a normal patient. The hatch lines outline the area of closure pressure and the dotted area represents the area of total urethral pressure.

bladder pressure and the urethral pressure), the functional length of the sphincteric unit (the length of the urethra which exhibits a positive pressure above the bladder pressure), the total urethral length (functional length plus the additional length to reach atmospheric pressure), and the anatomical length of the urethra as defined by radiopaque markers on the catheter. Normally, the anatomical length and the functional length are approximately equal. In a variety of diseases they start to separate and become different.

Several techniques are available to record urethral closure pressure profiles. Perfusion techniques utilize gas or water. The gas or water slowly and constantly emerges through an open side hole in the catheter (Figure 7.6). The recording reflects the resistance to perfusion of gas or water through the urethra. Non-perfusion techniques include catheters with pressure sensitive membranes or microtransducers which record any pressure applied to its surface.

Extensive comparative studies of these four parameters reveal that gas perfusion is the least reliable, least reproducible and the least accurate. Water is probably acceptable within certain limits. It lacks rapid responsiveness and it does not measure the pressure at one particular level of the urethra as the pressure profile implies. In reality it measures

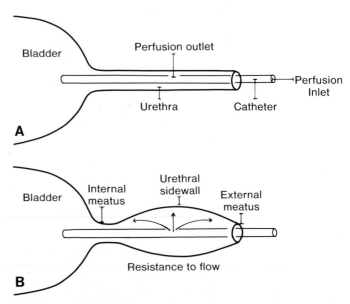

Figure 7.6. The perfusion urethral closure pressure profile. (A) The catheter in the urethra prior to infusion. (B) During perfusion there is resistance to flow at the internal and external urethral meatus as well as from the urethral sidewall.

the overall total resistance to the escape of the perfused water from the open side hole of the catheter to the outside through the external meatus or to the inside of the bladder through the urethrovesical t– junction (Figure 7.6).

The membrane catheter is very sensitive and quite accurate, gives reproducible results and measures localized intraurethral pressures (Figure 7.7). The disadvantages are the relative difficulty in the actual use of the technique, the necessity for specially constructed catheters, and the experience required for the personnel for calibrating, adjusting and applying the technique.

In all probability the microtransducer is best (Figure 7.8); it is very sensitive and very accurate. The only problems are the expense and the delicateness of the instrument. With appropriate modifications to increase its durability and the mounting of the transducers on a proper catheter, it will be

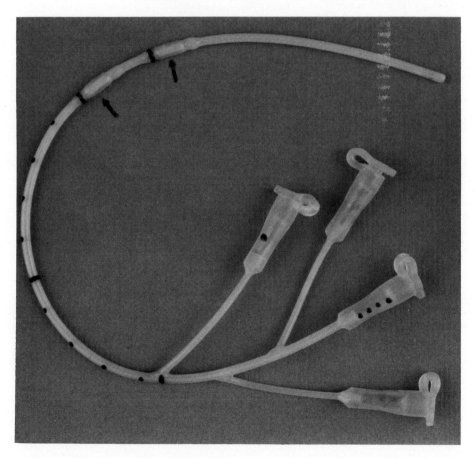

Figure 7.7. The membrane catheter. This catheter has four channels. Two open at the end of the catheter for intravesical pressure measurements and for intravesical perfusion during the CMG. The two balloons (arrows) measure intraurethral pressures.

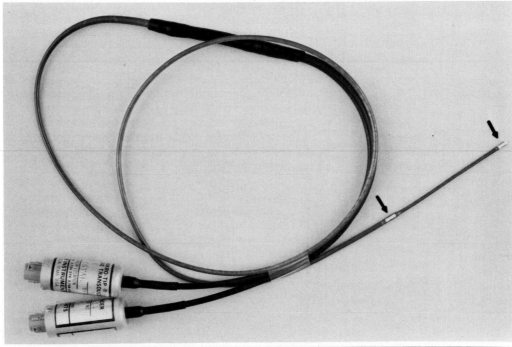

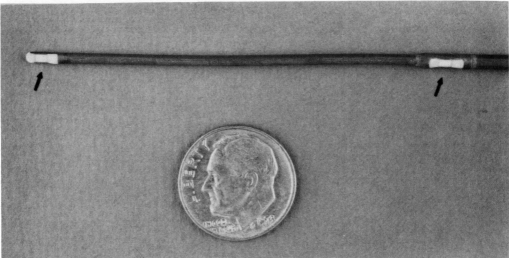

Figure 7.8. The microtransducer catheter. The two microtransducers (arrows) measure intravesical and intraurethral pressures.

the technique of choice. We plan to develop a single catheter containing both a pressure sensitive membrane and a microtransducer.

Our technique employs the membrane catheter. It is a four-channel silicone catheter with a 6 French outside diameter (Figure 7.7). It has radiopaque markers at the level of the membranes which are about $1\frac{1}{2}$ cm apart, and the first membrane is about 7 cm from the tip of the catheter. It contains additional markings at 1 cm intervals with a heavier mark every 5 cm. These radiopaque markings allow visualization radiologically and fluoroscopically, thus providing an accurate record of the actual level of pressure in the urethra. Two lumens exit from the catheter tip. One is for bladder filling and the other one is for recording bladder pressure. The two balloons are sensitive to urethral pressure; one is for the smooth or involuntary sphincter (U1) and the other for the voluntary or skeletal sphincter (U2).

This catheter allows the recording of simultaneous pressures in two areas of the urethra and also in the bladder with or without simultaneous bladder filling. Simultaneous intra-abdominal pressure recordings by using an intrarectal recording catheter allows subtraction of the intra-abdominal pressures from the intravesical pressure to provide an indication of the true detrusor pressure (Figure 7.1). Similarly, subtraction of peak urethral pressure (U2) from intravesical pressure provides for simultaneous recording of urethral closure pressure (Figure 7.9). This technique also includes measurements of urine flow rate and urine volume as well as a radiographically derived video image with sound recordings (Figure 7.10). Simultaneous recording is important to allow a meaningful study of the lower urinary tract in the individual patient.

The unit includes a specially designed remote control rotating toilet chair. Under the chair is a container to collect the urine for measurement of flow rates as well as the total volume voided. The x-ray machine and the image intensifier are in front. A television camera picks up the picture from the fluoroscopic image. The recorded pressures go to a channel mixer and then to the recorder; a second TV camera records the pressures and projects them on a video monitor screen. The channel mixer allows the simultaneous viewing of bladder and urethral fluoroscopy, including the catheter itself in the center of the screen, and the various pressures and flow rates appear simultaneously on either side. Videotape recording as well as a movie camera provide permanent records.

After placement of the catheter all the way into the bladder, gradual withdrawal allows a recording of the urethral closure pressure profile. Figure 7.9 is a recording of a normal pressure profile of an adult female.

The pressure sensitive membrane moves from the urethrovesical junction through the urethra to the external meatus, giving an accurate continuous pressure measurement along the entire length of the urethra. This recording shows that the maximum closure pressure is not at the level of the

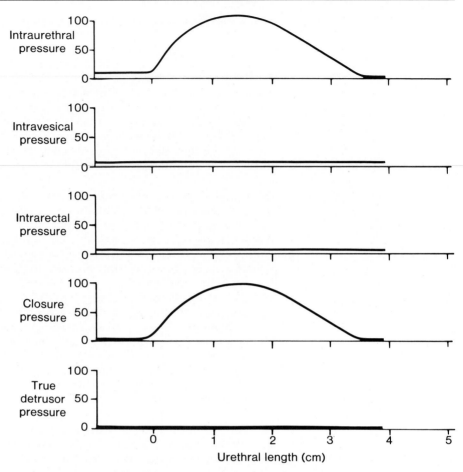

Figure 7.9.   The urethral closure pressure profile in the normal female. Subtraction of intravesical pressure from simultaneously measured intraurethral pressure provides a recording of the urethral closure pressure.

internal meatus; it is actually in the midsegment of the urethra where the overlapped voluntary sphincter surrounds the smooth muscle sphincteric unit (Figure 7.9).

One line of the tracing is the bladder pressure, recorded simultaneously during the profile by the tip of the catheter which is always in the bladder cavity. The difference between the bladder pressure and the urethral pressure is the closure pressure. This total squeeze around the pressure sensitive membrane defines the urethral closure pressure profile as the difference between the bladder pressure and the urethral pressure at any particular level.

Another important point of information provided by the urethral closure pressure profile is the distribution of the closure pressure along the anatomical length. That is, it defines the relation of the maximum point of closure pres-

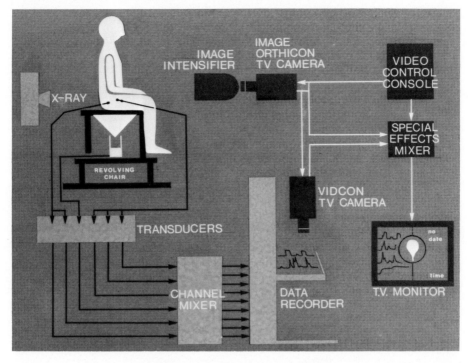

Figure 7.10. The urodynamic recording method. The urodynamic data and the video image are mixed and displayed on the television monitor.

sure to the bladder and the location of the weakest segment of the sphincteric mechanism in relation to urethral length. This technique allows a relatively precise localization of areas of specific weakness or overactivity of either the voluntary or involuntary sphincters. For example, if the smooth sphincter is lost the record shows decreased closure pressure in the proximal segment of the sphincteric mechanism (Figure 7.11). Knowledge of the anatomical location of theses two sphincteric components allows their separation for individual study. In the female the location of the maximum activity of the voluntary sphincter is in the midurethral segment.

DYNAMIC FUNCTION OF THE URETHRAL SPHINCTERIC MECHANISM

A functional assessment of the dynamics of the sphincteric unit is possible by the superimposition of a variety of voluntary activities on the urethral closure pressure profile. For example, we can study the transmission of pressure to the bladder and the urethra and can also appreciate the effectiveness of the contraction of the voluntary and involuntary sphincters around the urethra during varying amounts of bladder filling and with changes in position. Figure 7.12 is an example of this method of testing the function of the urethral sphincteric mechanism during these voluntary activities. The recording reflects bladder pressure and peak urethral pressure. For example, coughing usually

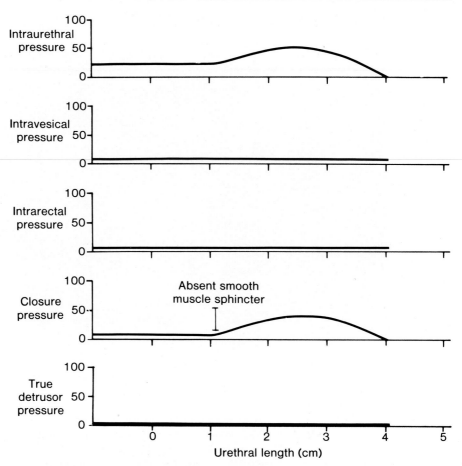

Figure 7.11. The UCPP in the incontinent patient. Characteristically, the closure pressure and functional urethral lengths are less than the normal patient.

produces a sharp increase in intra-abdominal pressure which brings about a corresponding increase in bladder pressure. At the same time the sphincter normally responds by accentuating its closure pressure even more. The ability of the sphincter to generate additional pressure occurs because of reflex mechanisms which become operative during any increased intra-abdominal pressure.

A similar response in both bladder and urethral pressure occurs with increases in intra-abdominal pressure during valsalva. However, the bladder and urethral pressure responds with a sustained pressure rise. The hold maneuver tests the ability of the voluntary sphincter to increase closure pressure on command. Its response is normally seen in the mid to distal urethra.

This ability of the sphincter mechanism to generate increased closure pressure during the stress of cough or

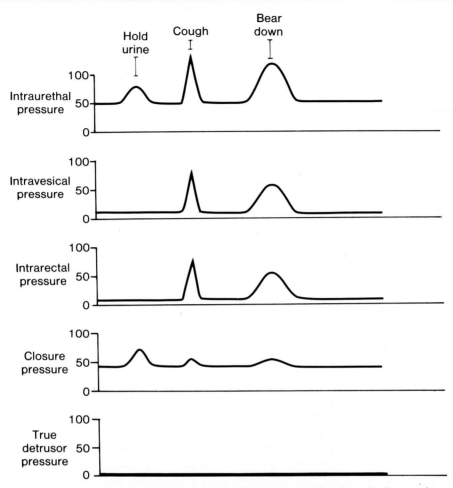

Figure 7.12. Dynamic assessment of the urethral sphincteric mechanism during various maneuvers in the normal patient. Closure remains positive during holding urine, straining and coughing.

valsalva or with voluntary holding decreases or becomes lost in a patient suffering from genuine stress incontinence (Figure 7.13). In effect, the compensatory mechanisms which normally increase urethral closure pressure and control urine loss during stress are no longer able to perform this function.

Some patients have excessively high intraurethral closure pressures. In Figure 7.14 the closure pressure is more than twice the average normal response reaching about 200 cm of water pressure. This excessively active voluntary sphincter activity exists without any rise in intra-abdominal or bladder pressure and indicates a spastic voluntary sphincter.

Positional changes definitely affect the closure pressure profile. With the normal patient in the sitting or supine

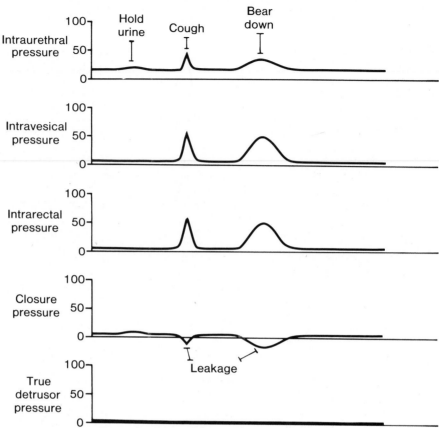

Figure 7.13. Dynamic assessment of the urethral sphincteric mechanism in the patient with genuine stress incontinence. The hold maneuver produces minimal or no pressure increase and the closure pressure becomes negative during coughing and straining with concomitant incontinence.

position the closure pressure profile is usually lower than when the patient assumes the upright position. When the patient stands, there is usually a 25 to 70% increase in the maximum closure pressure, primarily in the area of voluntary sphincter (Figure 7.15). Frequently, increases in functional length also occur. These changes in pressure and length augment the occlusive effect of the urethra to guard against urine loss during a rise in intra-abdominal pressure and during the increased stress involved in this change of position. This is the expected response in the normal female.

Patients with genuine stress incontinence lose this compensatory mechanism with position change. This is one of the most consistent findings in patients with this condition (Figure 7.16).

Various changes occur in the closure pressure profile during varying degrees of bladder distention (Figure 7.17). In the

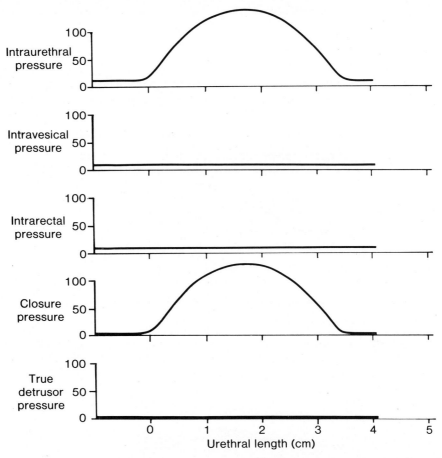

Figure 7.14.   Abnormally high urethral closure pressure. Closure pressure exceeds 140 cm H_2O.

normal patient with the bladder relatively empty, the closure pressure is quite adequate with only minor decreases during stress. The same occurs with the full bladder. In the patient with genuine stress incontinence no leakage occurs and the closure pressure remains positive with an empty bladder (Figure 7.18). Similarly, with a partially full bladder there is a rise in bladder pressure with an equal rise in urethral pressure. With stress, closure pressure nears zero but remains positive and no leakage occurs. With the bladder fully distended, the bladder pressure exceeds the urethral pressure and clinically apparent urine leakage occurs. This sequence emphasizes the importance of studying the patient during stressful maneuvers with a full bladder.

The study of the relationship of the activity of the sphincter with various bladder volumes becomes quite instructive in evaluating urethrovesical dynamics in patients with genuine stress incontinence. The basic features of genuine stress

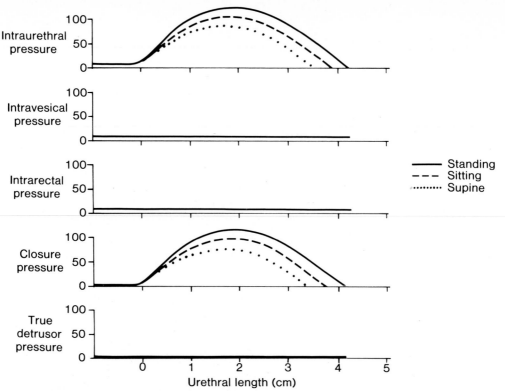

Figure 7.15. Superimposed UCPPs in the supine, sitting and standing positions in the normal patient. Characteristically, closure pressure and/or functional length increases with assumption of a more upright position.

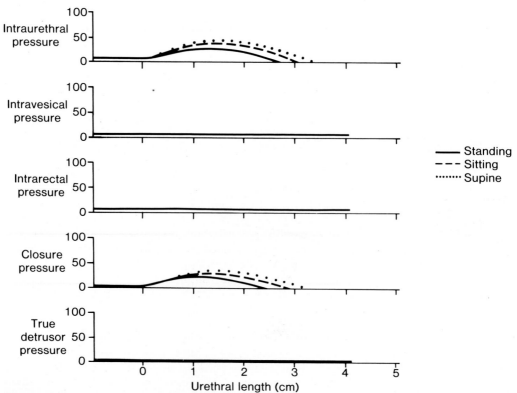

Figure 7.16. Superimposed UCPPs in the supine, sitting and standing positions in the patient with genuine stress incontinence. Characteristically, there is a decrease of closure pressure and/or functional length.

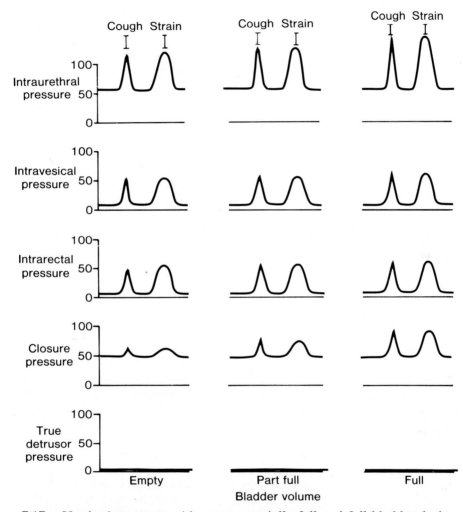

Figure 7.17. Urethral pressures with empty, partially full and full bladder during stress in the normal patient. There is positive transmission of the intra-abdominal pressure to the urethra which exceeds the actual pressure increase measured in the bladder and rectum. Closure pressure remains positive throughout.

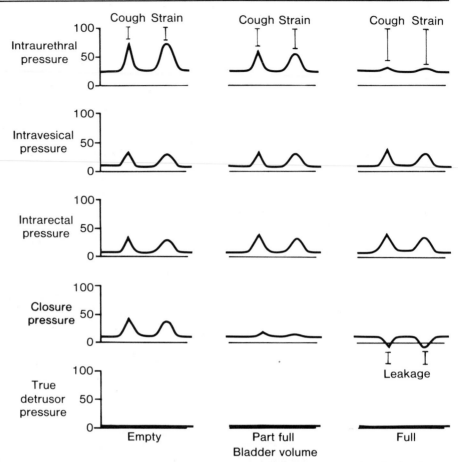

Figure 7.18. Urethral pressures with empty, partially full and full bladder during stress in the patient with genuine stress incontinence. Actual pressure transmission to the urethra decreases as the bladder fills, leading to negative closure pressures and urine loss through the urethra.

incontinence are low closure pressure, short functional length and loss of effectiveness of the proximal segment of the sphincteric mechanism. Most importantly, there is an abnormal response of the sphincteric mechanism to stress, to assumption of the upright position and to bladder filling. In each situation closure pressure and functional length usually decrease. There is also a weak hold manuever with testing for voluntary sphincter activity. Table 7.3 summarizes these features.

SUMMARY

The properly studied and properly analyzed cystometrogram and urethral closure pressure profile are valuable for the dynamic evaluation of bladder function and the sphincteric activity of the urethra. With subdivision of the sphincteric mechanism into its two muscular elements, the smooth as well as the voluntary component, it is possible to quantitate the extent of the sphincteric weakness as well as to

Table 7.3. Dynamic Function of the Urethral Sphincteric Mechanism in Normal Women and in Patients with Genuine Stress Incontinence

	Closure Pressure Response	
	Type of Patient	
	Normal	Stress incontinent
Changes with urethral closure pressure profile in response to:		
Cough	Increased	Minimal to none
Valsalva	Increased	Minimal to none
Holding urine	Increased	Minimal to none
Contraction of perineal muscles	Increased	Minimal to none
Bladder distention[a]		
Empty	—	—
Partially full	Increase	Minimal to none
Full distention	Further Increase	Minimal to none
Position[a]		
Supine	—	—
Sitting	Increase	Minimal to none
Standing	Further Increase	Minimal to none

[a] Response in pressure, length or both.

identify the basic etiology for the abnormality. As such, these are valuable tools in the urodynamic evaluation of the lower urinary tract.

References

1. **Abrams, P.H., Martin, S., Griffith, D.J.** The measurement and Interpretation of Urethral Pressures Obtained by the Method of Brown and Wickham. *Br. J. Urol.* 50:33, 1978.
2. **Andersen, J.T., Bradley, W.E.** Cystometry: Detrusor Reflex Activation, Classification and Terminology. *J. Urol.* 118:623, 1977.
3. **Awad, S.A., Downie, J.W.** Relative Contributions of Smooth & Striated Muscles to the Canine Urethral Pressure Profile. *Br. J. Urol.* 48:347, 1976.
4. **Brown, M., Wickham, J.E.A.** The Urethral Pressure Profile. *Br. J. Urol.* 41:211, 1969.
5. **Bruschini, H., Schmidt, R. A., Tanagho, E.A.** Effect of Urethral Stretch on Urethral Pressure Profile. *Invest. Urol.* 15:107, 1977.
6. **Drouin, G., McCurry, E. H.** Catheters for Studies of Urinary Tract Pressure. *Invest. Urol.* 8:195, 1970.
7. **Edwards, L., Malvern, J.** The Urethral Pressure Profile: Theoretical Considerations and Clinical Application. *Br. J. Urol.* 46:325, 1974.
8. **Gershon, C.R., Diokno, A.C.** Urodynamic Evaluation of Female Stress Urinary Incontinence. *J. Urol.* 199:787, 1978.
9. **Gleason, D.M., Bottaccini, M.R., Reilly, R.J.** Comparison of Cystometrograms and Urethral Profiles with Gas and Water Media. *Urology* 9:155, 1977.
10. **Harrison, N.H., Constable, A.R.** Urethral Pressure Measurement: A Modified Technique. *Br. J. Urol.* 42:229, 1970.

11. **Jonas, U., Tanagho, E.A.** Studies on Vesicourethral Reflexes: I. Urethral Sphincteric Responses to Detrusor Stretch. *Invest. Urol.* 12:357, 1975.

12. **Jonas, U., Tanagho, E.A.** Voiding Pressure As It Relates to Outlet and/or Sphincteric Resistance. *Invest. Urol.* 13:372, 1976.

13. **McGuire, E.J.** Combined Radiographic and Manometric Assessment of Urethral Sphincter Function. *J. Urol.* 118:632, 1977.

14. **Schmidt, R.A., Witherow, R., Tanagho, E.A.** Recording the Urethral Pressure Profile. *Urology* 10:390, 1977.

15. **Tanagho, E.A., Meyers, F.H., Smith, D.R.** Urethral Resistance: Its Components and Implications. I. Smooth Muscle Component. *Invest. Urol.* 7:136, 1969.

16. **Tanagho, E.A., Myers, F.H., Smith, D.R.** Urethral Resistance: Its Components and Implications. II. Striated Muscle Component. *Invest. Urol.* 7:195, 1969.

17. **Tanagho, E.A., Miller, E.R.** Initiation of Voiding. *Br. J. Urol.* 42:175, 1970.

18. **Tanagho, E.A., McCurry, E.H.** Pressure and Flow Rate as Related to Lumen Caliber and Entrance Configuration. *J. Urol.* 105:583, 1971.

19. **Tanagho, E.A.** Simplified Cystography in Stress Incontinence. *Br. J. Urol.* 74:295, 1974.

20. **Tanagho, E.A., Jonas, U.** Membrane Catheter: Effective for Recording Pressure in Lower Urinary Tract. *Urology* 10:173, 1977.

21. **Tanagho, E.A.** Urinary Stress Incontinence. *Urol. Arch.* (Belgrade) 8:17, 1977.

22. **Tanagho, E.A.** The Anatomy and Physiology of Micturition. In *Clinics in Obstetrics and Gynaecology*, edited by Stuart L. Stanton. W.B. Saunders, London, 1978.

8 Urodynamics: Integration of Electromyography with Cystometry and Urethral Pressure Profiles

William E. Bradley, M.D.

Most of the urodynamic techniques for the evaluation of incontinent patients represent new dimensions in the analysis of this common medical problem. These techniques and their applications are still in a process of continual evolution. Fortunately, through a history of collaboration of engineers with clinical investigators, urodynamic technology and instrumentation is more reliable now than ever before.

Two schools of thought regarding the problem of incontinence developed concomitantly with the development of this new instrumentation. The first is the endoscopic-uro-dynamic-radiographic-anatomic approach, which is the time honored concept for documentation of anatomical and functional derangements. The second, and still evolving, method is the neurobiologic method, which studies incontinence in terms of neuromuscular innervation, using the electrophysiological approach.

The neurobiologic method necessitates that the investigator have a thorough knowledge of neuroanatomy and a basic familiarity with the methods of electrophysiologic diagnosis requiring extensive training and a basic knowledge of methodological shortcomings. This electrophysiological approach is important in the evaluation of cerebral dysfunction using electroencephalography with signal tracing and evoked response techniques. These same techniques allow a precise evaluation of peripheral neuromuscular disorders and have potential value in the study of incontinent patients. Unfortunately, they are not techniques which the practicing urologist or gynecologist can use in his daily practice and remain a subject for future specialized training programs.

The available electrophysiologic techniques include electromyography (EMG), electromyelography and electroencephalography. Electromyography records the electrical activity of individual skeletal muscle cells through a recording electrode placed in the muscle. Unfortunately, present techniques do not allow a study of similar events in autonomically controlled smooth muscle. Electromyelography is a signal tracing technique which is available to study both autonomic and somatic innervation of the bladder and urethra.

Although electroencephalography is a technique for future consideration, it is one of the few rational ways to investigate the cerebral control of micturition. Many patients with apparent stress incontinence have lesions of Loops I or IV. In reality, these patients do not have an anatomical reason for their incontinence but have lost cerebral control of the detrusor reflex.

ELECTROMYOGRAPHY OF MOTOR UNITS

Electromyographic techniques include several choices of specific methodologies. Analysis of individual motor units is the time honored technique of the electromyographer who studies peripheral skeletal neuromuscular disease. He inserts a needle electrode into the skeletal musculature or applies a surface electrode and looks for evidence of peripheral denervation (Figure 8.1). The electromyographic signs of peripheral denervation are well known and are unequivocable.

Unfortunately, the actual technique of insertion of needle electrodes into urethral sphincteric muscle produces a number of problems. The insertion process itself produces an injury potential from local trauma with a release of potassium and a change in the excitability of the surrounding muscle. When combined with muscle tightening from the pain of needle insertion, these effects produce considerable artifactual confusion.

Needle recording has another disadvantage in that it only provides information concerning a localized sampling of muscular activity, rather than a summation of the total net activity of the skeletal sphincteric mechanism.

Another way to analyze electromyographic activity is to record electrophysiological patterns by summation and electronic integration of the total net output of either the

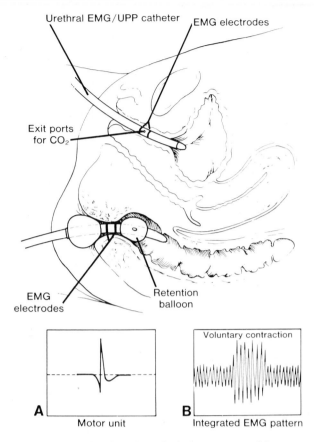

Figure 8.1. The urethral and anal electromyographic surface and needle recording devices in place in the urethra and the anus. The individual motor unit obtained during contraction of the normal pelvic floor is shown (**A**) as well as the integrated pattern (**B**). An increase in activity occurs during voluntary contraction of the pelvic floor (**B**).

periurethral striated muscle or the anal sphincter with surface or needle electrodes (Figure 8.1B). This provides a total net record of sphincteric activity. When done concurrently with cystometry it provides important information regarding the integration of sphincteric activity with detrusor reflex function.

Since the anal sphincter and the periurethral striated muscle have a common source of innervation and behave functionally as a unit, either muscle is suitable for most recording purposes. Some controversy still exists regarding whether the activity in the anal sphincter muscle accurately reflects periurethral striated sphincter activity. Usually, the two produce similar recordings but disparities are common in patients with a prior history of urethral surgery, with certain cauda equina lesions and probably in patients with anatom-

ical reasons for incontinence. Since genuine stress incontinence results mostly from disease of the periurethral striated
muscle, it is more efficient to record directly at the suspected
location of primary pathology.

When the electromyographer places a needle electrode he
looks for evidence of denervation. If the normal patient
contracts skeletal muscle a recruitment pattern results. That
is, a normal buildup in motor unit activity occurs. On the
other hand, if there's denervation, then not only is the
recruitment pattern absent, but there's production of low
amplitude isolated electrical activity called fibrillation potentials which have a characteristic sound on a loudspeaker.
With myopathic disease of the pelvic floor, characteristically many scattered low amplitude potentials occur with a
much higher frequency than fibrillation potentials. With
acute denervation, fibrillation potentials appear within 2 to
3 weeks. Subsequently, nerve regeneration occurs and polyphasic reinnervation potentials replace the fibrillation
potentials. The original motor unit potential does not reap-
pear at any time during the regenerative process. In older
patients with anterior horn cell disease of the sacral cord an
increased synchronization of the motor unit potentials occurs, the so called giant potentials. Frequently, saw toothed
degeneration potentials intermingle with the low amplitude
short duration fibrillation potentials.

Fasciculation potentials of high amplitude and long duration occur with denervating lesions. Unfortunately, these
are non-specific findings. All of these potentials indicate
acute denervation with the exception of the polyphasic
potentials which are evidence of a long-standing chronic
denervation process with subsequent regeneration.

In many patients with anatomical incontinence myelography reveals evidence of both acute and chronic denervation.
Unfortunately, the exact significance of these findings is
unclear due to the absence of information on the frequency
of these findings in age matched controls.

**ELECTROMYO-
GRAPHIC PATTERN
RECORDING**

Electromyographic pattern recordings indicate the net electrical activity of the skeletal sphincter and the width of the
open excursion on the record reflects the frequency of
individual motor unit potentials. The greater the pen excursion, the larger the number of potentials occurring in the
muscle. This provides an electronically generated summation of muscular electrical activity. The major drawback of
this technique is that it is incapable of distinguishing normal
from abnormal individual motor unit potentials. Its major
advantages are its simplicity and potential for widespread
clinical use. Pattern recordings use surface electrodes
mounted on a suitable urethral catheter or anal plug. Figure
8.1 demonstrates an anal catheter with an intrarectal pres-

sure recording device and surface electrodes. The two balloons retain it in position. This device is preferable to the Teflon anal plug, which tends to fall out in older patients with genuine stress incontinence. The figure also shows a similar arrangement on a catheter designed for urethral electromyographic pattern recording.

Pattern recording provides information regarding the normalcy of sphincteric activity. Figure 8.2 shows a patient with a normal cystometrogram and normal EMG activity and a normal EMG response during the terminal detrusor contraction. Figure 8.3 shows a patient with detrusor hyperreflexia during a gas cystometrogram. When asked to contract the periurethral striated muscle during the same interval, she provides EMG evidence of muscular activity. This indicates that the corticospinal tract to the periurethral striated muscle (Loop IV) is intact and that this patient has

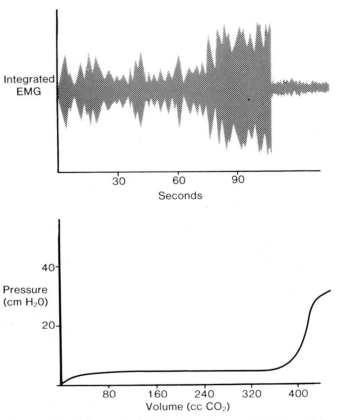

Figure 8.2. Normal combined tracing of EMG activity during the cystometrogram. There is a gradual increase in electromyographic activity. The patient successfully suppresses all detrusor activity until the end of the evaluation when a detrusor contraction occurs and EMG activity of the pelvic floor ceases.

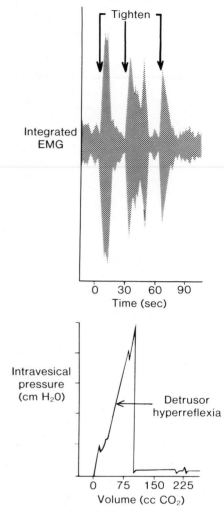

Figure 8.3. Detrusor hyperreflexia with normal pelvic floor EMG. The detrusor contraction occurs at low CO_2 volume and precedes the decrease of EMG activity in the urethral sphincter. The patient cannot inhibit this event.

a lesion of the detrusor reflex pathways with sparing of the innervation of the periurethral striated muscle.

Sphincteric abnormalities are of two forms, detrusor sphincter dyssynergia or uninhibited reflex sphincter relaxation (Figures 8.4 and 8.5). The former occurs when the skeletal sphincter and detrusor contract at the same time, whereas the latter indicates an abnormal pattern of sphincter relaxation which is beyond the volitional control of the patient. Figure 8.4 displays the record of a patient who has detrusor hyperreflexia during a gas cystometrogram; the patient also has an uncontrollable suppression of activity in the peri-

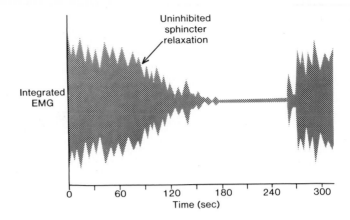

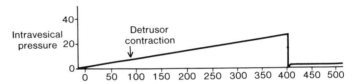

Figure 8.4. Uninhibited or reflex urethral sphincter relaxation. The detrusor contraction occurs at a very low volume of CO_2 and precedes the decrease of EMG activity in the urethral sphincter. The patient cannot inhibit this event.

urethral striated muscle. Figure 8.5 demonstrates the opposite pattern of clonic activity in the periurethral striated muscle during a normal detrusor contraction which may serve as an impediment to voiding. Some patients demonstrate both abnormalities, depending upon whether they are in the supine or erect position. Since many reflex disturbances are only evident in the upright position, it is important to study the patient in several postures. The fact that a single patient occasionally demonstrates both of these patterns explains the apparent conflicts noted in the medical histories of these individuals.

Some patients evidence a holding pattern with an increased tightening of the periurethral striated muscle during cystometry (Figure 8.6). A distinction from detrusor sphincter dyssynergia due to neurological disease is the presence of an abnormal extensor plantar response in the latter.

ELECTROMYELOG-RAPHY

Electromyelographic techniques document abnormalities of the autonomic nervous system which is an etiologic factor in many patients with incontinence. The application of an electrical stimulus to the proximal portion of the urethra stimulates the afferent sensory autonomic innervation through the hypogastric nerves (Figure 8.7). The stimulus passes back to the spinal cord and evokes a response in the

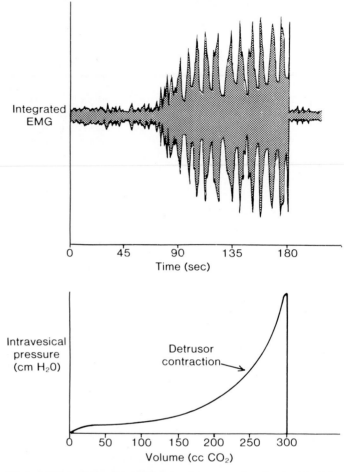

Figure 8.5.   Detrusor sphincter dyssynergia. As the bladder fills pelvic floor EMG activity increases and continues during the detrusor contraction.

pudendal motor neurons. The same current applied in the distal urethra stimulates the pudendal or somatic sensory innervation which evokes a response in these same neurons. The end result is the generation of efferent motor impulses which pass out to the anal sphincter and cause it to contract. An anal plug or an indwelling anal catheter records the contraction on an EMG amplifier and strip chart recorder.

In the normal volunteer the transit time from stimulus to anal sphincter response is between 50 and 70 msec (Figure 8.8A). This technique allows the identification of asymptomatic peripheral neuropathies which commonly occur in diabetic patients.

Autonomic neuropathy produces a diphasic response which has a latency or transit time in excess of 100 msec (Figure

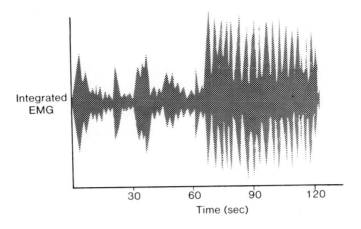

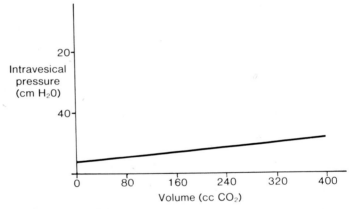

Figure 8.6. The EMG holding pattern during the CMG. Increased EMG activity occurs during the CMG. (Compare with Figure 8.4.)

8.8B). The autonomic neuropathic change slows conduction in the axon due to changes in the distance between the nodes of Ranvier (Figure 8.9). The normal motor axon innervating the periurethral striated muscle or the sensory axons innervating the detrusor muscle have a myelin coating interrupted at regular intervals by nodes of Ranvier. The conduction velocity is proportional to the internodal distance.

Autonomic neuropathy in diabetic patients characteristically demonstrates Wallerian degeneration, a demyelinating type of neuropathy with destruction of the nerve. An alternative form is a segmental demyelination.

With repair and reconstitution of the myelin, a shorter internodal distance results which slows conduction velocity (Figure 8.9). Some patients with bladder instability caused by change in posture demonstrate a slowing or actual

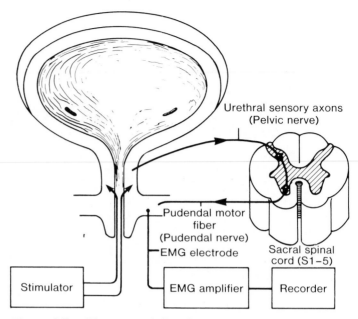

Figure 8.7. Electromyelographic stimulatory technique. A stimulus applied to the urethra travels via the pelvic nerve to the sacral cord where it causes activation of the pudendal motor nerve. Pelvic floor contraction results.

disappearance of the evoked response. This is evidence that the patient not only has a central neuropathic disturbance causing an abnormality in detrusor reflex innervation or volitional control, but also has impairment of the peripheral innervation of the detrusor.

ELECTROENCEPHALOGRAPHY

Electroencephalography is an effective technique for diagnosis of childhood enuresis and has potential for the evaluation of adult incontinence. After sleep deprivation the physician inserts an intravesical catheter and performs a cystometrogram during sleep. Deep sleep evokes high voltage slow waves (Figure 8.10A). If the cystometrogram elicits a detrusor reflex, this activity ceases, indicating intactness of the central pathways from the bladder to the brain. On the other hand, if an epileptiform abnormality appears, this indicates the need for management with anticonvulsants (Figure 8.10B).

ELECTROMYOGRAPHY AND THE URETHRAL CLOSURE PRESSURE PROFILE

The combination of the urethral closure pressure profile and electromyography provides information regarding the source of the lack of compensation in the profile during bladder filling or changing to a standing position. It is important to know whether this is dysfunction of smooth muscle, the periurethral striated muscle, or an abnormality of the peripheral innervation.

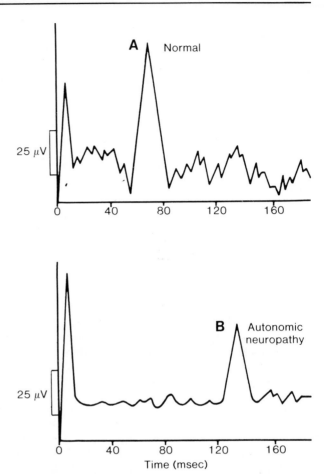

Figure 8.8. Electromyelography of the urethral sphincter. A stimulus applied to the urethra in the normal patient reaches the pelvic floor in less than 70 msec (**A**); the transit time is more than 100 msec in a patient with autonomic neuropathy (**B**).

Using a special catheter (Figure 8.1) it is possible to simultaneously record the electromyographic activity of the skeletal muscle component of the urethral sphincteric mechanism with the urethral pressure profile. If the patient has a decrease of the urethral closure pressure under the stress of bladder filling or assuming a more upright position, it is important to know whether this is dysfunction of urethral smooth muscle or the periurethral striated muscle. In addition, when combined with electromyelography, it is possible to determine whether this pressure decrease is due to an abnormality of the peripheral innervation.

The actual electrodes consist of stainless steel wrapped around the recording catheter. The carbon dioxide exit

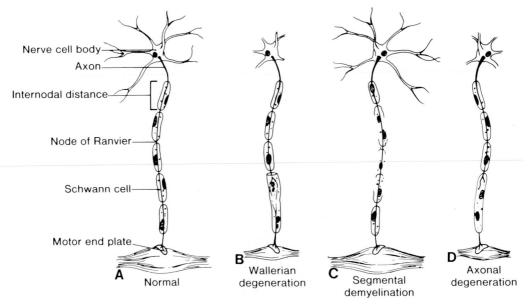

Figure 8.9. Internodal distances. Nodes of Ranvier are farther apart in normal patients (**A**) as opposed to patients with neuropathy (**B–D**). (Redrawn from Adams, R. And Victor, M. *Textbook of Neurology.* W.B. Saunders Co., Philadelphia, 1978.)

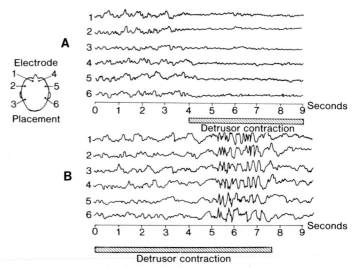

Figure 8.10. Electroencephalogram during sleep. (**A**) Normal high voltage slow waves which cease when a detrusor contraction occurs. (**B**) Epileptiform activity during a detrusor contraction.

ports are approximately 0.25 ml in diameter to accommodate the high flow rates of gas, which must be in excess of 100 ml per minute to obtain an accurate index of the urethral closure pressure. During catheter withdrawal this catheter records the distal periurethral striated muscle electromyographic activity as well as the urethral pressure profile (Figure 8.11, A and B). In order to achieve reproducibility of results and to preserve the concept of functional urethral length, constant velocity machine catheter withdrawal is best.

The effect of bladder filling on the healthy volunteer is to increase the urethral closure pressure (Figure 8.12). This compensatory pressure increase with bladder filing is absent in the patient with genuine stress incontinence. The effect of alpha adrenergic blockade is to decrease urethral pressure except in the distal third, where the periurethral striated muscle accounts for most of this pressure. The alpha blockade probably exerts its major effect on the submucosal vascular plexuses of the urethra.

In the patient with stress incontinence there is a smooth parabolic urethral closure pressure curve (Figure 8.13A). With bladder filling on assumption of a more upright position there is decay of the profile consisting of a shortening of the functional urethral length, which is due to an autonomic neuropathy. In this same patient after a bladder neck suspension, it is interesting that we do not increase the

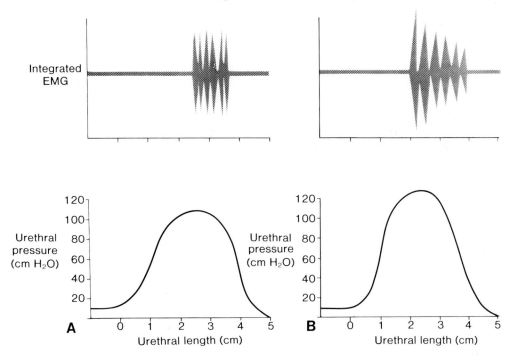

Figure 8.11. The combined electromyographic and urethral pressure profiles. In the normal patient peak electromyographic activity of the pelvic floor occurs nearly synchronously with peak urethral pressure (**A**), whereas there is a generalized increase in pelvic floor activity with spasticity (**B**).

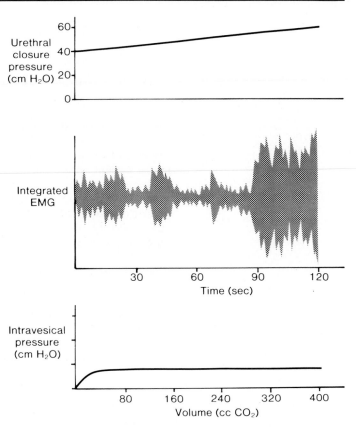

Figure 8.12. Combined cystometry, urethral pressure and EMG recording. In this normal patient urethral closure pressure and pelvic floor EMG gradually increase with bladder filling.

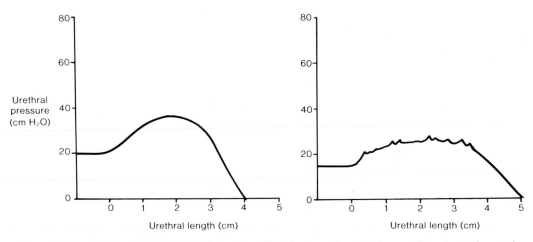

Figure 8.13. Urethral closure pressure profiles in a patient with genuine stress incontinence. A comparison of the preoperative curve (**A**) with the postoperative curve (**B**) reveals a lessened closure pressure but an elongated functional length.

amplitude of the closure pressure postoperatively (Figure 8.13B). Rather, there is an increase in the functional urethral length and thereby an increase in intraurethral resistance.

The result of adding these electrophysiologic techniques to the analysis and investigation of the patient with stress incontinence is to show that stress incontinence may originate in an associated neurologic disease process. This is a neuropathic disorder of the urethra, which evidences itself in the urethral pressure profile as decreased urethral pressure with bladder filling or assumption of a more upright position. The electromyographic techniques show that there is an associated nerve conduction slowing due to the superimposition of an autonomic neuropathy on the primary conditions of multiparity and aging.

SUMMARY

The application of these electrophysiologic techniques to the clinical investigation of the patient with incontinence shows that "stress incontinence" is not always due to purely anatomical reasons. Neuropathic changes in the detrusor muscle and abnormalities of the central innervation of the detrusor muscle and its reflex pathways produce incontinence by facilitating uninhibited bladder contractions. The presence of neuropathic changes in the urethra as defined by electromyographic techniques emphasizes the need to include the autonomic neuropathies associated with diabetes, multiparity and/or aging in the differential diagnosis of incontinence. The technique is new, yet promises to be of great value in the study of the incontinent patient.

References

1. **Andersen, J.T., Bradley, W.E.** Early Detection of Diabetic Autonomic Neuropathy. *Diabetes* 25:1100, 1976.
2. **Andersen, J.T., Bradley, W.E.** Electromyographic and Gas Urethral Pressure Profile. *Urology* 7:561–565, 1976.
3. **Andersen, J.T., Bradley, W.E.** Cystometric Sphincter and Electromyelographic Abnormalities in Parkinson's Disease. *J. Urol.* 116:75–78, 1976.
4. **Andersen, J.T., Bradley, W.E.** Postural Detrusor Hyperreflexia. *J. Urol.* 116:228–230, 1976.
5. **Andrew, J., Nathan, P.W.** Lesions of the Anterior Frontal Lobes and Disturbances of Micturition and Defecation. *Brain* 87:233–262, 1964.
6. **Bors, E.** Neurogenic Bladder. *Urol. Surv.* 7:177–250, 1957.
7. **Bors, E., Comarr, A.E.** *Neurological Urology.* University Park Press, Baltimore, 1971.
8. **Bors, E., Porter, R.W.** Neurosurgical Considerations in Bladder Dysfunction. *Urol. Int.* 25:114–133, 1970.
9. **Bowen, J.M., Bradley, W.E.** Some Contractile and Electrophysiological Properties of the External Anal Sphincter Muscle of the Cat. *Gastroenterology* 65:919–928, 1973.
10. **Bowen, J.M., Timm, G.W., Bradley, W.E.** Some Contractile and Electrophysiological Properties of the Periurethral Striated Muscle of the Cat. *Invest. Urol.* 13:327–330, 1976.

11. **Bradley, W.E.** Cystometry and Sphincter Electromyography. *Mayo Clin. Proc.* 51:329–335, 1976.
12. **Bradley, W.E., Andersen, J.T.** Techniques for Analysis of Micturition Reflex Disturbances in Childhood. *Pediatrics* 59: 546, 1977.
13. **Bradley, W.E., Timm, G.W.** Cystometry. VI. Interpretation. *Urology* 7:231–235, 1976.
14. **Bradley, W.E., Logothetis, J.L., Timm, G.W.** Cystometric and Sphincter Abnormalities in Multiple Sclerosis. *Neurology* 23: 1131–1139, 1973.
15. **Bradley, W.E., Timm, G.W., Scott, F.B.** Cystometry. V. Bladder Sensation. *Urology* 6:654–658, 1975.
16. **Bradley, W.E., Chou, S.N., Markland, C., Swaim K.** Biochemical Assay Technique for Estimation of Bladder Fibrosis. *Invest. Urol.* 3:59–64, 1965.
17. **Bradley, W.E., Timm, G.W., Rockswold, G.L., Scott, F.B.** Detrusor and Urethral Electromyelography. *J. Urol.* 114:891–894, 1975.
18. **Brown, M., Wickham, J.E.A.** The Urethral Pressure Profile. *Br. J. Urol.* 41:211, 1969.
19. **Eickenberg, H.V., Amin, M., Klompus, W., Lich, R.** Urologic Complications Following Abdominoperineal Resection. *J. Urol.* 115:180–182, 1976.
20. **Enhorning, G.** Simultaneous Recording of Intravesical and Intraurethral Pressure. A Study of Urethral Closure in Normal and Stress Incontinent Women. *Acta. Chir. Scand.* 270:1–68, 1961.
21. **Ellenberg, M.** Diabetic Neurogenic Vesical Dysfunction. *Arch. Intern. Med.* 117:348–354, 1966.
22. **Ellenberg, M., Weber, H.** The Incipient Asymptomatic Diabetic Bladder. *Diabetes* 16:331–335, 1967.
23. **Jonas, S., Brown, J.** Neurogenic Bladder in Normal Pressure Hydrocephalus. *Urology* 5:44–50, 1975.
24. **Lapides, J., Friend, C.R., Ajemian, E.P., Reus, W.S.** Denervation Supersensitivity as a Test for Neurogenic Bladder. *Surg. Gynecol. Obstet.* 114:241–244, 1962.
25. **Scott, F.B.** Uroflowmeter in the Evaluation of Voiding Disorders. *Med. Rec. Ann.* 60:263, 1967.
26. **Scott, F.B., Bradley, W.E., Timm, G.W.** Treatment of Urinary Incontinence by an Implantable Prosthetic Urinary Sphincter. *J. Urol.* 112:75, 1974.
27. **Timm, G.W., Bradley, W.E.** Technologic and Biologic Considerations in Neuro-Urologic Prosthesis Development. IEEE *Trans. Biomed. Eng.* BME-20:208–212, 1975.

9 Urodynamics: Uroflowmetry and Female Voiding Patterns

Emil A. Tanagho, M.D.

NORMAL VOIDING ACT

Normal voiding requires coordination between contraction of the detrusor and relaxation of the urethral sphincteric mechanism. The detrusor contracts, producing adequate and sustained intravesical pressure until emptying is complete. Concomitantly, the sphincter relaxes sufficiently for bladder pressure to exceed urethral pressure. This results in the initiation of urine flow. During physiologic voiding the first event is urethral relaxation, followed in 2 to 3 seconds by detrusor contraction (Figure 9.1). Initial detrusor contraction produces a pressure increase of not more than 30 or 40 cm of water, which decreases later on. The initially high sphincteric pressure drops at the beginning of micturition. This closing pressure remains low until the voiding act terminates, at which time it returns to prevoiding levels. This results in a peak flow rate of 25 cc per second (Figure 9.1). This example demonstrates the classic pattern of normal micturition, with a sharp start, a strong sustained flow and a sharp ending.

FLOW RATE

In women the normal urinary flow rate is about 25 to 30 ml per second. This rate of flow is the product of combined detrusor contraction and outlet resistance created by the urethral sphincteric mechanism. If outlet resistance is reasonably low, or if it decreases to minimal levels during micturition, detrusor contraction with minimal pressure generates an adequate flow rate. If outlet resistance remains high, however, the magnitude of detrusor contraction must increase in order to deliver the same flow rate.

103

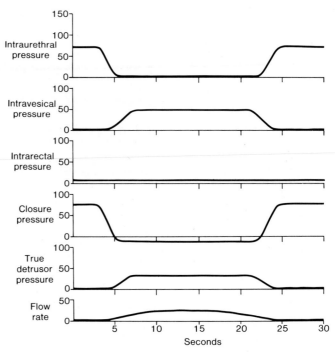

Figure 9.1. Diagrammatic representation of the normal female voiding act. Urethral relaxation precedes the vesical contraction which continues for about 20 seconds and is associated with a normal flow rate of greater than 20 cc per second. All pressures on the graphs in this chapter are in cm of H₂O.

Outlet resistance has two main features: the effect of the surrounding musculature and the potential caliber of the urethral lumen. Two minor features are the abundance of infoldings of the urethral mucosa and the adequacy of periurethral vascularity. These minor features are estrogen dependent components of the urethral sphincteric mechanism. In normal situations, outlet resistance is primarily a function of the voluntary and involuntary musculature of the sphincteric unit. The urethral lumen is normally adequate and has the capacity to expand to a large caliber during micturition. Resistance to flow largely results from the muscular activity or tonus of the sphincteric unit. This resistance determines the maximum urine volume that passes through the urethral lumen.

A fixed relationship exists between the caliber of the urethral lumen and the detrusor pressure required to deliver a given flow rate. Surprisingly, in a static system, very low pressures and rather narrow lumens accommodate large volumes of urine. Lumen size is not a critical factor in determining flow rate. With a lumen of 14 French the pressure necessary to deliver a 40 cc flow rate is about 18 cm of water. An average detrusor pressure of 20 cm of water against an 8 French urethral lumen easily delivers a flow rate of 15 cc per second. Under the same pressure, a lumen of 11 French handles 35 cc per second.

Mechanical factors in outlet resistance are of little significance in the female. Only major encroachments on the urethral lumen by stricture, kink or obstruction impede the flow of urine to any significant degree if voiding pressures are normal. Kinking of the urethra at the urethrovesical junction occurs in association with mechanical obstructions in the female.

A more important determinant of flow rate is the configuration of the bladder outlet. When there is a rather sharp transition between the intravesical cavity and the origin of the urethra, the flow rates are about 25% less than when the bladder outlet funnels (Figure 9.2).

The essential factor influencing flow rate is the voluntary part of the sphincteric mechanism. In women the smooth sphincter rarely contributes to functional obstruction. Invariably, it is the voluntary sphincter that is the impeding factor, just as with normal detrusor function it is the major determinant of flow rate.

It is necessary to delineate and to separate the functional causes from the neuropathic causes of urethral obstruction. Further subdivisions in the functional group include those due to infection, irritation for any reason, and the very

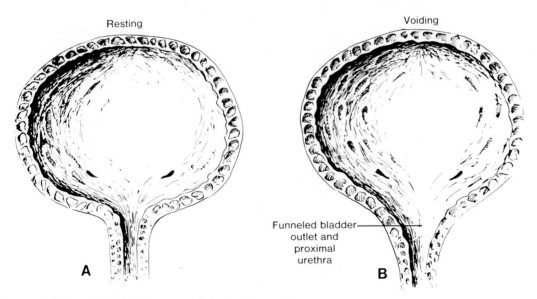

Resting

Voiding

Funneled bladder outlet and proximal urethra

A

B

Figure 9.2. Configuration of the bladder outlet. (**A**) At rest. No funnelling is present. (**B**) During voiding. The proximal urethra funnels.

common psychogenic group. The latter group of patients lack the ability to relax the sphincteric unit during voiding.

FUNCTIONAL OBSTRUCTION

Voluntary sphincteric activity and the resistance it produces during voiding is due to two factors, either lack of relaxation or an actual overactivity. Both of these are quite significant. To detect these changes two pressures are important: the sphincteric pressure and the true detrusor pressure.

LACK OF SPHINCTERIC RELAXATION

This creates a relatively high resistance which becomes obstructive (Figure 9.3). In this example the sphincteric pressure stays the same except that there is an increase at the end of voiding. During the voiding act, there is a strong detrusor contraction of 100 to 105 cm of water pressure without urethral sphincteric relaxation. Under these circumstances the flow rate is only 6 cc per second. This patient failed to relax her sphincter and tried to overcome this resistance by overactivity of the detrusor which generated three times normal intravesical voiding pressures to deliver only about one-fourth the normal flow rate.

SPHINCTERIC OVERACTIVITY

The worst variety of sphincteric overactivity is called detrusor sphincter dyssynergia (Figure 9.4). Dyssynergia exists

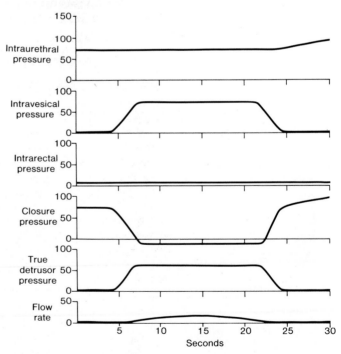

Figure 9.3. An obstructive voiding pattern. No decrease in intraurethral pressure occurs with voiding and closure pressure approaches zero due to an abnormally high intravesical pressure. A normal flow rate occurs even though this is an abnormal voiding pattern.

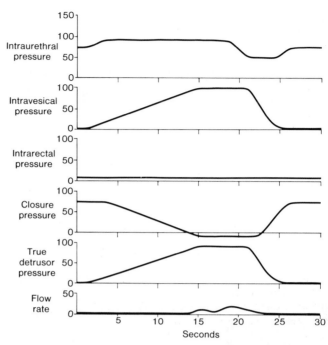

Figure 9.4. Obstructive voiding with detrusor sphincter dyssynergia. The detrusor pressure increases during a series of voiding attempts, but micturition doesn't occur due to a positive closing pressure. Finally, poor urethral relaxation allows an intermittent pattern of flow.

when a detrusor contraction stimulates a simultaneous contraction of the sphincteric unit. In this group of patients with no sphincteric relaxation the sphincter sustains or augments its closure pressure during a detrusor contraction. This results in a serious blockage of the urethra. In this example, since there are no corresponding pressure increases in the intra-abdominal pressure recording, these increases in pressure are genuine detrusor contractions (Figure 9.4). Each of these contractions of 50 to 75 cm of water pressure coincides with similar increases in voluntary sphincteric activity. As a result, no voiding occurs since urethral closure pressure never becomes negative. In this same patient the sphincter finally relaxes and some urine flow results. The relaxation, however, is not enough and the detrusor contraction is weak, so the flow rate is still poor with an intermittent pattern.

VOIDING WITHOUT DETRUSOR CONTRACTION

With Valsalva. Another group of patients has a normal flow rate without any detrusor activity whatsoever (Figure 9.5). This is due to appreciable sphincteric relaxation assisted by increasing intra-abdominal pressure by straining. The example appears to show a good, strong detrusor contraction. However, the intra-abdominal pressure tracing indicates that all of this pressure increase is only an apparent pressure

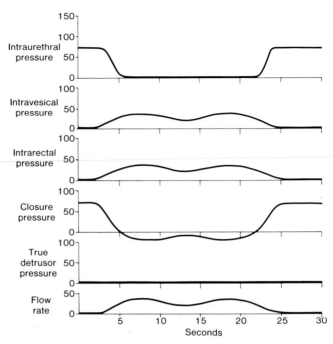

Figure 9.5. Voiding without detrusor contraction. Normal flow rate results from urethral intravesical relaxation with pressure augmentation from valsalva.

increase due to straining. This emphasizes the importance of simultaneous intrarectal pressure recordings in order to avoid misinterpretation of these voiding patterns.

Without Valsalva. Another group of patients void primarily by total, sharp sphincteric relaxation alone (Figure 9.6). This example shows a flow rate averaging 25 cc per second due solely to urethral relaxation combined with a minimum amount of straining, allowing complete emptying of the bladder.

Patients with urinary incontinence commonly void by urethral relaxation alone. Since it is frequently impossible to elicit a detrusor contraction, detrusor atony is a concern in this group of patients. Another concern is the end result after the surgeon rebuilds the sphincter and increases this patient's outlet resistance. Does residual urine and bladder outlet obstruction result from the patient's inability to develop a detrusor contraction? Fortunately, these patients develop normal voiding mechanisms postoperatively with normal detrusor contractions.

SUMMARY

The normal female voids with a variety of mechanisms (Table 9.1). The normal and the most common mechanism is a mild detrusor contraction with intravesical pressures

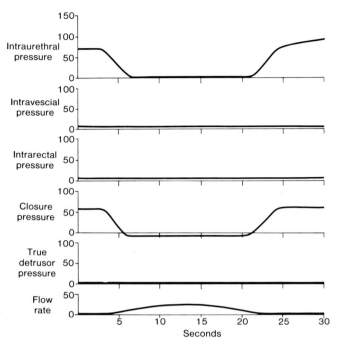

Figure 9.6. Voiding without detrusor contraction. Normal flow results from urethral relaxation alone.

Table 9.1. Normal Female Voiding Mechanisms

Pressure Changes		
Urethra	Bladder	Abdomen
1. Complete relaxation	Mild increase	Absent
2. Complete relaxation	None	Absent
3. Complete relaxation	None	Present

Table 9.2. Abnormal Female Voiding Mechanisms

Pressure Changes		
Urethra	Bladder	Abdomen
1. No Change	Increase	Absent
2. Increase	Increase	Absent

not exceeding 20 to 40 cm of water pressure preceded by an associated complete sphincteric relaxation. Normal flow rates of 20 to 30 cc per second result. Alternative normal voiding mechanisms include the absence of a detrusor contraction in association with excellent perineal relaxation with or without voluntary straining.

Abnormal voiding patterns include those where the detrusor contraction occurs without urethral relaxation or an actual increase in sphincteric contraction (Table 9.2). These are obstructive patterns producing relatively low flow rates.

The combination of urinary flow rate with recordings of intraurethral and intra-abdominal pressures as well as a determination of true intravesical pressure effectively evaluate female voiding mechanisms.

References

1. **Andersen, J.T.** Detrusor Hyperreflexia in Benign Intravesical Obstruction. Cystometric Study. *J. Urol.* 155:532, 1976.
2. **Anikwe, R.M.** Direct Recording of Urethral Resistance Using "Urethroresistance." *J. Urol.* 119:643, 1978.
3. **Asmussen, M., Ulmsten, U.** Simultaneous Urethrocystometry and Urethral Pressure Profile Measurement with a New Technique. *Acta Obstet. Gynecol. Scand.* 54:385, 1975.
4. **Gleason, D.M., Bottaccini, M.R., Reilly, R.J., Byrne, J.C.** Urethral Compliance and its Role in Female Voiding Dysfunctions. *Invest. Urol.* 11:83, 1973.
5. **Hojsgaard, A.** The Urethral Pressure Profile in Female Patients with Meatal Stenosis. *Scand. J. Urol. Nephrol.* 10:97, 1976.
6. **Low, J.A., Kao, M.S.** Intravesical and Intraurethral Pressure as a Measure of Sphincter Function. *Obstet. Gynecol.* 40:627, 1972.
7. **Nanninga, J.B., Kaplan, P.** Experience with Measurement of Bladder Electrical Activity. *J. Urol.* 120:82, 1978.
8. **Tanagho, E.A., Miller, E.R., Meyers, F.H., Corbett, R.K.** Observations on the Dynamics of the Bladder Neck. *Br. J. Urol.* 38:72, 1966.
9. **Tanagho, E.A., Smith, D.R., Meyers, F.H.** The Trigone: Anatomical and physiological considerations. 2. In Relation to the Bladder Neck. *J. Urol.* 100:633, 1968.
10. **Tanagho, E.A., Meyers, F.H., Smith, D.R.** Urethral resistance: Its Components and Implications. I. Smooth Muscle Component. *Invest. Urol.* 7:136, 1969.
11. **Tanagho, E.A., Meyers, F.H., Smith, D.R.** Urethral Resistance: Its Components and Implications. II. Striated Muscle Component. *Invest. Urol.* 7:195, 1969.
12. **Tanagho, E.A., Miller, E.R.** Initiation of Voiding. *Br. J. Urol.* 42:175, 1970.
13. **Tanagho, E.A., McCurry, E.** Pressure and Flow Rate as Related to Lumen Caliber and Entrance Configuration. *J. Urol.* 105:583, 1971.
14. **Tanagho, E.A.** Interpretation of the physiology of Micturition. In *Hydrodynamics of Micturition*, edited by F. Hinman, Jr. Charles C. Thomas, Springfield, Ill., 1971, pp. 18–45.
15. **Tanagho, E.A., Miller, E.R.** Functional Considerations of Urethral Sphincteric Dynamics. *J. Urol.* 109:273, 1973.
16. **Tanagho, E.A.** The Anatomy and Physiology of Micturition. In *Clinics in Obstetrics and Gynaecology*, edited by Stuart L. Stanton. W.B. Saunders, London, 1978.
17. **Van Gool, J., Tanagho, E.A.** External Sphincter Activity and Recurrent Urinary Tract Infection in Girls. *Urology* 10:348, 1977.
18. **Yalla, S.V., Blunt, K.J., Fam, B.A., Constantinople, N.L., Gittes, R.F.** Detrusor-urethral Sphincter Dyssynergia. *J. Urol.* 118:1026, 1977.

10 Aspects of Continence, Incontinence and Micturition in Women Based On Simultaneous Urethral Cystometry

Mogens Asmussen, M.D.

This chapter summarizes the modern technique of simultaneous urethral cystometry (SUCM) using microtransducer catheters and further explores the current status of scientific information derived from the clinical and research application of this technique. This chapter also indicates areas in need of further study in order to increase our knowledge of the function of the lower urinary tract in women.

INTRODUCTION

The bladder and the urethra form a functional unit in which the bladder is a reservoir and the urethra is the outlet or biological valve. When the pressure in the urethra at any one point, at any time and under any condition of stress or change of position is the same or exceeds the pressure within the bladder, no urine can pass through the urethra. In order for urine to pass through the urethra, the bladder pressure must exceed the maximal urethral pressure (13). This simple physiological fact is important for a complete understanding and also for a thorough comprehension of the etiology, diagnosis and treatment of urinary incontinence and disturbances of micturition.

Recent technical advances allow exact permanent records to be made of intravesical and intraurethral pressures at any anatomical location in the urethra, at any time and under any condition of stress or change of position by the patient. These recordings produce accurate information

111

regarding not only the intraurethral pressure and the intravesical pressure, but also the static and dynamic relationships between the simultaneously recorded pressures in these two organs. Such exact pressure recordings from normal patients and from patients suffering from urinary incontinence and micturition disturbances provide us with a new diagnostic dimension in the management of incontinence in women.

DEFINITIONS

In 1979 the International Continence Society published its latest standardization of terminology of lower tract function, dysfunction and evaluation (8). Although the author strictly follows these norms, this chapter introduces a number of new definitions regarding the static and dynamic events in the lower urinary tract. Appendix I details the recommendations of the International Continence Society (8).

Integrated urethral pressure: The integrated area under the total urethral pressure profile (see Figure 10.6).

Integrated urethral closure pressure: The integrated area under the urethral closure pressure portion of the total urethral pressure (see Figure 10.6).

Continence: A condition where the maximal urethral pressure (MUP) is the same or exceeds the bladder pressure at rest and with all conditions of stress.

Incontinence: A condition with involuntary loss of urine when the intravesical pressure exceeds the maximal urethral pressure in the absence of detrusor activity.

Micturition: The ability to completely empty the bladder through the urethra when the natural urge occurs. The normal individual is also able to stop micturition when desired.

Controlled provoked micturition: Controlled provoked micturition: The occurrence of micturition or overflow during a constant bladder filling with the patient at rest. Usually the physician measures maximal urethral pressure in relation to the bladder pressure during this test.

Urge: A strong desire to void at any bladder volume but without loss of urine. It is abnormal when the sensation occurs at an unacceptably low bladder volume.

Urge incontinence: The inability to prevent loss of urine through the urethra in combination with a strong desire to void at an unacceptably low bladder volume.

Unstable urethra: Oscillating urethral pressure variations not synchronous with cardiac rate and without significant bladder pressure variations (see Figure 10.13). Striated muscle activity most likely causes these oscillations.

Detrusor sphincter dyssynergia: A simultaneous increase in urethral and intravesical pressures without straining, with or without the sensation of urge and with or without the loss of urine.

Bladder transmission capacity: That part of the intra-abdominal pressure which transmits to the bladder.

Urethral transmission capacity: That part of the intra-abdominal pressure which transmits to the urethra.

Pressure transmission capacity ratio: The bladder transmission capacity in relation to the urethral transmission capacity. Subtraction of the intravesical pressure from the intraurethral pressure during stress, such as during a cough urethral pressure profile provides this information (see Figure 10.7).

Urethral pulsations: Variations in the urethral pressure, usually seen in the midurethra, which are synchronous with the cardiac rate. The filling and emptying of the submucosal periurethral vascular bed causes these pulsations (2,13). This is not the same condition as the unstable urethra.

True intravesical pressure: Identical to the intravesical pressure. The bladder is the best organ available to indicate the intra-abdominal pressure when not measuring directly in the intra-abdominal cavity. Measuring the intrarectal pressure only excludes artifact since it has its own intrinsic pressure variations. Calculating the true intravesical pressure by subtraction of the rectal pressure from the bladder pressure often gives negative pressure values which cannot truly reflect actual intravesical pressure.

PRESENT TECHNIQUE AND METHODOLOGY

Standardized simultaneous urethral cystometry (SUCM) includes urethral pressure profile measurements, which record the intraurethral and intravesical pressures with great accuracy (1–3, 5–7, 13, 20, 22). Two microtransducers placed 6 cm apart in a specially designed 7F, thin, semi-flexible, smooth Dacron catheter record the intraurethral and intravesical pressures (Figure 10.1). The catheter connects to a differential amplifier and a paper recorder which provides a permanent record of the signals from the microtransducers and also simultaneously and separately traces the differences between the two pressures (Figure 10.2 and 10.3). This simultaneous electronic subtraction facilitates the evaluation of the results, especially during a rapidly occurring event, such as the stress of coughing.

A mechanical withdrawal instrument standardizes the ure-

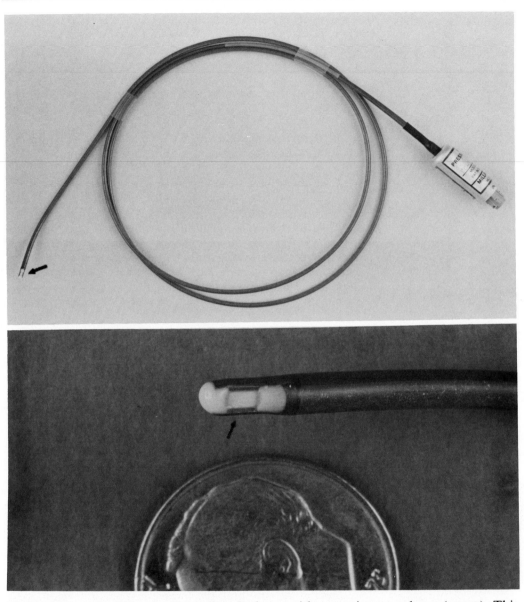

Figure 10.1. The Microtip Recording Catheter with one microtransducer (arrow). This may be used to record rectal pressure in conjunction with the double microtip transducer catheter shown in Figure 7.8, Chapter 7. (Millar Instruments, Inc., Houston, Texas.)

thral pressure profile measurement (Figure 10.2). This mechanical device withdraws the catheter through the urethra with a constant speed. During withdrawal through the urethra the most proximally located transducer records the intraurethral pressure from the urethrovesical junction to the external meatus of the urethra. The distal transducer simultaneously measures the intravesical pressure (Figure 10.3). Reproducible measurements require a smooth and free withdrawal of the catheter through the urethra with the transducers consistently oriented toward the right or left urethral sidewall. This system has a distinct advantage over most currently available commercial urodynamic equipment, since the entire measuring system can be precisely calibrated statically as well as dynamically by use of a special calibration unit before and after each examination (Figure 10.4). This calibration unit also simultaneously sterilizes the catheter. Furthermore, the reproducibility and responsiveness of the microtransducers far exceeds that which is necessary to measure even the fastest dynamic event in the lower urinary tract. Double lumen fluid filled catheters do not fulfill this important criterion.

The urodynamic measuring system determines the following parameters with great accuracy (1,2,5–7; Figures 10.5 and 10.6): the functional length of the urethra (FL); the total length of the urethra (TL); the maximum urethra

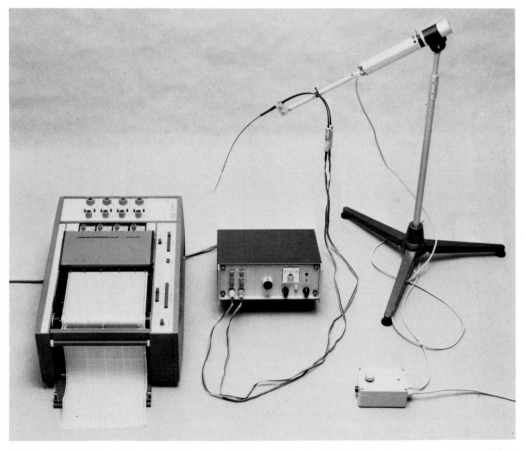

Figure 10.2. The Pressure Recorder (left) and Catheter Withdrawal Apparatus (right). The withdrawer holds the microtip catheter, which is attached to its control mechanism (center). (Vingmed, A/S, Oslo, Norway.)

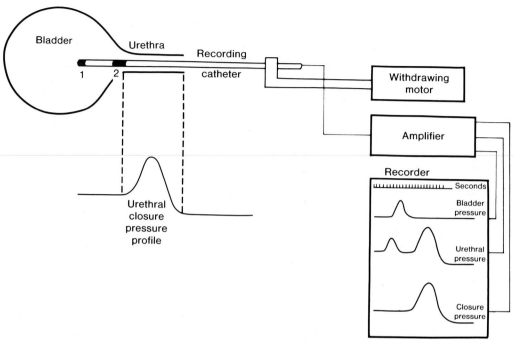

Figure 10.3. The recording methodology. This is a schematic drawing of the equipment used for simultaneous urethrocystometry and urethral pressure profile measurements. The upper left part of the figure demonstrates the recording catheter with tranducer 1 at the tip and transducer 2 located 6 cm proximally. when the catheter is withdrawn at a constant rate, transducer 2 registers the pressure along the urethra. Microtransducer 1 remains in the bladder registering the intravesical pressure. Since both the paper speed of the recorder and the withdrawal speed of the catheter are identical, this allows direct measurement of urethral length.

pressure (MUP); urethral closure pressure (UCP); intravesical pressure (IVP); integrated urethral pressure (IUP); and integrated urethral closure pressure (IUCP).

In this standardized procedure the recommendation is to measure and calculate these urethral closure pressure parameters as an average of three consecutive curves (2). The technique also allows analysis of the intraurethral pressure in relation to the bladder pressure at any desired location, at any time and under any static or dynamic condition. Dynamic measurements provide information regarding the pressure transmission capacity ratio, which is the algebraic sum of urethrovesical pressure relationships during stress and are directly indicated on the subtraction curve. The cough urethral pressure profile is an example of this type of measurement (Figure 10.7). The technique allows examination of the patient in any desired position, such as, supine, sitting, semisitting or standing.

During actual cystometry, a thin, soft catheter delivers fluid to the bladder at a constant rate. Its placement alongside the measuring catheter does not significantly affect intra-urethral pressure. This filling catheter is 1 mm in diameter and 60 mm long and connects to an intravenous drip system. With a bottle of normal saline at body temperature placed 50 cm above the bladder, this simple system delivers approximately 50 ml per minute into the bladder, without any need for sophisticated mechanized instillation. SUCM during filling until either overflow or micturition occurs with the patient at rest is termed "controlled provoked micturition." Cystometry and the subsequent simultaneous measurement of urethral closure pressure and intravesical pressure during micturition provide the most complete urodynamic information about the voiding act, especially when combined with either simultaneous intrarectal pressure measurements to approximate true detrusor pressure or simultaneous radiographic videofilming (1,2,29) (see Chapters 7 and 13).

Electromyographic studies of the striated pelvic floor musculature and urinary flow studies provide important additional information (27) (see Chapter 8 and 9).

The microtransducer is an expensive delicate instrument which requires extremely careful handling and storage. However, when used properly, this instrument has a life span of more than 1000 examinations, thus giving a low instrumental cost per examination.

LOWER URINARY TRACT PHYSIOLOGY

The intravesical pressure depends upon the amount of fluid in the bladder, the tension of the bladder wall on this fluid from both muscular activity of the detrusor muscle and from the passive elastic components of the bladder wall, and that part of the intra-abdominal pressure which transmits to the bladder.

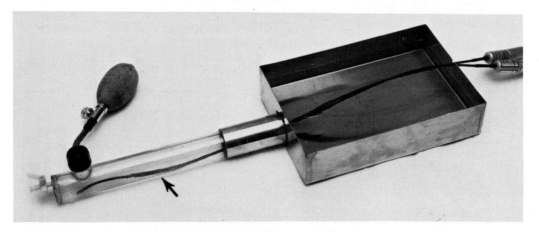

Figure 10.4.   The microtransducer Calibration Unit. Pressurization of the chamber (arrow) allows simultaneous calibration of the transducers and sterilization. (Vingmed, A/S, Oslo, Norway.)

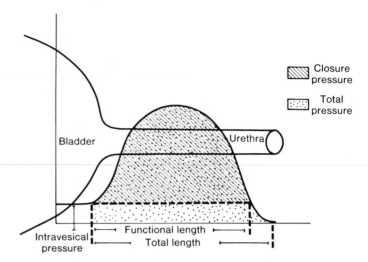

Figure 10.5. The urethral closure pressure profile. Functional urethral length is that distance along the urethra where intraurethral pressure exceeds the simultaneously measured intravesical pressure. Total length adds the additional distance to reach atmospheric pressure. Urethral closure pressure is the difference between the urethral pressure and the simultaneously measured intravesical pressure. Maximum urethral pressure is closure pressure plus intravesical pressure.

The intraurethral pressure, however, is more complex. The urethra is a 2- to 4-cm, short biological tube with no actual lumen most of the time. The urethra has a lumen only during voluntary micturition or with urinary incontinence. The urethral closure pressure profile defines the composite amount of urethral pressure and has several active and passive components. These components include the striated muscle fibers within the urethral wall and surrounding its exterior; the smooth musculature within the urethral wall and also within the walls of the blood vessels around the urethral lumen; vascular congestion in the submucosal plexus of veins; the elasticity of the urethral wall; and that part of the intra-abdominal pressure transmitted to the urethra (Figure 10.8). The urethra has a rich autonomic innervation compared to the bladder and an especially plentiful number of sympathetic receptors (25). At the site of the maximal urethral pressure the middle third of the urethra contains many of these receptors within the blood vessel walls (33).

The different parameters contributing to the urethral pressure profile vary considerably in relation to age (Figure 10.9 and 10.10), number of childbirths, body weight, anatomical urethral position and the influence of various medications in both normal and stress incontinent women (Tables 10.1 and 10.2). Women whose incontinence is due to anatomical reasons have shorter functional and total urethral lengths as determined by the urethral pressure profile. In both continent and incontinent women the functional and total lengths of the urethra are greater in the supine position than in the erect position (see Chapter 7).

Confusion exists regarding the relative importance of the contributions of the voluntary and involuntary components of the urethral sphincteric mechanism to the urethral pressure profile in women. The medical literature contains many studies designed to answer this question. Most use various autonomically active drugs to determine the relative contributions of the sympathetic and parasympathetic neurons. Unfortunately, the effect of drugs on the urethral pressure profile and on the bladder pressure is difficult to estimate and calculate. It is important to consider the systemic effects of these drugs, such as the resulting intra-arterial pressure alterations when the investigator uses ther-

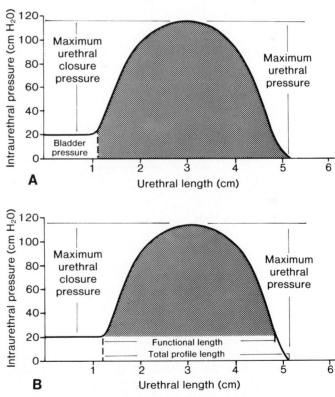

Figure 10.6. The integrated urethral closure pressure profile. The shaded area under the upper curve constitutes the integrated *total* urethral pressure (**A**). The shaded area under the lower curve indicates the integrated urethral *closure* pressure (**B**).

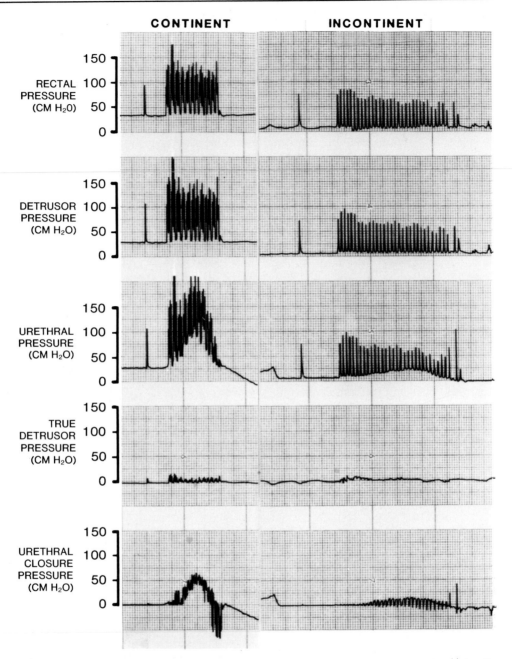

Figure 10.7. The cough urethral pressure profile. As the recording catheter is gradually withdrawn through the urethra, the patient coughs continuously. The continent patient (left) has an area of positive pressure under the curve which prevents urine leakage. The incontinent patient (right) lacks any areas of positive pressure. The change in closure pressure during coughing directly indicates the pressure transmission capacity ratio.

apeutic dosages. These drugs profoundly influence the per-iurethral vascular bed and, therefore, also influence urethral pressure. For example, alpha stimulating drugs cause augmentation of urethral closure pressure, and alpha blocking drugs cause urethral relaxation with a decrease of the maximal urethral pressure and maximal urethral closure pressure (12). Both types of drugs also have profound cardiovascular effects, which must also affect the vascular congestion in the urethra, an important contributing factor to urethral pressure (30).

Using simultaneous urethral cystometry and intra-arterial pressure recordings during curarization anesthesia for radical hysterectomy, with clamping of the common iliac arteries, the authors found that the intraurethral pressure at rest consists of several different components (30). Each of these contributes about one-third to the total urethral pressure and includes intrinsic and extrinsic striated muscle activity, congestion of the blood vessels in the urethra and the miscellaneous components, such as smooth muscle activity in the urethral wall and the urethral elastic elements. The fact that the vascular contribution is so great emphasizes the need to monitor and account for the effect of changes in arterial pressure during pharmacological studies of urethral function. Unfortunately, difficulties arise in the precise estimation of the relative contributions of each of

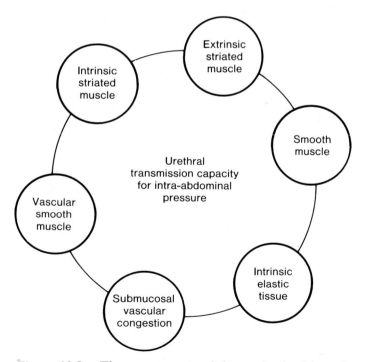

Figure 10.8. The components of the urethral sphincteric mechanism.

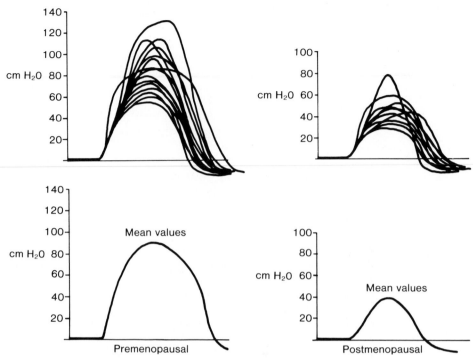

Figure 10.9. The urethral closure pressures in pre- and postmenopausal women. This figure gives the individual urethral closure pressure profiles from 15 premenopausal women and 10 postmenopausal women. The lower curve of each group gives the mean values for the curves. The urethral closure pressures are lower in the postmenopausal women than in the premenopausal women.

these different components of the composite urethral pressure. Similarly, their interdependence emphasizes that under various specific circumstances any one component might influence any or all of the other components with resultant changes in their relative contributions to urethral pressure (Figure 10.8).

The normal urethra demonstrates oscillations synchronous with the cardiac rate which are most apparent in the area of peak urethral pressure (Figure 10.11). The prominence of these pulsations changes with age, periurethral vascular integrity, anatomical support and estrogen status. These vascular effects are potentially important in the study of urethral function. For example, in a recent study the reestablishment of the urethral blood supply after bilateral common iliac occlusion caused an increase in the amplitude of the urethral pulsations more than expected from the actual increase in urethral pressure. In the awake patient, interruption of micturition causes an immediate increase in urethral pressure and the return of a pulsation pattern which is similar to that seen after reestablishment of aortic blood flow in the study described above (Figure 10.12).

Alpha stimulating drugs increase the amplitude of the pulsations more than expected from the change in urethral pressure and blood pressure. Also, alpha blocking drugs decrease the pulsations more than expected from the change in urethral pressure and blood pressure. Similarly, bilateral pudendal blockade reduces the amplitude of the urethral pulsations proportionately more than expected from the decrease in urethral pressure. This occurs in spite of an adrenalin induced rise in intra-arterial pressure and pulse rate. For these reasons, it is evident that alterations in blood pressure change the urethral pressure and that somatic and autonomic factors also contribute to this change in intra-urethral pressure. These facts emphasize the importance of periurethral vascularity in the maintenance of continence.

In spite of the clinical response of patients with incontinence to oral and topical estrogens, an unpublished study shows that no statistically significant alterations in the urethral and bladder pressure occurred after treatment of women with high doses of estrogen or progesterone (30). The observed clincal response is, therefore, due to factors other than measurable pressure. Most likely, the effect is from the positive effects of estrogen on the submucosal urethral vascularity and on the urethral mucosa itself.

In a recent study using nifedipine, a calcium antagonist, no alterations in the bladder or urethral pressure, nor any change in bladder capacity occurred (28). However, the study patients developed a significant increase in residual urine, suggesting an inhibition of contractile activity of the detrusor muscle (14). Others noticed the same effect with intramuscular administration of emepromium bromine (4).

ANATOMICAL CONSIDERATIONS

The bladder rests posteriorly on the anterior vaginal wall and laterally approaches the pelvic sidewall. The urethrovesical junction and the urethra also rest on the anterior vaginal wall, and the urethra perforates the urogenital diaphragm just distal to the location of the maximal urethral pressure (29,30). The pubourethral-vesical ligament com-

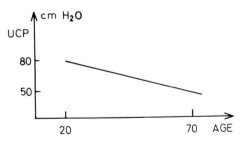

Figure 10.10. The urethral closure pressure in relation to age. There is a gradual decrease in closure pressure with advancing age.

Table 10.1.   Urethral Pressure Parameters in Normal Pre- and Postmenopausal Women[a]

	Premenopausal	Postmenopausal
Average age	30	65
Parity	1.3	1.4
Urethral length (cm)		
Functional	2.6	2.3
Total	3.0	2.9
Urethral pressure (Cm H_2O)		
Closure	81	43
Maximal	90	59
Bladder pressure (Cm H_2O)	9	17
Mean urethral pulsations (Cm H_2O)	15	4

[a] From Asmussen, 1975 (2).

plex anchors the bladder neck and the urethra to the symphysis (24). These ligaments also have smooth muscle components (18) (see Chapter 1). A correct normal anatomical fixation of the urethrovesical junction and the urethra intra-abdominally by the help of these ligaments is an important factor in the optimal physiological functioning of the different components which contribute to the urethral

MICTURITION

Micturition Patterns. A normal micturition occurs when the individual has the ability to completely empty the bladder through the urethra whenever there is a natural desire to do so. In most cases the individual is also able to stop the flow of urine when desired (2,20,31). It is important to stress that the urethra and the bladder comprise a functional unit at all times. In order to obtain a complete evaluation of the static and dynamic events in the lower urinary tract, the physician measures intraurethral, intravesical and intrarectal pressures simultaneously. This is especially important to determine the individual patient's micturition pattern.

The most common micturition pattern begins with a decrease in intraurethral pressure, followed 2 or 3 seconds later by an increase in the intravesical pressure, causing a negative closure pressure (Figure 10.12 and see Chapter 9). A second normal micturition pattern involves a decrease in intraurethral pressure, causing a negative closure pressure without alteration of the bladder pressure. In essence, the woman pulls out the drain plug by dramatically decreasing her urethral resistance. The short length of the female urethra, the weight of the urine and the effects of advancing age make this voiding mechanism possible.

Other techniques for accomplishing micturition involve a combination of the first two methods with abdominal straining. Thus, with or without a detrusor contraction, the bladder pressure exceeds the maximal urethral closure pressure because of increased intra-abdominal pressure, due to voluntary straining.

Another uncommon and distinctly pathological micturition pattern occurs when there is no alteration in the urethral pressure and the urination is due to a high pressure detrusor contraction. A true voiding dyssynergism exists when the urethra contracts synchronously with the detrusor contraction.

Controlled Provoked Micturition. During controlled provoked micturition nearly all normal and symptomatic women show one of these micturition patterns. However, many of these examinations also show an unstable urethra associated with a strong urge to void at some time before the actual urination (Figure 10.13). The relevance of this urgency under these testing conditions is unclear but is probably due to increased striated muscle activity which serves to prevent urine loss. Patients with multiple sclerosis or other neurological diseases involving the lower urinary tract often show normal micturition patterns which are uncontrollable and occur at abnormally low bladder volumes.

Well performed urodynamic studies indicate that a detrusor contraction always occurs coincidentally with a pressure change in the urethra; there is usually a decrease in the urethral pressure which precedes the detrusor contraction. Sometimes, however, this decrease of urethral pressure is of insufficient magnitude to produce negative closure pressure or leakage of urine. A strong desire to void often occurs with this event. Both normal and symptomatic women inhibit impending urine loss by voluntarily increasing urethral closure pressure. This is an example of detrusor-sphincter dyssynergy.

Table 10.2. Ranges of Maximal Urethral Pressures and Urethral Closure Pressures by Age Groups[a]

Age	Urethral Pressure (Cm H_2O)	
	Maximal	Closure
<21	84–111	65–92
21–30	83–112	63–93
31–40	73–110	53–90
41–50	73–92	54–73
51–60	74–89	53–68
61–70	57–73	37–53
>70	57–67	37–47

[a] Modified from Rud et al. (30).

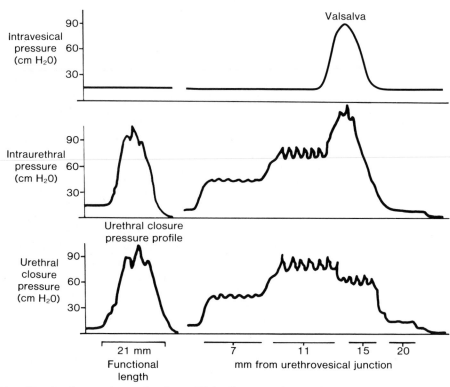

Figure 10.11. Urethral vascular pulsations. This diagram shows the relative intensity of vascular pulsations at 7 mm, 11 mm, 15 mm and 20 mm from the internal meatus in a healthy woman. Marked urethral pulsations occur at the area of maximal urethra pressure. The closure pressure and the intensity or the vascular pulsations changed minimally during valsalva at 15 mm.

The relative contributions of each of the specific components of the urethral sphincteric mechanism to the decrease in urethral resistance during the initiation of micturition is unknown. EMG studies show that the periurethral striated muscles relax (see Chapter 8). It also seems logical to conclude that the smooth muscle component behaves similarly. It is known, however, that when women initiate micturition, the urethral vascular pulsations decrease and disappear (Figure 10.12). Similarly, during valsalva, the intraurethral pressure immediately increases to a certain magnitude and the vascular pulsations disappear (Figure 10.11). After this maneuver, the intraurethral pressure rapidly decreases to below the previous baseline and then slowly increases. During this time the vascular pulsations gradually return, indicating filling of the submucosal vascular channels. This vascular filling takes about 10 to 20 seconds, which is the same period of time required for the urethral pressure to increase and to stabilize following reestablishment of the arterial blood supply to the urethral after aortic occlusion (30).

In the absence of both a valsalva maneuver and a detrusor contraction some patients show an overflow pattern of voiding during controlled provoked micturition. The bladder pressure increases because of stretching of the fibroelastic elements in the bladder wall during filling. In women, overflow incontinence rarely occurs, except in complete retention due to psychiatric causes or in patients subsequent to extended radical hysterectomy or other pelvic

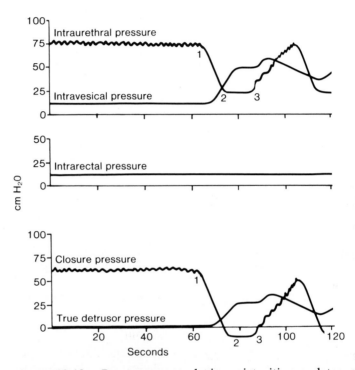

Figure 10.12. Pressure events during micturition as determined by simultaneous urethral cystometry. This pressure tracing is from a healthy women volunteer before, during and after micturition. Vascular pulsations highlight the premicturition urethral pressure. When the volunteer responds to the request to urinate (**1**), an instantaneous fall in the urethral pressure occurs with loss of vascular pulsations. After another 3 seconds a rapid increase of the true detrusor pressure (bladder pressure minus rectal pressure) takes place, indicating intrinsic detrusor activity. When the urethral closure pressure (the urethral pressure minus the bladder pressure) becomes zero or negative, urine escapes from the uethra (**2**). When requested to hold urine (**3**), the patient increases her urethral pressure and the closure pressure becomes positive with a slow return of vascular pulsations. The rectal pressure measurements exclude artifacts due to alterations in intra-abdominal pressure, facilitating estimation of actual intrinsic detrusor activity.

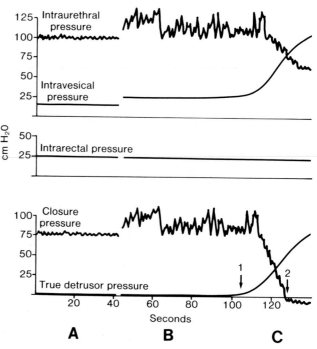

Figure 10.13. A urodynamic diagram from a patient with urgency incontinence. The left part of the diagram (Section A) shows the pressures after infusion of 100 ml saline. Note the stability of both the urethral and the bladder pressures as well as the regular urethral vascular pulsations evident in both the urethral and closure pressure tracings. Intrinsic rectal muscular activity causes the changes in rectal pressure with inverse changes in true detrusor pressure (bladder pressure minus detrusor pressure). Section B shows the oscillating pressure variations within the urethra and the bladder after infusion of 150 ml saline. The patient now has the desire to urinate. Note the instability of the urethral pressure which is characteristic of the unstable urethra. In Section C, the patient now has a strong desire to urinate. The bladder volume is 200 ml. The patient cannot hold urine any longer and produces a constant negative closure pressure at the point indicated by the second arrow where voiding beings. The first arrow indicates the onset of a detrusor contraction.

surgery causing denervation of the lower urinary tract. These patients must learn to void by straining (26).

STRESS INCONTINENCE

Stress incontinence is a sign or a symptom associated with involuntary loss of urine from the bladder through the urethra by a sudden increase of intraabdominal pressure without a detrusor contraction.

Stress incontinence is common in women. However, only when the stress becomes so severe that it causes the individual to be uncomfortable or interferes with her usual social activity does the symptom and sign constitute a disease which requires treatment. Stress incontinence occurs more often in older women and in parous women. It is also frequent in obese women and bears little relationship to urogenital prolapse. Various theories purport to explain the etiology of stress incontinence. One such theory relates a defect in anatomical position and size of the posterior urethrovesical angle as the most significant findings in stress incontinent women. This theory emphasizes that the preferred surgical procedure corrects the angle and the anatomical position (15,19). Another theory blames the too short female urethra as the cause of stress incontinence, producing a low pressure at rest; surgery stretches the urethra and increases the pressure (21). Further studies indicate that stretching of the urethra by surgery increases the intraurethral pressure since the smooth muscle then works at a more optimal compliance, thus, the reason for surgical cure (9,32).

A third theory states that the main cause of stress incontinence is a low pressure transmission capacity to the proximal urethra during stress because of its extra-abdominal position (13) (Figure 10.14).

The aim of surgery is to restore the urethra to its normal intra-abdominal position, thus correcting this defect.

A fourth theory based on SUCM emphasizes the estimation of the pressure transmission capacity ratio. This is the ratio of the amount of transmitted intra-abdominal pressure to the bladder as compared to the urethra at any given instant and location in the urethra. If this ratio, under any condition of stress, gives a positive or zero maximal closure pressure (1), the patient is continent regardless of the magnitude of any other urethral pressure parameter (Figure 10.7 and 10.15). This ratio gives a negative closure pressure in stress incontinent women, and the purpose of any treatment is to gain an optimal pressure transmission capacity ratio (Figure 10.15).

Damage to the pubourethral ligament complex most commonly occurs after traumatic birth and makes the bladder neck and the urethra excessively mobile (24). Since the actual movement of the urethrovesical junction results in a loss of much of the energy from the intra-abdominal pressure rise, this mobility gives a low pressure transmission ratio. Similarly, a poor pressure transmission ratio results from the periurethral fibrosis following traumatic deliveries, irradiation therapy, operations for prolapse, stress incontinence and urethral diverticula. Proper surgical fixation of the urethra and urethrovesical junction to the pelvic liga-

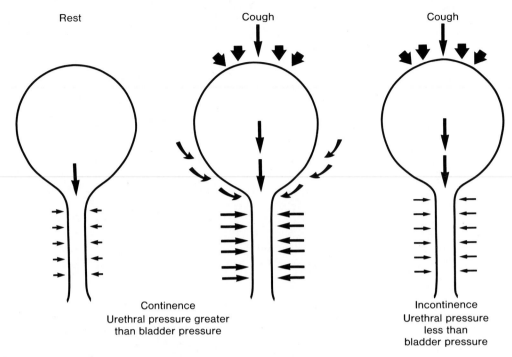

Figure 10.14. The pressure transmission patterns of the bladder and the urethra. At rest, the urethral pressure exceeds the intravesical pressure and no urine leakage occurs. The number and length of the arrows indicate the relative amount of pressure due to coughing. The normal woman's bladder and urethra both receive the same force with little net difference because of a good pressure transmission capacity ratio. This occurs when the urethra is an intra-abdominal organ. When the urethra loses its anatomical supports, it becomes an extra-abdominal organ. In this abnormal position it receives less pressure than the bladder. Thus, there is more force applied to the bladder than to the urethra. When this force exceeds urethral resistance, incontinence occurs due to an insufficient pressure transmission capacity ratio.

ments and the pelvic musculature gives an optimal pressure transmission ratio. This occurs even though suprapubic surgical procedures for female stress incontinence produce little or no alteration in the resting intra-urethral pressure (17). Successful surgery frequently actually decreases the urethral closure pressure somewhat, probably because of the traumatization of the periurethral tissues during the operation. These findings indicate that surgical treatment affects the dynamic and not the static mechanisms important in the genesis of genuine stress incontinence. The most likely explanation is a better transmission capacity ratio due to equalization of pressure impinging upon the bladder and the proximal urethra during stress.

Therapy of postmenopausal stress incontinent women with standard dosages of estradiol or estriol fails to alter either the urethral closure pressure or the length of the urethra in any consistent or significant manner (30). The reason for

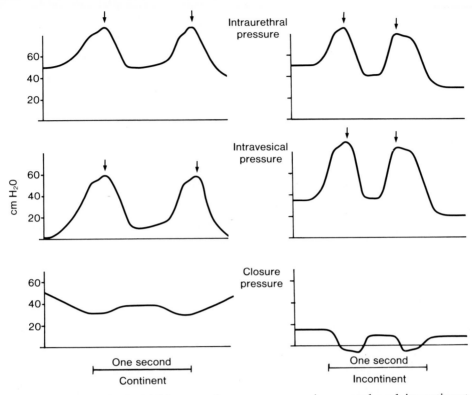

Figure 10.15. The effect of coughing on closure pressures in normal and incontinent women. The distal transducer is in the bladder and the proximal one is at the site of peak urethral pressure. On the left are the pressure recordings during two coughs (arrows) occurring in less than 1 second in a normal continent woman. Closure pressure remains positive. On the right are the pressure recordings during two coughs (arrows) in an incontinent woman. Closure pressure becomes negative during each cough, indicating an inefficient pressure transmission capacity ratio.

improvement of the stress incontinence in this study was a better pressure transmission capacity ratio.

SUMMARY AND CONCLUSIONS

Simultaneous urethrocystometry provides a reliable technique to fully evaluate women complaining of urinary incontinence. The results readily indicate those patients who will benefit from a surgical procedure. Most often those patients with genuine stress incontinence have an altered pressure transmission capacity ratio due to the abnormal anatomical position of the urethra and urethrovesical junction. Once the physician decides to operate, he must recognize that the purpose of the operation is to reestablish the natural intra-abdominal fixation to the urethra to allow an optimal pressure transmission capacity ratio, without disturbing the natural function of the urethra. The physician is careful to preserve the normal periurethral tissue, the urethral blood supply and the nervous innervation to this sensitive and delicate organ. Strict avoidance of all periurethral tissues during the dissection and the use of modified retropubic procedures accomplishes this purpose (10,11,23,32). Similarly, these operations allow simultaneous correction of uterine prolapse and mild to moderate degrees of cystocele. Unfortunately, vaginal operations of any kind do not fulfill these important surgical criteria, especially that of avoidance of periurethral tissues to minimize periurethral scarification. In postmenopausal women, the combination of surgery with estrogen therapy has a definite benefit to the patient.

The often used precept pertaining to incontinence surgery which states: "Do a vaginal procedure first, then go above," is no longer appropriate. To plan the next operation by choosing the first is contrary to modern gynecological surgical practice.

References

1. **Asmussen, M., Ulmsten, U.** Simultaneous Urethrocystometry and Urethra Pressure Profile Measurement with a New Technique. *Acta Obstet. Gynecol. Scand.* 54:385–386, 1975.
2. **Asmussen, M.** Urethro-Cystometry in Women. Development and Clinical Application of a New Standardized Technique for Simultaneous Intravesical-intraurethral Pressure Recording, Including Measurements of the Urethral Pressure Profile. Thesis. Malmo, Sweden, 1975.
3. **Asmussen, M., Lindstrom, K., Ulmsten, U.** A Catheter-manometer Calibrator—A New Clinical Instrument. *Biomed. Eng.* 13:175–180, 1975.
4. **Asmussen, M., Ulmsten, U.** Unpublished data.
5. **Asmussen, M.** Intraurethral Pressure Recording. Scand. J. Urol. Nephrol. 10:1–6, 1976.
6. **Asmussen, M., Ulmsten, U.** A New Technique for Measurements of the Urethra Pressure Profile. *Acta Obstet. Gynecol. Scand.* 55:167–173, 1976.
7. **Asmussen, M., Ulmsten, U.** Simultanous Urethro-cystometry with a New Technique. *Scand. J. Urol. Nephrol.* 10:7–11, 1976.
8. **Bates, P. et al.** The Standardization of Terminology of Lower Urinary Tract Function. *J Urol.* 121:551–554, 1979.
9. **Bruschini, H., Schmidt, R. A., Tanagho, E. A.** Effect of Urethral Stretch on Urethral Pressure Profile. *Invest. Urol.* 15:107–111, 1977.
10. **Burch, J.C.** Urethrovaginal Fixation to Cooper's Ligament for Correction of Stress Incontinence, Cystocele, and Prolapse. *Am. J. Obstet. Gynecol.* 81:281, 1961.
11. **Burch, J.C.** Urethrovaginal Fixation to Cooper's Ligament in the Treatment of Cystocele and Stress Incontinence. *Prog. Gynecol.* 4:591, 1963.
12. **Ek, A.** Innervation and Receptor Functions of the Human Urethra. Thesis. Lund, Sweden, 1977.
13. **Enhorning, G.** Simultaneous Recording of Intravesical and Intraurethral Pressure. *Acta Chir. Scand.* Suppl. 276, 1961.
14. **Forman, A., Andersson, K. E., Henriksson, L., Rud, T., Ulmsten, U.** Effects of Nifedipine on the Smooth Muscle of the Human Urinary Tract in Vitro and in Vivo. *Acta Pharmacol. Toxicol.* 43:111–118, 1978.

15. **Green T.** Urinary Stress Incontinence. Differential Diagnosis, Pathophysiology and Management. *Am. J. Obstet. Gynecol.* 122:368–399, 1975.

16. **Henriksson, L.** Studies on Urinary Stress Incontinence in Women. Thesis. Malmo, Sweden, 1977.

17. **Henriksson, L., Asmussen, M., Lofgren, O., Ulmsten, U.** A Urodynamic Comparison Between Abdominal Urethrocystopexy and Vaginal Sling Plasty in Female Stress Incontinence. *Urol Int.* 33:111–116, 1978.

18. **Huisman, A.B.** Morfologie van de vrouwelijke Urethra. Thesis. Groningen, Netherlands, 1979.

19. **Jeffcote, T.N.A., Roberts, H.** Observations on Stress Incontinence of Urine. *Am. J. Obstet. Gynecol.* 64:721–738, 1952.

20. **Karlsson, S.** Experimental Studies on the Function of the Female Bladder and Urethra. *Acta Obstet. Gynecol. Scand.* 32:285, 1953.

21. **Lapides, J., Ajemian, E. P., Bruce, H.S., Lichtward, J.R., Breakey, B.A.** Physiopathology of Stress Incontinence. *Surg. Gynecol. Obstet.* 3:224–231, 1960.

22. **Millar, H.D., Baker, L.E.** A Stable Ultraminiature Catheter-tip Pressure Transducer. *Biomed. Eng.* 11:86, 1973.

23. **Murnaghan, G.F.** Colposuspension in the Management of Stress Incontinence. *Br. J. Urol.* 47:236, 1975.

24. **Olesen, K.P., Grau, V.** The Suspensory Apparatus of the Female Bladder Neck. *Urol. Int.* 31:33–37, 1976.

25. **Owman, C.H., Sjoberg, N.O.** The Importance of Short Adrenergic Neurons in the Seminal Emission Mechanism of Rat, Guinea Pig and Man. *J. Reprod. Fertil.* 28:379–397, 1972.

26. **Palm, L.** Bladder Function in Women with Disease of the Lower Urinary Tract. An Evaluation Based On Micturition Cystourethrography and Simultaneous Pressure-flow Measurements. Thesis. Muskgaard, Copenhagen, 1971.

27. **Petersen, I., Sterner, I., Sellden, U., Kollberg, S.** Investigation of Urethral Sphincter in Women with Simultaneous Electromyography and Micturition Urethrocystography. *Acta Neurol. Scand.* 38, Suppl. 3, 145, 1962.

28. **Rud, T., Andersson, K.-E., Ulmsten, V.** Effects of Nifedipine in Women with Unstable Bladders. *Urol. Int.* 34:421–429, 1979.

29. **Rud, T., Westby, M., Ulmsten, U.** Initiation of Micturition: A Study of Combined Urethrocystometry and Urethrocystography in Healthy and Stress Incontinence Females. *Scand. J. Urol Nephrol.* 13:82, 1979.

30. **Rud, T., Asmussen, M., Andersson, K.E., Hunting, A., Ulmsten, U.** Factors Maintaining the Intra-urethral Pressure in Women *Invest. Urol.* 17:343, 1980.

31. **Tanagho, E. A., Miller, E.R.** Initiation of Voiding. *Br. J. Urol.* 42:175, 1970.

32. **Tanagho, E.A.** Colpocystourethropexy: The Way We Do It. *J. Urol.* 116:751, 1976.

33. **Ulmsten, U., Sjoberg, N.O., Alm. P., Andersson, K.E., Owman, C.H., Walles, B.** Functional Role of an Adrenergic Sphincter in the Female Urethra and the Guinea Pig. *Acta Obstet. Gynecol. Scand.* 56:387, 1977.

11 Dynamic Urethroscopy

Jack R. Robertson, M.D.

The female urethra is a neglected structure. Physicians seldom recognize its importance in the genesis of pelvic or lower urinary tract symptoms. Now, gynecologic urologists realize the true role of the urethra in pelvic pathology and view its interior with the 0° urethroscope. All physicians who deal with the symptomatic lower urinary tract should develop facility in the use of the urethroscope.

Modern urethroscopic technique is dynamic in its approach. It stresses not only visualization of the interior of the urethra and the base of the bladder, but also the response of the urethral sphincteric mechanism to bladder filling and to various commands and stressful maneuvers. This emphasis on dynamic urethral function adds a new and important dimension to the evaluation of the functional integrity of the lower urinary tract.

HISTORICAL PERSPECTIVE

Bozzini developed the first endoscope about 1805. A candle provided a sufficient light source to allow visualization of the interior of the bladder. His pioneering efforts led to his expulsion from the local medical society.

At Johns Hopkins Hospital Howard Kelly established the first residency training program in gynecology where gynecologists became genitourinary surgeons for women. Kelly developed a cystoscope consisting of a tube with a handle and used a head mirror for the light source. He discovered

135

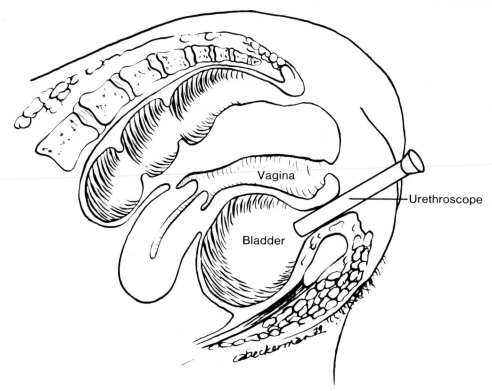

Figure 11.1. Ballooning of the bladder in the knee-chest position for endoscopy.

that the bladder ballooned with air when the patient assumed the knee-chest position (Figure 11.1). Using this position he examined the interior of the bladder and became the first person to pass ureteral catheters under direct vision.

About this time Nitzke developed the new indirect water endoscope, and urologists recognized the advantages of lower urinary tract endoscopy. They built a medical specialty around this instrument. This male-oriented panendoscope is inadequate for female urethroscopy due to its 30° view which limits urethral visualization.

The Robertson TM urethroscope is about 8 inches long with a sleeve that locks over the outside (Figure 11.2). There is an inlet for gas which is essential for urethroscopic examination.

TECHNIQUE OF URETHROSCOPY

The technique for female urethroscopy uses a single channel gas cystometer as the source of carbon dioxide. The tip of the urethroscope is 24 French in diameter and tapered. Table 11.1 outlines the procedure for the clinical evaluation of patients who have genuine stress incontinence or other genitourinary problems.

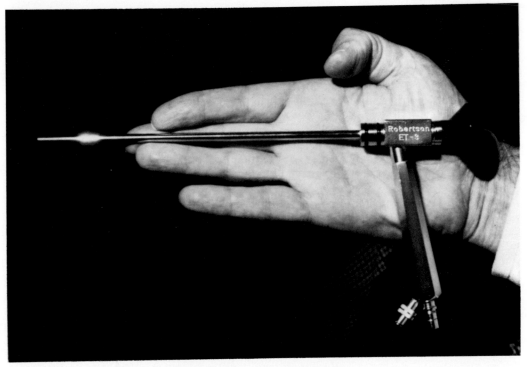

Figure 11.2. The urethroscope.

Table 11.1. The Sequence of Endoscopic Evaluation of the Urethra and Trigone

1. Urethral opening pressure.
2. Urethral visualization from external meatus to urethrovesical junction.
3. Trigonal and ureteral orifice visualization.
4. With observation of the urethrovesical junction
   A. During bladder filling
   B. With hold command
   C. With valsalva and cough
5. Observation of urethra for exudate and abnormal orifices.
   A. Posterior urethral glandular exudate
   B. Diverticula
   C. Fistula
6. Continued urethral observation
   A. Occlusion of urethrovesical junction.
   B. Urethral palpation for expression of exudate.

Under direct endoscopic view and with the carbon dioxide flowing at 150 cc per minute, the physician obtains an opening urethral pressure (Figure 11.5). This is not a urethral closure pressure profile but simply that pressure necessary to open the urethra. The gas is the obturator and provides a less traumatic entry.

Since the manipulation of the urethroscope in the urethra causes erythema, it is important to visualize the interior of the urethra during the initial introduction of the instrument. After visualization of the urethra, the urethroscope enters the bladder through the urethrovesical junction. Evaluation of the trigone follows with visualization of the ureteral orifices.

The endoscopist withdraws the instrument to the urethrovesical junction and views this area during bladder filling and during other superimposed dynamic activities. An evaluation of the responsiveness of the urethrovesical junction to the command of "hold urine," and to the stress of valsalva and cough when the bladder is nearly full, follows.

A search for the orifices of diverticula or fistulas and exudate from the posterior urethral glands or diverticula completes the urethral visualization sequence. A continuous flow of CO_2 and the occlusion of the urethrovesical junction aid in the search for abnormal orifices within the urethra, enabling better visualization of the area. Simultaneous urethral palpation and massage frequently express exudate under direct visualization.

ENDOSCOPY OF THE NORMAL URETHRA

Endoscopically, the normal urethra has a lush pink epithelium (Figure 11.3, top left). The urethrovesical junction is round and symmetrical (Figure 11.3, top right) and the trigone is pale pink with smooth epithelium and slit-like ureteral orifices (Figure 11.3, middle left).

DYNAMIC URETHROSCOPY IN THE NORMAL PATIENT

In the course of doing a carbon dioxide cystometrogram with endoscopic control, various changes occur in the urethrovesical junction. As the bladder fills the inverted U-shaped urethrovesical junction closes (Figure 11.4). With further bladder filling there is further urethral tightening ahead of the endoscope. This represents the increased tone of the periurethral striated muscle which develops as the bladder fills.

During bladder filling the endoscopist uses various challenge maneuvers to test the integrity of the urethrovesical junction. These challenges include asking the patient to hold urine, to bear down and to cough. In the normal patient these challenges cause further tightening of the vesical neck which remains stationary. It is not possible to stimulate a vesical contraction without the volitional agreement of the patient. If a vesical contraction does occur the normal patient always suppresses it.

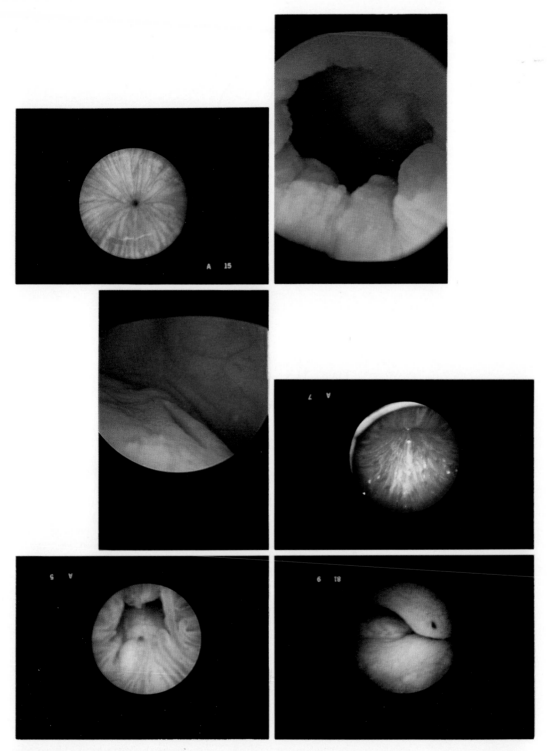

Figure 11.3. Urethroscopic views of the female urethra. The normal urethra (top left). The normal urethrovesical junction (top right). The normal trigone with one of the ureteral orifices (middle left). The red urethra in a patient with urethritis (middle right). Urethral inflammatory polyps and fronds at the urethrovesical junction (lower left). A urethral diverticular orifice (lower right).

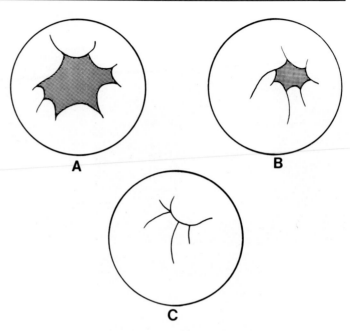

Figure 11.4. Diagram of the normal urethrovesical junction and its changes with bladder filling: **(A)** empty, **(B)** partially full and **(C)** full bladder.

OPENING PRESSURES IN NORMAL AND INCONTINENT PATIENTS

The urethral opening pressure in the normal patient registers between 70 and 90 cm water, and the urethroscope easily enters the urethra at an angle from 0° to 45° with the horizontal (Figure 11.5). Figure 11.6 diagrammatically demonstrates the urethrovesical junction in patients with genuine stress incontinence. These patients have vesical necks with minimal anatomical support. During stress the vesical neck behaves like an inelastic rubber band. After three or four vigorous coughs the vesical neck opens (funnels) and descends. It is very slow to reform and to return to its normal position. Similarly, the vesical neck reacts sluggishly, if at all, to the "hold" command.

URETHROSCOPY AND THE UNSTABLE BLADDER

The patient with an unstable bladder demonstrates an increase in intravesical pressure with a cough and several seconds later, the vesical neck opens and urine escapes from the external meatus (Figure 11.5). In some patients bladder filling stimulates this reaction; in others, one of the detrusor activating procedures causes vesical contraction. These patients cannot suppress these detrusor contractions.

URETHROSCOPY IN THE URETHRAL SYNDROME

Those patients in whom the urethral syndrome is the cause of their incontinence characteristically have a red urethra with exudate from the posterior periurethral glands, particularly with visualization during urethral massage (Figure 11.3, middle right). Commonly, the inflamed urethra contains polyps and fronds, particularly at the urethrovesical junction (Figure 11.3, lower left).

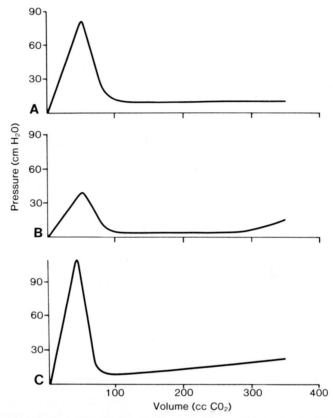

Figure 11.5. Urethral opening pressures. **(A)** normal, **(B)** genuine stress incontinence and **(C)** detrusor instability patients.

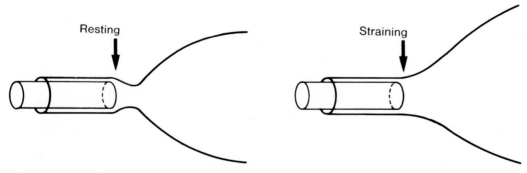

Figure 11.6. Diagram of the urethrovesical junction in the patient with genuine stress incontinence. The end of the urethroscope is located at the junction of the mid and upper third of the urethra (arrows). With straining funnelling is characteristic.

Table 11.2. Urethroscopy of Normal and Abnormal Patients

Dynamic Function of the Urethro-vesical Junction During:	Normal	Genuine Stress Incontinence	Unstable Bladder
Empty bladder		Closed	Closed
Partially full bladder	Closed	Slowly opens	Closed if no vesical contraction
Full bladder			
Holding	Closes	Sluggish closure	Closes
Straining	Remains closed	Opens	Remains closed if no vesical contraction
Coughing			
Vesical contraction	Opens, then closes, with suppression		Open and remains open due to inability to suppress
Ability to suppress a vesical traction	Present	Present	Absent

URETHROSCOPY AND DIVERTICULA

The endoscopist attempts to visualize urethral diverticula during urethral distention (Figure 11.3, lower right). Urethral palpation frequently reveals puffs of exudate which help to localize diverticular orifices.

URETHROSCOPY OF THE ECTOPIC URETER AND FISTULA

Although the ectopic ureter is rare, the characteristic spurts of urine reveal its identity. Urethrovaginal fistulas also have a characteristic appearance.

SUMMARY

The direct visualization of urethral-trigonal anatomy and pathology with the 0° urethroscope reveals the existence of previously unrecognized pathological entities. The dynamic nature of the technique also provides a method of evaluation of the functional integrity of the urethral sphincteric mechanism during bladder filling and with superimposition of varying commands and stressful situations (Table 11.2). The localization of diverticular orifices, ectopic ureters and fistulas is also possible. Finally, when coordinated with urodynamic techniques, it completes the essential composite evaluation of normal and abnormal urethrovesical function.

References

1. **Bozzini, P.** Lichteiter, Eine Erfindung Zur Anschung Innerer Theile, Und Krankheiten Nebst Abbildung. *J. Pract. Arzeykunde* 24:107, 1806.
2. **Kelly, H.A.** *Bull. John Hopkins Hosp.* November 1893.
3. **Nitzke, M.** Eine Neue Balbachtungs-und Untersuchunigsmethods fur Harnrohre, Harnblase and Rectum. *Wein. Med. Wochenschr.* 24:649, 1879.
4. **Robertson, J.R.** Ambulatory Gynecologic Urology. *Clin. Obstet. Gynecol.* 17:255, 1974.
5. **Robertson, J.R.** Gas Cystometrogram with Urethral Pressure Profile. *Obstet. Gynecol.* 44:72, 1974.
6. **Robertson, J.R.** *Genitourinary Problems in Women*, Charles C. Thomas, Springfield, Ill., 1978.
7. **Robertson, J.R.** Gynecologic Urethroscopy. *Am. J. Obstet. Gynecol.* 115:986, 1973.

12 The Preoperative Evaluation of Patients for Incontinence Surgery*

Donald R. Ostergard, M.D.
C. Paul Hodgkinson, M.D.

The most important elements of incontinence surgery are not the technical problems in the operative procedure itself, but how one decides when to do it, when not to do it, and which procedure to use. The preoperative studies and their interpretation are crucial in this decision making process.

PREOPERATIVE DIAGNOSTIC STUDIES USING ELECTRONIC URETHROCYSTOMETRY

The need for improvement of the standard water cystometrogram (CMG) for evaluation of detrusor function led to the development of the direct electronic urethrocystometric technique. This technique employs two water-filled 3-mm polyethylene tubes. One tube is open-ended and is placed into the bladder. To the end of the other tube is attached a small thin-walled Latex balloon which is placed into the midurethra (Figure 12.1). The catheters are held there by a harness permitting the patient to stand and walk. The tubes are about 10 feet long with the proximal end attached to a transducer and a recording machine with the paper running at 1 mm per second.

Figure 12.2 shows a typical example of a normal standard non-electronic cystometric study done by retrograde instillation of water. As the patient's bladder fills, there is a gradual increase in pressure. By comparison, Figure 12.3 is an electronic CMG done with retrograde water filling. Little or no pressure increase occurs.

---

* See Preface for origin of this chapter.

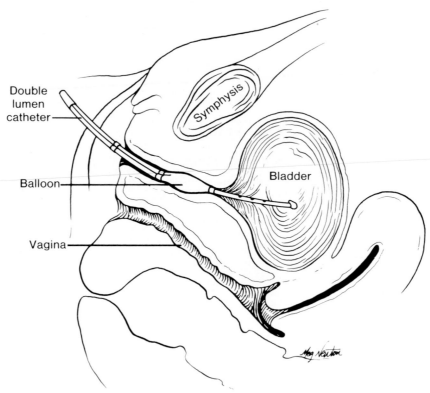

Figure 12.1   Diagram of the urethrocystometric catheter and its placement in the bladder and urethra.

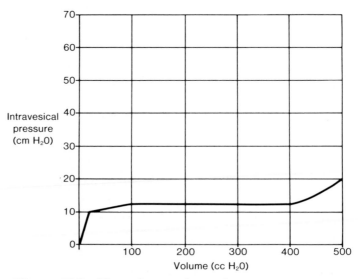

Figure 12.2   Normal non-electronic water cystometrogram. A gradual pressure increase occurs with bladder filling.

During direct electronic cystometry provocative tests are important to detect uninhibited detrusor contractions. The first is performed at the start of the test when the bladder is empty and at the second when the bladder is subjectively full. Coughing and heel bouncing are two of these provocative tests (Figure 12.4). With coughing at 30-second inter-

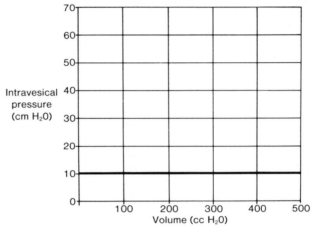

Figure 12.3 A typical normal segment of an electronic CMG. Vesical pressure increase with filling is almost imperceptible.

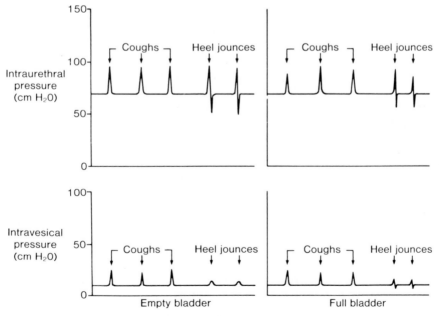

Figure 12.4 Provocative tests of coughing and heel bouncing at the start and end of the CMG. In this normal patient intraurethral pressure consistently exceeds intravesical pressure.

vals, there is a sudden sharp rise in pressure in both the bladder and the urethra lasting about 1 to $1\frac{1}{2}$ seconds. In the normal patient the pressure then immediately falls to the baseline and there is no evidence whatsoever of a detrusor contraction. With the patient standing on her toes, she jounces firmly on her heels, producing similar pressure recordings (Figure 12.4).

After performing these tests with an empty bladder, the patient's bladder is allowed to fill normally after previous hydration and chlorothiazide administration. One of the most important features with this kind of cystometry is that normal patients and those with anatomic (genuine) stress incontinence never demonstrate any increase in bladder pressure during bladder filling. Also, the urethral lead often shows a slight decrease in intraurethral pressure in patients with anatomic (genuine) stress incontinence because their urethras are relatively unresponsive to the stimulus for reflex contraction which usually occurs during bladder filling. When the bladder reaches subjective fullness, coughing and heel bouncing again provoke the detrusor. These do not provoke detrusor contractions in the patient with a stable bladder.

The next part of the test is a recording of bladder and urethral pressures during voiding. An electronic bedpan indicates qualitatively the precise moment urine flow starts and also roughly quantitates urine output. With this type of cystometry the bladder capacity usually exceeds that found with standard water cystometry.

Testing concludes with an evaluation of heat and cold sensation in the detrusor.

DETRUSOR DYSSYNERGIA

Incontinent patients with uninhibited detrusor contractions frequently show undulating curves or increases in pressure occurring as the result of spontaneous detrusor contractions and coincidental urine loss (Figure 12.5). This is detrusor dyssynergia, Type II. Although it is highly suspect for an association with neuromuscular disease it hardly ever results in the diagnosis of either specific urological or neurologic disease. These patients never completely fill their bladders, nor do they completely empty them, as indicated by residual urine volumes of 75 to 100 cc. Cystoscopy usually reveals fine trabeculation of the bladder, apparently because of the relative physiologic obstruction to urine flow. The important consideration is the differentiation of this type of urine loss from genuine stress incontience.

Abnormal bladder activity as a result of various provocative tests is detrusor dyssynergia, Type I (Figure 12.6). In these

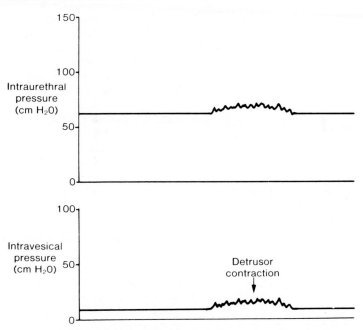

Figure 12.5 Detrusor dyssynergia, Type II. A detrusor contraction occurs without any form of prior stimulation.

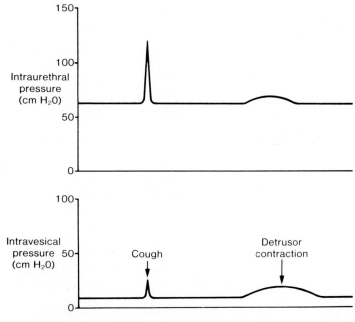

Figure 12.6 Detrusor dyssynergia, Type I. A detrusor contraction follows stimulation by coughing.

patients coughing produces a pressure increase which immediately decreases to baseline. However, approximately 20 seconds later a detrusor contraction occurs which the patient cannot inhibit, producing the loss of a small amount of urine. By history alone this type of incontinence is indistinguishable from genuine stress incontinence. If the question is asked, "Do you lose urine if you cough or sneeze?" the only possible answer is "Yes." Yet, her urine loss is not due to increased intra-abdominal pressure, a specific characteristic of genuine stress incontinence; she loses urine because of an uninhibitable detrusor contraction.

CLINICAL MEDICAL HISTORY

All patients complete a questionnaire prior to surgery (Table 12.1). Group I questions detect intrinsic disease of the bladder. Any positive response in this group of questions indicates the need for a urological consultation.

Group 2 questions detect neuromuscular dysfunction. Of particular importance is the question, "Does the sound, sight or feel of running water cause you to lose urine?" Most people with detrusor dysfunction answer "yes" to this question.

The next group of questions relates to various physical factors. Patients with anatomical incontinence always answer "yes" to the question regarding loss of urine immediately after coughing. The patient with genuine stress incontinence never has detrusor autocontractility. She always loses urine precisely at the time of increased intra-abdominal pressure. The direct transmission of increased intra-abdominal pressure to the bladder is not similarly transmitted to the urethra due to her altered anatomy. This allows the pressure in the bladder to exceed the intra-urethral pressure, thereby producing a negative urethral closure pressure which allows urine loss.

PREOPERATIVE CHAIN CYSTOGRAM

The chain cystogram provides information regarding the pathology of the perivesical and periurethral supporting tissues and the adaptability of the bladder and urethra to the altered anatomy of these supporting tissues. Although these radiographs allow measurement of the posterior urethrovesical angle, this angle is no longer as important in the pathophysiology of genuine stress incontinence as was previously thought. The physician obtains more significant preoperative information from these radiographic evaluations than by the estimation of angles alone.

Patients with uterovaginal prolapse practically never have genuine stress incontinence (Figure 12.7). When this patient strains down, the bladder rolls downward and backward, and the urethra remains relatively well supported. In these

Table 12.1. Incontinence Questionnaire

GROUP I: INTRINSIC DISEASE

1. Have you had treatment for urinary tract disease, such as stones, kidney disease, infections, tumors, injuries?	YES	NO
2. Have you had repeated bouts of pyelitis?	YES	NO
3. Is your urine ever bloody?	YES	NO
4. Is the volume of urine you usually pass large, average, small, very small? (please check)		
5. When you lose your urine accidently, are you ever *not* aware that it is passing?	YES	NO
6. Do you always have a severe sense of urgency before you lose your urine?	YES	NO
7. Do you lose urine as a constant drip from the vagina?	YES	NO
8. Did you have difficulty holding urine as a child?	YES	NO
9. Is it usually painful or difficult to pass your urine?	YES	NO

GROUP II: NEUROMUSCULAR DYSFUNCTION

1. As a child did you wet the bed?	YES	NO
2. Do you wet the bed now?	YES	NO
3. Have you ever had paralysis, polio, multiple sclerosis, a serious injury to your back, cyst or tumor on your spine, tuberculosis, a stroke, syphilis, diabetes, pernicious anemia?	YES	NO
4. Does the sound, the sight or the feel of running water cause you to lose urine?	YES	NO
5. Is your loss of urine a continual drip so that you are constantly wet?	YES	NO
6. Are you ever not aware that you are losing, or are about to lose, control of your urine?	YES	NO
7. Is your clothing slightly damp, wet, soaking wet, or do you leave puddles on the floor? (If yes, check proper one.)		
8. Have you had an operation on your spine, brain, or bladder?	YES	NO
9. Do you find it frequently necessary to have your urine removed by means of a catheter because you are unable to pass it?	YES	NO

GROUP III: PHYSICAL FACTORS

1. Do you lose urine by spurts during coughing, sneezing, laughing, lifting?	YES	NO
2. Do you lose urine when you are lying down?	YES	NO
3. Do you lose urine when you are sitting or standing erect?	YES	NO
4. When you are urinating, can you usually stop the flow?	YES	NO
5. Did your urine difficulty start after delivery of an infant?	YES	NO
6. Did it follow an operation?	YES	NO
7. Check the type of operation:		
Hysterectomy, abdominal incision		_____
Hysterectomy, removed through the vagina		_____
Removal of a tumor, abdominal incision		_____
Vaginal repair operation		_____
Suspension of the uterus		_____
Cesarean section		_____

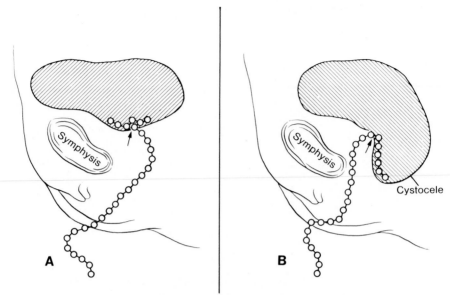

Figure 12.7   Chain cystogram of uterovaginal prolapse. With straining it is evident that the urethra is not attached to the most dependent portion of the bladder (arrows) and (**B**) a large cystocele becomes evident.

patients the maximum loss of support of the pelvic floor is not at the urethrovesical junction but is posterior to the urethrovesical junction. Since the urethra remains in a relatively normal anatomical position, the posterior rotation of the bladder actually tends to mechanically close off the urethra rather than open it.

In patients with genuine stress incontinence, a different type of urethrovesical configuration occurs (Figure 12.8). Downward pressure from above depresses the urethrovesical junction to the very lowest level of the bladder. The combination of a dependent urethrovesical junction and the hydrodynamic effect of intravesical urine produces a situation where the urethra tends to open from within.

There are those who criticize the chain cystogram on the basis that the urethrovesical relationships of the normal patient and those with anatomical incontinence are not very different and, therefore, the changes become non-specific. This is a true appraisal and the following comparison between canine and human anatomical relationships describes why. The canine urethra joins the bladder high on its posterior surface with the bladder dependent in the abdomen (Figure 12.9). Stress from increased intra-abdominal pressure depresses the bladder further downward and increases the acuteness of the urethrovesical angle. The female patient with genuine stress incontience who assumes

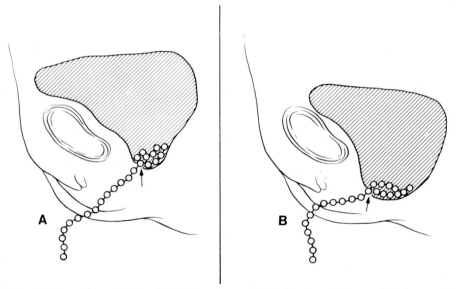

Figure 12.8   Chain cystogram of genuine stress incontinence. The urethra is attached to the most dependent portion of the bladder (arrows) in both the non-straining (**A**) and straining (**B**) views.

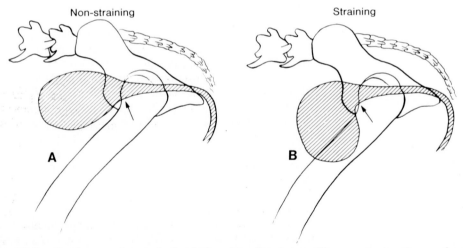

Figure 12.9   Canine urethrovesical relationship. Straining (**B**) accentuates the urethrovesical angle (arrows).

the canine position on her elbows and knees has a similar urethrovesical relationship (Figure 12.10). The urethrovesical junction is more or less supported from below by the symphysis. If this patient remains in the canine position she does not experience incontinence even with stress. With assumption of the upright position these relationships change completely with the urethrovesical junction now

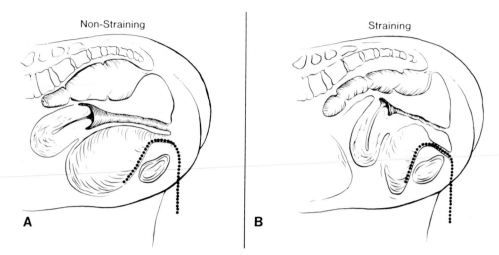

Non-Straining   Straining

A   **B**

Figure 12.10 Urethrovesical relationship in the human female with genuine stress incontinence. At rest in the canine position urethrovesical relationships are normal (**A**). With stress the angle becomes more acute and incontinence is prevented. Compare with the upright position shown in Figure 12.8.

located at the lowest, most dependent, level of the bladder (Figure 12.8).

A distinct advantage of the chain cystogram is in the comparison of pre- and postoperative urethrovesical configurations. The preoperative chain cystogram of Figure 12.8 shows a typical configuration of genuine stress incontinence. After a vaginoplastic procedure the urethrovesical junction's position is now at a higher level in comparison to the symphysis with some additional posterior rotation of the bladder.

Unfortunately, not all patients receive the proper operation. When the urethrovesical junction is at the level of the symphysis without straining and when straining descends minimally, vaginal surgery produces minimal elevation of the urethrovesical junction and a predictably unfavorable surgical result because of selection of the wrong operation. This emphasizes the errancy of doing a vaginoplastic operation merely on the basis of obstetric and gynecologic custom. The adage of "Do a vaginoplastic operation first, and then if it fails do a retropubic procedure," is not proper modern treatment.

Another point of emphasis is that errors are common when attempting to estimate relationships on clinical examination. Even when a complete prolapse of the anterior vaginal wall exists, frequently the urethra and bladder remain in a high retropubic position. The chain cystogram allows a precise determination of these urethrovesical relationships.

Urethrovesical x-rays are very important in the selection of patients for the proper surgical procedure. The fundamental part of any operation for cure of genuine stress incontinence is a thorough evaluation of the anatomy of the urethrovesical junction at rest and with stress. If the degree of stress incontinence incapacitates the patient, it is wrong to do a primary vaginoplastic operation in most instances since retropubic urethropexy procedures are much more successful than vaginoplastic operations.

For example, with vaginoplastic operations Jeffcoate stated a 60% cure rate and Lowe reported only 48% success rate. Most studies of retropubic urethropexy procedures report a cure rate in the range of 85 to 90%. There is no difficulty combining the procedure with repair of cystocele, rectocele or prolapse or with abdominal or vaginal hysterectomy.

SUMMARY

The selection of patients for surgical incontinence procedures requires an extensive historical evaluation and an equally complete study of urethrovesical function and anatomical relationships. The electronic recording of urethrovesical pressure relationships and the chain cystogram are important aids in this process. The gynecologic custom of first performing a vaginoplastic operation followed by a retropubic procedure in the event of failure is no longer valid.

References

1. **Crisp, W. E.** Letter to the Editor: What's the Angle? *Obstet. Gynecol.* 26:918, 1965.
2. **Hodgkinson, C.P.** Relationships of the Female Urethra and Bladder in Urinary Stress Incontinence. *Am. J. Obstet. Gynecol.* 65:560, 1953.
3. **Hodgkinson, C.P., Drukker, B.H., Hershey, G.J.C.** Stress Incontinence in the Female. VIII. Etiology, Significance of Short Urethra. *Am. J. Obstet. Gynecol.* 86:16, 1963.
4. **Lazarevski, M., Lazarov, A., Novak, J., Dimcevski, D.** Colpocystography in Cases of Genital Prolapse and Urinary Stress Incontinence in Women. *Am. J. Obstet. Gynecol.* 122:704, 1975.
5. **Hodgkinson, C.P., Cobert, N.** Direct Urethrocystometry. *Am. J. Obstet. Gynecol.* 79:648, 1960.

13 Radiological Techniques for the Evaluation of the Bladder and Urethra

Stuart L. Stanton, F.R.C.S., M.R.C.O.G.

INTRODUCTION

Radiological techniques are of great value in the evaluation of the lower urinary tract. These procedures range from the simple plain film of the pelvis to the extremely sophisticated, dynamic evaluations of the urethra and bladder with simultaneous pressure and urine flow recordings. Additional specialized techniques also provide specific information regarding the urethra, especially in the detection of diverticula (see Chapter 18). This chapter reviews those radiographic techniques which assess the anatomical relationships of the urethra and bladder and the dynamic function of the lower urinary tract.

PLAIN FILMS

Bony abnormalities of the pelvis frequently accompany developmental defects of the lower urinary tract. For example, separation of the symphysis pubis accompanies epispadias (Figure 13.1) and bladder exstrophy (Figure 13.2). These result from a failure of fusion of the primitive somites in the midline with lack of mesodermal support to the endoderm and ectoderm. In epispadias there is defective formation of the bladder neck leading to sphincteric incompetence and separation of the clitoris into two halves. Bladder exstrophy represents a greater degree of abnormality with failure of the development of the anterior bladder and abdominal walls. Acquired separation of the symphysis pubis occurs following symphysiotomy and trauma (Figure 13.3).

155

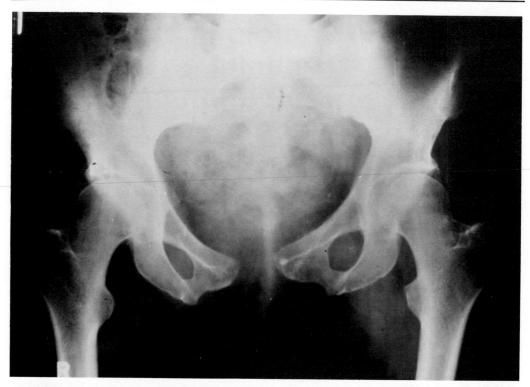

Figure 13.1   Epispadias. There is an abnormal separation of the symphysis pubis. (Reproduced with permission of the author and the editor. *American Journal of Obstetrics and Gynecology.*)

Congenital abnormalities of the sacrum may cause urinary complaints because of associated neurological defects. These include spina bifida occulta (Figure 13.4) and sacral agenesis (Figure 13.5). Acquired conditions of the lumbosacral spine causing symptoms include spondylolisthesis between L4 and L5, and L5 and S1, and prolapsed intervertebral discs at these levels. These produce predominantly lower motor neuron effects on the bladder and urethra.

INTRAVENOUS PYELOGRAM

The intravenous pyelogram (IVP) is an essential component of the investigation of patients with continuous incontinence either due to a congenital abnormality or to a fistulous tract. The IVP discloses the presence of ectopic ureters (Figure 13.6) and ureteric and occasionally vesicovaginal fistulas. The presence of a significant postmicturition residual alerts the clinician to exclude a voiding disorder.

STATIC CYSTOGRAM

The introduction of a radiopaque dye into the bladder via the urethra provides information about the morphology of the bladder, bladder neck and urethra. It demonstrates urinary/contrast leakage either through the urethra or

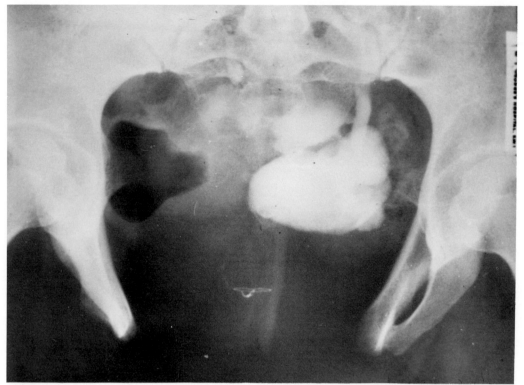

Figure 13.2   Bladder exstrophy. This x-ray demonstrates the failure of formation of the symphysis pubis.

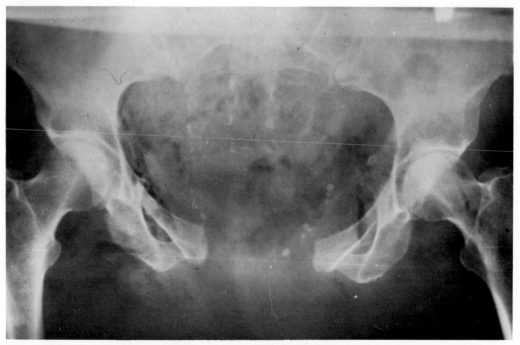

Figure 13.3   Traumatic separation of the symphysis pubis with associated old fractures of the pelvic ring. The traumatic event displaced the urethra by rupturing the ligaments and supports of the bladder neck producing stress incontinence.

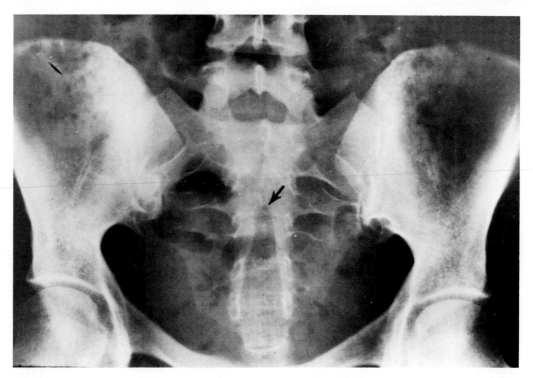

Figure 13.4 Spina bifida occulta. The arrow indicates the site where bifurcation begins. This patient had tethering of her filum terminale which led to urinary frequency and eventual overflow incontinence. (Reproduced with permission of S.L. Stanton, F.R.C.S., from *Female Urinary Incontinence*. Lloyd-Luke Medical Books, London, 1977.)

through any fistulous connection into the vagina or abdomen (Figure 13.7).

The cystogram also provides information regarding location of the urethrovesical junction relative to the posterior aspect of the symphysis pubis at rest and on straining. Normally, the urethrovesical junction resides posteriorly and superiorly to the lower edge of the symphysis (Figure 13.8). In patients whose urinary incontinence has an anatomical basis, the junction descends below this level. Use of a beaded chain helps delineate the urethra, bladder neck and bladder base. The posterior urethrovesical angle is no longer of importance in the incontinent patient and requires no further discussion.

MICTURATING CYSTOGRAM

The micturating cystogram is a method of radiological screening of the bladder and urethra during voiding and is a dynamic investigation. It demonstrates the pathophysiology of the urethrovesical junction during coughing and voiding. Opaque media of different viscosities appropriately modify the technique. A useful modification is the intro-

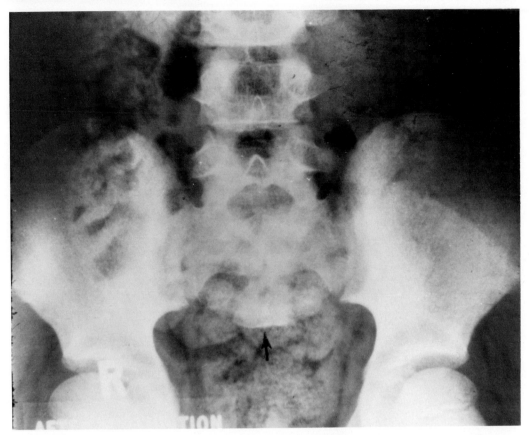

Figure 13.5   Sacral agenesis. The arrow indicates the end of the bony spinal column.

duction of a heavy barium paste into the urethra, followed by a lighter radiopaque dye. The barium paste outlines the urethrovesical junction and the base of the bladder, while the more viscous dye outlines the remainder of the bladder (Figure 13.9). Outlining the vagina and rectum with barium paste provides information on their relative positions.

**VIDEOCYSTO-
URETHROGRAPHY**

Videocystourethrography (VCU) combines all aspects of the micturating cystogram with fluoroscopy and simultaneous recordings of intravesical and intrarectal pressures and urine flow rates (see Chapter 6, Figure 6.4). Video mixing techniques record the information on video tape for instant or later replay and discussion.

The procedure is as follows: the patient lies supine on a tilting radiologic table. After measurement of the residual urine by sterile catheterization using a 12 Foley catheter (Figure 13.10), the physician fills the bladder by gravity with 25% diodone at a rate of 100 ml per minute. A weighing transducer measures the rate of filling. A 1-mm

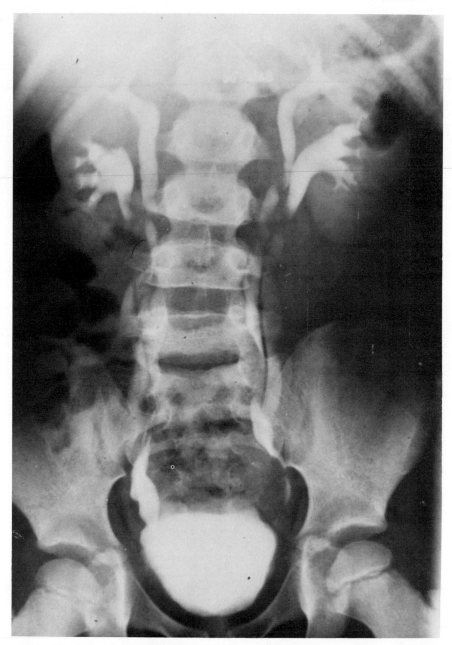

Figure 13.6 Ectopic ureter. This intravenous urogram shows a duplex system on both sides. The ectopic ureter opened into the vagina and the patient had incontinence since birth.

diameter fluid filled catheter placed alongside the filling catheter connects to a pressure transducer to measure the intravesical pressure. Protected from fecal blockage by a finger cot, a 2-mm fluid filled catheter inserted a short

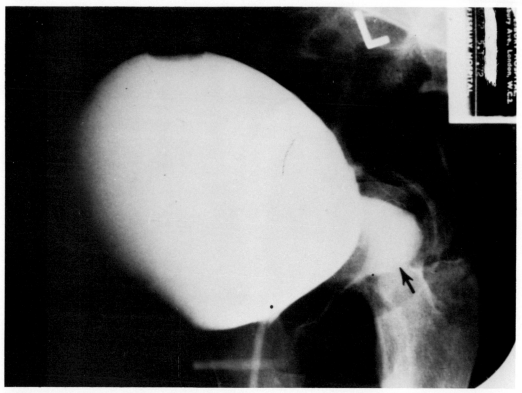

Figure 13.7 Vesicovaginal fistula. An erect lateral micturating cystogram shows a vesicovaginal fistula with contrast in the vagina (arrow).

distance into the rectum measures the rectal (abdominal) pressure. Electronic subtraction of the abdominal pressure from the intravesical pressure gives the detrusor pressure, an exact index of detrusor activity. During filling, the investigating team notes first sensation and full bladder capacity. When the patient complains of subjective bladder fullness, the physician removes the filling catheter and stands the patient upright and radiologically screens the patient in the erect oblique position noting leakage or bladder base descent. The patient then voids and subsequently interrupts her stream. A uroflowmeter records peak urine flow rate and volume voided; simultaneously, a transducer records the maximum voiding pressure and the physician observes the patient's ability to "milkback" urine from the urethra to the bladder during the stop-void command. The patient resumes voiding and after emptying her bladder, fluoroscopy reveals the presence or absence of residual urine. About 15% of women have difficulty in voiding when erect. When this occurs, the patient transfers with pressure lines and transducer connections to an adjacent side room where she sits on a commode with a uroflowmeter in place and voids in privacy.

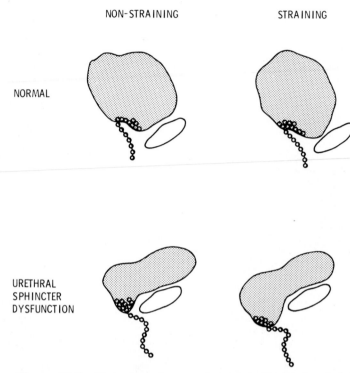

Figure 13.8 Drawings from a lateral radiograph of the bladder with the base of the bladder and urethra outlined by Hodgkinson's metallic bead chain. It indicates the appearance in the normal woman and in the woman with urethral sphincter dysfunction. (Reproduced with permission of C.P. Hodgkinson et al. and the editor, *Clinical Obstetrics and Gynecology.*)

A television camera, positioned above the recorder and with a mixing device, projects three of the six recorded channels alongside the radiographic image of the bladder on a television monitor. The recorded parameters include the intravesical pressure, the detrusor pressure and the flow rate. Videotape records this combined picture with a sound commentary (Figure 13.11).

As voiding begins in the normal patients, the pelvic floor relaxes, the urethral pressure falls and the bladder neck opens, followed by a rise in detrusor pressure. This variable detrusor pressure rise is usually below 70 cm of water (Figure 13.12). In order to determine whether the patient has voluntary control of micturition, the physician asks the patient to stop voiding. Immediately, the voluntary striated muscular component of the urethral sphincteric mechanism contracts and effectively closes off the urethra, thus stopping the flow of urine (Figure 13.13). Milkback now occurs

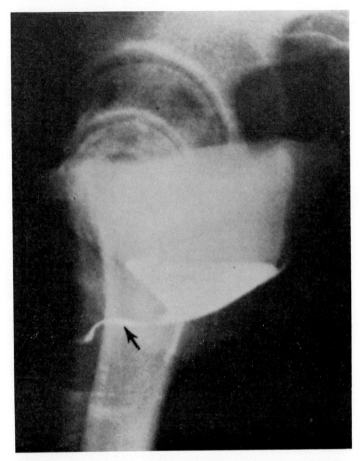

Figure 13.9   Erect lateral micturating cystogram showing lower bladder and urethra (arrow) outlined using opaque media of different contrast. (Reproduced with permission of J.E. Morgan and G. Farrow and the editor of the *British Journal of Urology*.)

which is the process by which the proximal urethra returns urine into the bladder. The maximum voiding detrusor pressure may rise abruptly (Figure 13.14). This represents isometric contraction of the slow acting detrusor in the presence of urethral closure as a result of a contracted voluntary striated component of the urethral sphincter. This is the isometric contraction phase of the detrusor. The detrusor pressure falls when the slower acting detrusor muscle relaxes. The bladder neck closes when the detrusor pressure falls to the premicturition level.

This examination sequence confirms whether or not the patient leaks urine and under what circumstances leakage occurs. It also provides information about her maximum

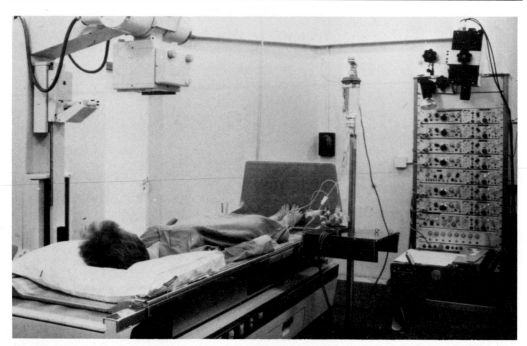

Figure 13.10 Patient and the radiologic table; Grass recorder with television camera and stand with transducers. (Reproduced with permission of the author and the editor of *Clinical Obstetrics and Gynecology*.)

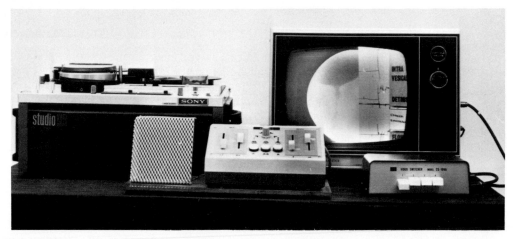

Figure 13.11 The videotape recorder, mixer and television monitor. (Reproduced with permission of the author and the editor, *Clinical Obstetrics and Gynecology*.)

voiding pressure, her peak flow rate, the effectiveness of milkback, the presence of residual urine, and whether or not she responds effectively to the command of "stop micturition." This technique exposes the patient to approximately 800 millirads, which is less than the exposure for an intravenous pyelogram.

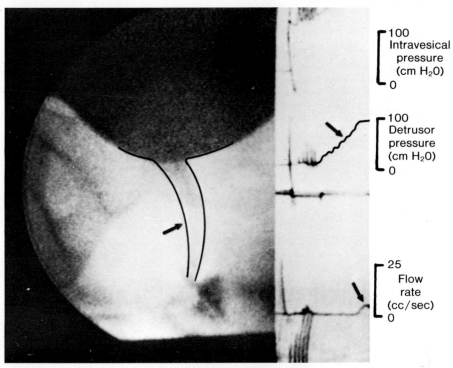

Figure 13.12 Final video image showing normal micturition. The opaque medium opacifies the urethra (arrow). Notice increased true detrusor pressure and the record of flow rate (arrows).

In the patient with urethral sphincter incompetence (genuine stress incontinence) and without detrusor instability, the bladder fills normally without detrusor contractions and with a pressure rise of less than 15 cm of water. On standing erect the detrusor pressure rise remains less than 15 cm of water and on coughing there is loss of contrast material through the urethra. The bladder neck often exhibits excess mobility and descent and may be open at rest without a rise in detrusor pressure (Figure 13.15). The patient may or may not be able to interrupt her urinary stream on command and subsequently voids to completion.

By contrast, with detrusor instability, there may be detrusor contractions or a steep detrusor pressure rise greater than 15 cm of water during filling and on standing (Figure 13.16). Stress incontinence may occur on coughing and may trigger a detrusor contraction (Figure 13.17). Often the contractions occur early during the filling phase prior to reaching full bladder capacity. Despite reports to the contrary, this author finds no relationship between the ability to voluntarily interrupt the urinary stream and the diagnosis of either urethral sphincter incompetence or detrusor instability.

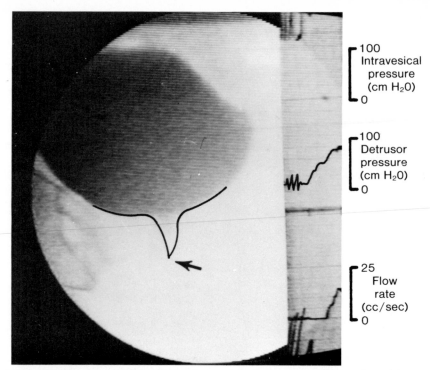

Figure 13.13. Video image showing voluntary interruption of the micturition stream at midurethra (arrow).

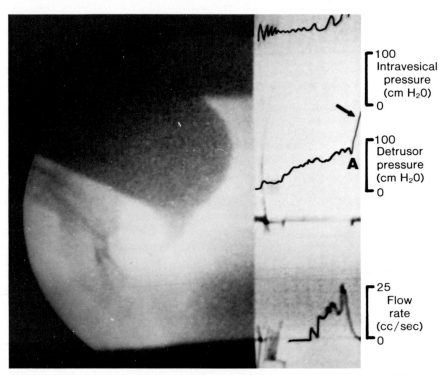

Figure 13.14 Video image showing detrusor isometric contraction phase. When asked to stop voiding at point A, the extrinsic voluntary component of the sphincter mechanism contracts and closes the urethra before the detrusor begins to relax. This results in a marked increase in detrusor pressure (arrow) which gradually falls to the prevoiding level, once relaxation of the detrusor occurs. At the same time, the bladder neck gradually closes.

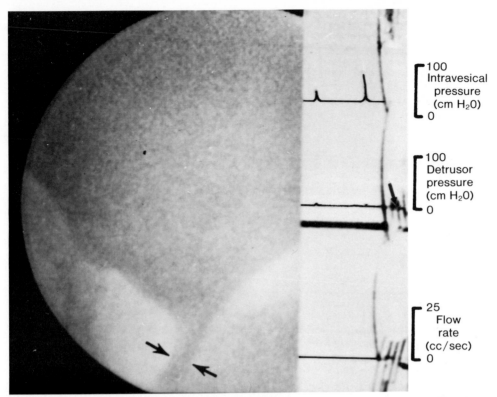

Figure 13.15 Video image demonstrating incontinence due to urethral sphincter incompetence. The detrusor pressure is at zero (arrow) and there is contrast media escaping via the bladder neck and urethra following a cough. The arrows outline the urethra.

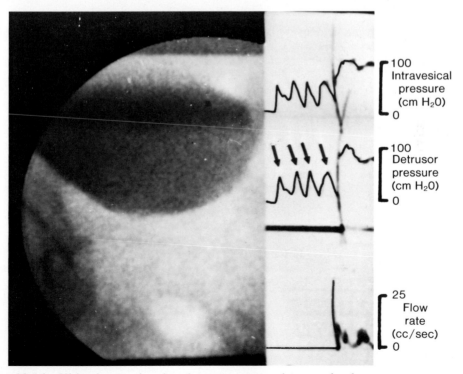

Figure 13.16 Video image showing detrusor contractions on the detrusor pressure tracing during bladder filling (arrows).

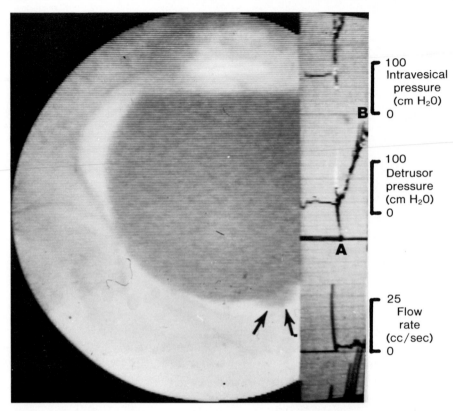

Figure 13.17 Video image demonstrating a rise in detrusor pressure. The patient stands upright at point A and begins to cough at point B. The bladder neck is partially open (arrows). (Reproduced with permisson of the author and the editor, *Clinical Obstetrics and Gynecology*.)

SUMMARY

Radiographic techniques provide information on anatomical relationships of the urethrovesical junction and its dynamic response to various stressful conditions. The combination of simultaneous video recording of pressure and flow data with the radiographic image allows a precise assessment of disordered function of the lower urinary tract.

References

1. **Cardozo, L., Stanton, S.L.** A Comparison between Genuine Stress Incontinence and Detrusor Instability. *Br. J. Obstet. Gynecol.* (in press).

14 Vesical and Urethral Denervation Sensitivity Testing

Thomas A. McCarthy, M.D.

INTRODUCTION

The cystometrogram (CMG) is the "reflex hammer" of the urologist. Like the reflex hammer the CMG tests reflex behavior of the bladder and diagnoses various types of neurogenic bladder dysfunctions. The greatest use of the CMG is in the identification of the bladder which demonstrates uninhibitable detrusor contractions. For bladders which are hyporeflexic or atonic, the most common cause is denervation. Until recently vesical denervation was a diagnosis of exclusion. The positive detection of bladder denervation is now possible using the CMG.

Coincident with recent advances in the field of urodynamics, the urethra is now a known cause of voiding dysfunction. The lowered urethral pressure associated with genuine stress incontinence is well known. The recognition that the urethra is also subject to neurogenic dysfunction in much the same way the bladder is and may be the result of chronic urethral denervation is a recent advance. Testing procedures for detecting urethral denervation are now available.

DENERVATION SENSITIVITY TESTING

The pioneering efforts and the ingenuity of Doctors Cannon, Lapides and Koyanagi provide us with ability to detect denervation of both the bladder and urethra. In 1939 Cannon popularized the concept of supersensitivity of denervated structures. This theory states that when an organ is chronically deprived of its motor innervation, it develops an increased sensitivity to its neurohumoral transmitter. This phenomenon is true for smooth muscle, striated muscle, ganglia and glands.

The physiologic cause for the phenomenon of denervation sensitivity is thought to be an increase in the size of the receptor area (Figure 14.1). No longer is depolarization limited to the motor end plate. Apparently, the entire surface area of individual denervated muscle fibers responds to transmitter substances. This results in an exaggerated response to the neurohumoral transmitter. The denervation sensitivity tests measure supersensitivity responses of the bladder or urethra to transmitter substances. These responses are greater than the usual response to the same dosage and route of administration of these substances.

CLASSICAL VESICAL DENERVATION SENSITIVITY TESTING

The technique for performance of the vesical denervation sensitivity test as developed by Lapides is as follows: (1) Perform CMG as control; (2) record pressure/volume relationships at 100 cc; (3) inject bethanecol chloride, 0.03 mg/kg (or 2.5 mg for average patient) S.Q.; (4) perform posttreatment CMGs at 10, 20 and 30 minutes after administration in exactly the same manner as the control CMG.

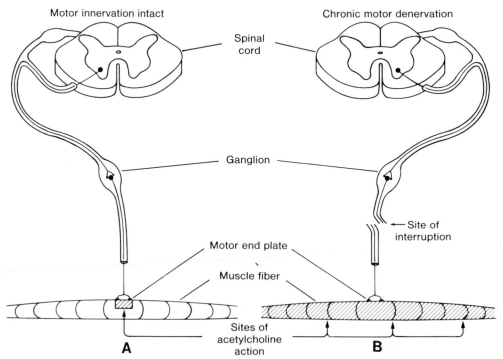

Figure 14.1. The phenomenon of denervation sensitivity. **(A)** The normal area for receptor response is shown with intact motor innervation. **(B)** After chronic denervation the area responding to the neurotransmitter markedly enlarges.

ALTERNATE TECHNIQUE FOR VESICAL DENERVATION SENSITIVITY TESTING

Glahn developed an alternate technique for bladder denervation sensitivity testing in order to decrease the potential sources of error inherent in the Lapides method. The Lapides method requires more than one CMG and measures pressure changes in an environment of changing volume. Glahn's method reduces exogenous stimuli to the chemical agent alone. A secondary benefit is a decreased time requirement.

The technique is as follows: (1) Fill bladder with 100 cc normal saline; (2) measure resting pressure and allow to equilibrate; (3) inject 2.5 mg bethanechol S.Q.; (4) record intravesical pressure each minute until the identification of the maximum pressure or the occurrence of definite pathological values; (5) discontinue observations after 30 minutes.

INTERPRETATION

With both techniques the normal bladder pressure rise after bethanechol administration is less than 15 cm H_2O above the control (Figure 14.2). Therefore, any pressure rise on CMG greater than 15 cm H_2O indicates chronic vesical denervation from disease of the autonomic (parasympathetic) lower motor neuron. Subsequent paragraphs discuss technical and interpretative precautions.

TECHNICAL PRECAUTIONS

The presence of asthma, cardiac disease or hyperthyroidism contraindicates the use of bethanechol. As a parasympathomimetic, bethanechol may induce bronchospasm, hypotension, and, in hyperthyroid patients, atrial fibrillation. Intravenous injection greatly increases side effects and toxicity.

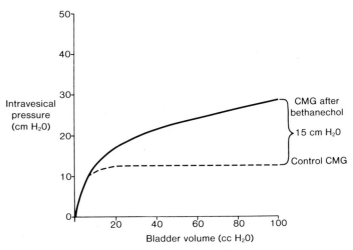

Figure 14.2. The Vesical Denervation Sensitivity Test. The positive test demonstrates an intravesical pressure increase of greater than 15 cm H_2O over the control CMG at 100 cc bladder volume.

Removal of the urethral catheter sometimes results in severe suprapubic pain which lasts as long as 5 to 10 minutes. Although the source of this reaction is unknown, slow and cautious handling of the catheter during the procedure minimizes this response.

INTERPRETIVE PRECAUTIONS

A variety of factors influence the results of denervation sensitivity testing which require consideration in the interpretation of test results.

If the patient has uninhibited bladder contractions, repeat the test under spinal anesthesia or ganglionic blockade, i.e., trimethaphan. If the bladder response to bethanechol is greater than 15 cm H_2O over the control CMG during adequate blockade of central impulses, the test is positive and the patient has vesical lower motor neuron denervation. A positive test result requires muscular integrity of the detrusor. Therefore, any suspicion of recent or chronic muscular damage places a negative test result in doubt. A single recent overdistension may interfere with normal myogenic function so that the test may be falsely negative.

A final precaution involves the presence of emotional stress which appears to intensify cholinergic stimulation of the bladder by up to 10 cm H_2O pressure.

URETHRAL DENERVATION SENSITIVITY TESTING

The technique for performance of the urethral denervation sensitivity test is as follows: (1) Obtain control urethral closure pressure profile and determine maximum urethral pressure; (2) inject ethylphenylephrine, 4 mg IV or an equivalent dose of an alpha stimulator; (3) five minutes

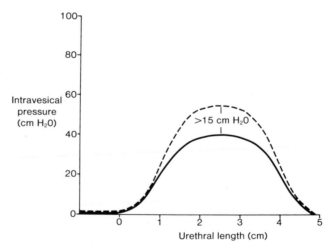

Figure 14.3. The Urethral Denervation Sensitivity Test. The positive test demonstrates an increase in maximal closure pressure of greater than 15 cm H_2O over the control pressures.

after injection, repeat urethral closure pressure profile and determine maximal urethral pressure.

INTERPRETATION

An increase of 15 cm H_2O or more in maximal urethral pressure indicates chronic urethral denervation (Figure 14.3).

COMMENT

The use of these denervation sensitivity tests in conjunction with standard urodynamic evaluations makes definitive diagnosis of complex problems easier and, therefore, provides for more appropriate clinical management. No longer is a lower motor neuron defect a diagnosis of exclusion. By judicious use of these tests, the diagnosis becomes one of relative certainty. The knowledge that chronic urethral denervation exists adds one more diagnostic possibility to consider prior to operative intervention for "stress incontinence."

References

1. **Cannon, W.B., Rosenbleuth, A.** *The Supersensitivity of Denervated Structures.* The Macmillan Co., New York, 1949.
2. **Diokno, A.C., Davis, R., Lapides, J.** Urecholine Test for Denervated Bladders. *Invest. Urol.* 13:233, 1975.
3. **Glahn, B.E.** Neurogenic Bladder Diagnosed Pharmacologically on the Basis of Denervation Supersensitivity. *Scand. J. Urol. Nephrol.* 4:13–27, 1970.
4. **Goodman, L.S., Gilman, A.** The Pharmacologic Basis of Therapeutics, 4th Ed. The Macmillan Co., New York, 1970.
5. **Kirwin, T.S., Hawes, G.A.** The Diagnostic Value of Residual Urine Estimation. *J. Urol.* 41:413, 1934.
6. **Koyanagi, T.** Denervation Supersensitivity of the Urethra to Alpha Adrenergics in the Chronic Neurogenic Bladder. *Urol. Res.* 6:89–93, 1978.
7. **Lapides, J., Friend, C.R., Ajemian, E.P., Reus, W.F.** Denervation Supersensitivity as a Test for Neurogenic Bladder. *Surg. Gynecol. Obstet.* 114:241, 1962.
8. **Plum, F.** Autonomous Urinary Bladder Activity in Normal Man. *Arch. Neurol.* 2:497, 1960.

15 Propantheline and Phentolamine Testing

Thomas A. McCarthy, M.D.

A precise determination of the etiology of lower urinary tract complaints allows initiation of definitive treatment to effect a cure. In most areas of medicine this is an achievable goal. However, complaints related to the female lower urinary tract frequently defy and frustrate diagnostic endeavors. The remarkable complexity of the storage and voiding function of the lower urinary tract contributes significantly to these limitations. The absence of a precise diagnosis limits the physician's ability to predict the effectiveness of a given pharmacologic treatment regimen. The inevitable result is the need for therapeutic trials of various medications. In recent years, significant advances in the understanding of the normal and pathologic function of the lower urinary tract allow more precise elucidation of pathophysiologic entities involving neurologic and physiologic functions of the bladder and urethra. Specialized pharmacologic testing procedures now allow advance prediction of success or failure with a given drug classification. This chapter presents two pharmacologic testing procedures for evaluation of proposed therapy for hypertonicity of the smooth muscular component of the urethral sphincteric mechanism and for therapy of uninhibited bladder contractions.

PHENTOLAMINE TEST

The urethral sphincteric mechanism consists of both smooth and striated musculature. The alpha adrenergic portion of the autonomic nervous system innervates the smooth muscle components. The striated portion obtains its innervation

175

from the peripheral nervous system. Complex central mechanisms ultimately control both elements. For normal voiding to occur, both elements must relax in harmony with detrusor contraction.

In some patients adequate relaxation does not occur and a relative outlet obstruction complicates detrusor function. This over-activity and/or lack of relaxation is neurologic in origin and results from either the smooth or striated component of the urethral sphincter. Alpha adrenergic blocking agents block the smooth muscle component of the urethra and affect relaxation. However, they are ineffective in blocking the striated component. Often, patients receive empiric alpha sympatholytic therapy. If a good response occurs, the physician assumes that the smooth muscular component is responsible. This method requires a 1- to 2-week pharmacologic trial with drugs which frequently have untoward side effects. The phentolamine test aids in the distinction of the relative contributions of the smooth and skeletal muscular components of the urethral sphincteric mechanism and predicts which patients will respond to therapy with alpha adrenergic blocking agents.

In males, the phentolamine test correlates with outpatient therapy and seems to be predictive. The basis of the male test lies in a comparison of urinary flow rates pre- and postinjection of phentolamine. In the female, however, the phentolamine test has not been correlated with outpatient therapy and the basis of the test is a comparison of the urethral closure pressure profile (UCPP) before and after injection of phentolamine.

Procedure

The method of performing the test in females is as follows: (1) Record baseline blood pressure, pulse and UCPP in supine position. (2) Give phentolamine mesylate 0.1 mg/kg IV bolus. (3) Record blood pressure and pulse every minute until a tachycardia of at least ten beats per minute occurs (usually 3 minutes after injection). (4) Repeat UCPP and compare maximum urethral pressures before and after phentolamine. (5) Observe the patient for 30 minutes for any adverse side effects of the phentolamine.

Interpretation

While no strict comparison exists between results of the phentolamine test and success of outpatient therapy in women, it is possible to make some assertions based on inferences from current knowledge. Under test conditions and in the dose described, phentolamine causes a fall of urethral pressure of at least 30% of baseline in patients with relative outflow obstruction (Figure 15.1). Also, in patients with neurogenic bladder dysfunction and increased bladder neck resistance, outpatient treatment with phenoxybenzamine restores a more normal voiding pattern.

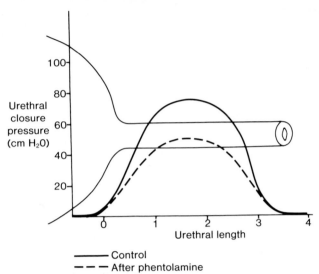

Urethral closure pressure (cm H₂O)

——— Control
— — — After phentolamine

Figure 15.1. The phentolamine test. The upper curve represents the control profile and the lower curve was obtained after drug administration. A decrease in maximal closure pressure of 30% or more denotes a positive test.

This information suggests that any patient showing a decrease of at least 30% of baseline in maximal urethral pressure after the injection of phentolamine is a good candidate for outpatient phenoxybenzamine therapy. A patient showing a lesser or absent response to phentolamine requires evaluation for external striated sphincter spasm.

PROPANTHELINE TEST

The other test used to predetermine drug efficacy is the propantheline test. In patients with uninhibited detrusor contractions propantheline suppresses this bladder activity. A 15-mg IV dose abolishes detrusor contractions in most patients with uninhibited contractions and frequently increases bladder capacity. A small study correlated this response with the subsequent response to outpatient anticholinergic therapy.

Procedure

(1) Perform a control cystometrogram. (2) Administer propantheline 15 mg IV and repeat the cystometrogram 10 to 25 minutes after the injection.

Interpretation

After administration of propantheline the uninhibited contractions seen on the control CMG generally disappear or, at least, decrease in amplitude and frequency in association with an increase in bladder capacity (Figure 15.2). This suppression of detrusor activity correlates with response to outpatient anticholinergic therapy. Available reports do not comment on false negative or false positive results.

One difficulty with the propantheline test is that while

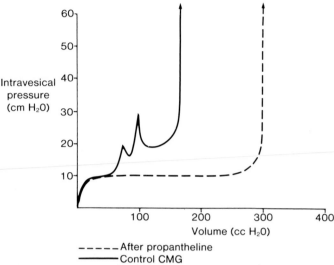

After propantheline
Control CMG

Figure 15.2. The propantheline test. The solid line represents the control CMG which shows an uninhibited bladder contraction. After propantheline administration the bladder capacity increases with a delayed terminal bladder contraction.

intravenous propantheline in a dose of 15 mg effectively controls uninhibited bladder contractions, an oral agent with similar efficacy in the absence of unacceptable side effects is not available. The oral effectiveness depends upon a balance of the anticholinergic effects of the drug with its side effects. Some patients tolerate oral propantheline and experience relief of symptoms. In others the side effects of dry mouth, blurring of vision and occasional tachycardia preclude its use. Hopefully, newer anticholinergic agents will produce the desired effect without the common unacceptable side effects.

SUMMARY

The propantheline and phentolamine tests allow selection of an effective method of outpatient management for uninhibited contractions and for overactivity of the smooth muscle component of the urethral sphincter. The propantheline test demonstrates good correlation between the test result and the effectiveness of subsequent outpatient management. Incomplete evaluation of the phentolamine test precludes effective routine clinical use at the present time. It is, however, a potentially useful test in the management of patients with uninhibited detrusor contractions.

References

1. **Awad, S.A., Downie, J.W., Lywood, D.W. et al.** Sympathetic Activity in the Proximal Urethra in Patients with Urinary Obstruction. *J. Urol.* 115:545, 1976.

2. **Bradley, W.E., Timm, G.W., Scott, F.B.** Cystometry I. Introduction. *Urology* 5:424, 1975.

3. **Diokno, A.C., Hyndman, C.W., Hardy, D.A. et al.** Comparison of Action of Imipramine (Tofranil) and Propantheline (Probanthine) on Detrusor Contraction. *J. Urol.* 107:42, 1972.

4. **Diokno, A.C., Lapides, J.** Oxybutynin: A New Drug with Analgesic and Anticholinergic Properties. *J. Urol.* 108:307, 1972.

5. **Gregory, J.G., Wein, A.J., Schoenberg, H.W.** A Comparison of the Action of Tofranil and Probanthine on the Urinary Bladder. *Invest. Urol.* 12:233, 1974.

6. **Krane, R.J., Olsson, C.A.** Phenoxybenzamine in Neurogenic Bladder Dysfunction II. Clinical Considerations. *J. Urol.* 110:653, 1973.

7. **Olsson, C.A., Siroky M.B., Krane, R.J.** The Phentolamine Test in Neurogenic Bladder Dysfunction. *J. Urol.* 117:481, 1977.

8. **Stockamp, K.** Treatment with Phenoxybenzamine of Upper Urinary Tract Complications caused by Intravesical Obstruction. *J. Urol.* 113:128, 1975.

9. **Susset, J.G., Picker, P., Kretz, M. et al.** Critical Evaluation of Uroflowmeters and Analysis of Normal Curves. *J. Urol.* 109:874, 1973.

10. **Whitfield, H.N., Doyle, P.T., Mayo, M.E. et al.** The Effect of Adrenergic Blocking Drugs on Outflow Resistance. *Br. J. Urol.* 47:823, 1976.

III PATHOLOGY AND TREATMENT OF LOWER URINARY TRACT ABNORMALITIES

16 The Urethral Syndrome

Donald R. Ostergard, M.D.

The urethral syndrome, a common malady of women, is one of the differential diagnoses whenever a patient presents with lower urinary tract symptoms in the absence of bacteriological evidence of infection. Although the urethral syndrome presents with varied and unpredictable symptomatology and physical findings, sufficient information regarding this condition is now available to warrant the formulation of an aggressive diagnostic and treatment plan.

DEFINITION AND DIAGNOSIS

The physician diagnoses the urethral syndrome after exclusion of urinary tract infection by culture when the patient complains of any combination of the following symptoms: frequency, urgency, dysuria, terminal dysuria, urge incontinence, apparent stress incontinence, pelvic pressure or tenesmus, failure of pain relief with bladder emptying, suprapubic pain, bleeding after urination, dyspareunia, urethral discharge or nocturia. Other causes of these symptoms include urethral diverticula, bladder stones, intraluminal suture from previous urethral or bladder surgery, along with other rarer forms of intrinsic urethral and detrusor pathology. Thus, the diagnosis of the urethral syndrome is by exclusion of those other diagnostic entities.

Synonyms for this syndrome in the medical literature are non-purulent urethritis, granular urethritis, cystalgia, irritable bladder, neuralgia of the bladder, cystospasm, trigonitis, cystitis coli, cystitis coli proliferans, rheumatic urethritis, cystourethritis and senile or chronic urethritis.

ETIOLOGY

The precise etiology of the urethral syndrome remains obscure. The suggested etiological factors in the medical literature are as follows: anxiety neurosis and other psychiatric disturbances, such as depression and stress reactions, infection of periurethral glands, stasis of periurethral gland secretion, periurethral soft tissue infection, estrogen deprivation, trigonal vaginal metaplasia, allergy, meatal stenosis, urethral polyps and urethral cysts.

PHYSICAL FINDINGS

The physical findings in the urethral syndrome are as myriad as the symptoms and may include any combination of the following: urethral tenderness, urethral induration, mucosal edema, mucosal hyperemia, mucosal atrophy, vaginal type of squamous epithelium in the trigone (trigonal vaginal metaplasia), granularity, urethral polyps or fronds, urethral exudate from posterior periurethral glands (see Chapter 1), trigonal granularity or exudate, urethral masses and urethral or trigonal mucosal cysts. Urethroscopic examination detects most of these (see Chapter 11).

TREATMENT

The treatment of the urethral syndrome is not in common agreement. Writers in the medical literature propose a variety of therapies with each therapy used singly, in variable succession with others, or in combination with most other therapeutic modalities. Each proposed treatment regimen results in similar percentages of "cures." The various suggested medical treatment modalites are: cranberry juice, vitamins A and D, urethral antibiotic and estrogen containing suppositories, periurethral steroid injection, systemic antibiotics, vaginal or oral estrogens, psychotherapy and antihistamines. The various surgical treatment modalities are: urethral fulguration with silver nitrate; electrocautery of the urethral mucosa, trigonal mucosa and polyps; resection of the distal one-third of the urethra, caruncles, polyps or periurethral glands; avulsion, sounding or unroofing of periurethral glands; urethral dilatation and internal or external urethrotomy. The following paragraphs describe the most commonly used treatment modalities.

Urethral dilatation is currently the treatment of choice for the urethral syndrome. Under topical urethral anesthesia or local bladder pillar block, dilatation continues to 38F or until discomfort or bleeding necessitates discontinuation. Bladder pillar block anesthesia is a new technique for urethral anesthesia. The injection of 5 cc of local anesthetic solution into each bladder pillar at 2 and 10 o'clock allows dilatation to 38F in 90% of patients. If the patient's uterus is absent, similar injections at 4 and 8 o'clock at the urethrovesical junction produce similar results. Using this anesthetic technique only about 10% of patients have sufficient discomfort to warrant discontinuation of the procedure before reaching 38F. The only other reason for stopping the procedure is the appearance of blood, indicating a mucosal tear which may scarify, particularly if extended by further dilatation. Most patients require repeat dilatations two or more times at two weekly intervals. Frequently patients experience no symptomatic benefit from the first or even the second dilatation. It is also not unusual for these individuals to have a temporary worsening of symptoms between treatments. An alternative treatment regimen is a single overdilatation up to 45F which requires regional or general anesthesia. The risks of urethral laceration and scarring limits the usefulness of this procedure.

Although the exact therapeutic mechanism of dilatation remains obscure, it probably exerts its therapeutic effect by expression of infected material from the periurethral glands. With meatal stenosis a streamlining of the previously turbulent pattern of urine flow through the urethra may produce the symptomatic relief.

The medical literature contains reports of the successful use of estrogen suppositories in the hypoestrogenic patient. Since the urethra and trigone are both estrogen dependent structures renewed hormonal support has therapeutic benefit. Since urethral estrogen suppositories are no longer commercially available, fortunately, topical vaginal estrogens have similar therapeutic value. Many investigators report that broad spectrum systemic antibiotic therapy is beneficial in the treatment of the urethral syndrome under the assumption that periurethral gland infection is the primary cause of this condition. Usually the physician prescribes long term therapy at low dosage, for example, ampicillin, 250 mg, twice a day prescribed for 3 months.

Periurethral steroids decrease the chronic inflammatory process around the urethra. Usually, 1 mg of triamcinolone or its equivalent is injected into the periurethral tissue along the entire length of the urethra bilaterally.

The small orifices of several major periurethral glands are visible through the urethroscope within 0.5 cm of the external meatus. With a wire cautery inserted into the gland orifice, the duct is unroofed into the urethra. This technique promotes continued drainage of the glandular material into the urethra.

External urethrotomy overcomes resistance to urine flow at the external meatus and lessens intraurethral turbulence during micturition.

If the patient's symptoms do not respond to the employment of these therapeutic regimens, it is necessary to search further to definitively exclude all other possible diagnostic entities. Cystoscopy is necessary in those patients with previous vesical or urethral surgery to rule out intravesical stones or sutures.

SUMMARY

Inconsistent and varied symptomatology and physical findings characterize the urethral syndrome. Its etiology is obscure. In spite of the proportion of the female population afflicted with this condition, a precise plan of consistently effective therapy remains to be described. In our experience, however, the majority of patients respond to urethral dilatation, particularly when bladder pillar block anesthesia allows serial dilatation to 38F. Most patients require repeated dilatation at two weekly intervals to achieve reasonably long-lasting therapeutic results. Urethral dilatation remains the treatment of choice for the urethral syndrome.

References

1. **Altman, B.L.** Treatment of Urethral Syndrome with Triamcinolone Acetonide. *J. Urol.* 116:583–584, 1976.
2. **Brooks, D, Mauder, A.** Pathogenesis of the Urethral Syndrome in Women and its Diagnosis in General Practice. *Lancet* 2:893, 1972.
3. **Eberhart, C.** The Etiology and Treatment of Urethritis in Female Patients. *J. Urol.* 79:293–299, 1958.
4. **Gallagher, D.H.A., Montgomerie, J.Z., North, J.D.K.** Acute Infections of the Urinary Tract and Urethral Syndrome in General Practice. *Br. Med. J.* 1:622, 1965.
5. **Henry, L, Fox, N.** Histological Findings in Pseudomembranous Trigonitis. *J. Clin. Pathol.* 24:605–608, 1971.
6. **Huffman, J.W.** The Development of the Periurethral Glands in the Human Female. *Am. J. Obstet. Gynecol.* 46:773–785, 1943.
7. **Jackson, E.A.** Urethral Syndrome in Women. *Radiology* 119:287, 1976.
8. **Kaufman, RE, Wiesner, P.J.** Nonspecific Urethritis. *N. Engl. J. Med.* 291:1175–1177, 1974.
9. **Leiter, E.** Management of Recurrent Cystourethritis in Women. *Urology* 1:111, 1973.
10. **Lewis, E.L., Griffith, T.H.** Recurring Cystourethritis in Women: Is An Effective Therapy Available? *J. Urol.* 110:544, 1973.
11. **Magamatsu, G.R.** Female Cystourethritis. Editorial. *Urology* 1:111, 1973.
12. **Mahoney, D.T., Laferte, R.O., Blais, D.J.** "Studies of Enuresis: VIII. Detrusor and Sphincter Instability caused by Overactivity of Integral Voiding Reflexes. *Urology* 9:590, 1977.
13. **Ostergard, D.R.** Bladder Pillar Block for Urethral Dilatation in Women. *Am. J. Obstet. Gynecol.* 136:187–188, 1980.
14. **Riba, L.W.** Point of View: The Urethritis Syndrome. *Urology* 8:97, 1976.
15. **Richardson, F.H., Stonington, O.G.** Urethrolysis and External Urethroplasty in the Female. *Surg. Clin. North Am* 49:1201–1208, 1969.
16. **Rieser, C.** A New Method of Treatment of Inflammatory Lesions of the Female Urethra. *J.A.M.A.* 204:86, 1968.
17. **Seddon, J.M., Bruce, A.W.** Cystourethritis. *Urology* 11:1–9, 1978.
18. **Smith, P.** Age Changes in the Female Urethra. *Br. J. Urol.* 44:667–676, 1972.

19. **Tanagho, EA, Lyon, R.P.** Urethral Dilatation Versus Internal Urethrotomy. *J. Urol.* 105:242–244, 1971.
20. **Tyler, D.E.** Stratified Squamous Epithelium in the Vesical Trigone and Urethra: Findings Correlated with the Menstrual Cycle and Age. *Am. J. Anat.* 3:319–325, 1962.
21. **Youngblood, V.H., Tomlin, E.M., Davis, J.B.** Senile Urethritis in Women. *J. Urol.* 78:150–152, 1957.
22. **Youngblood, V.H., Tomlin, E.M., Williams, J.O., Kimmelstiel, P.** Exfoliated Cytology of the Senile Female Urethra. *J. Urol.* 79:110–113, 1958.
23. **Zinskind, P.D., Mannes, H.A.** Approach to Bladder Neck and Urethral Obstruction in Women. *Surg. Clin. North Am.* 53: 571–580, 1973.
24. **Zufall, R.** Treatment of the Urethral Syndrome in Women. *J.A.M.A.* 184:894–895, 1963.

17 Urinary Fistulas

Jack R. Robertson, M.D.

Vesicovaginal fistulas are uncommon. The most common cause in developed countries is surgical, especially following hysterectomy. Obstetrical causes for these fistulas occur in lesser developed countries. Unless there is ureteral involvement, posthysterectomy vesicovaginal fistulas are repairable through the vagina due to their location at the vault apex, just anterior to the site of vaginal cuff closure (Figure 17.1). This location decreases the need for the standard technique of direct dissection and closure of the fistulous tract and allows the use of the much simpler Latzko or partial colpocleisis procedure.

STANDARD PRINCIPLES OF FISTULA REPAIR

The most important standard principles of fistula repair include excision of the fistulous tract, extensive mobilization of all layers and closure without tension. The typical location of the vesicovaginal fistula is just anterior to the vaginal cuff incision line (Figure 17.1A). Placement of a Foley catheter through the fistulous tract for traction to bring the fistula into the operative field facilitates the procedure (Figure 17.1B). The circumferential vaginal incision isolates the fistulous tract for excision down to the vesical mucosa (Figure 17.1C). If the physician removes the scar tissue on the vesical mucosal side of the fistula, hematoma formation is likely with breakdown of the operative repair. Extensive undermining of the surrounding vaginal and vesical mucosa allows later closure without tension (Figure 17.2A). After excision of the fistulous tract (Figure 17.2B) transverse

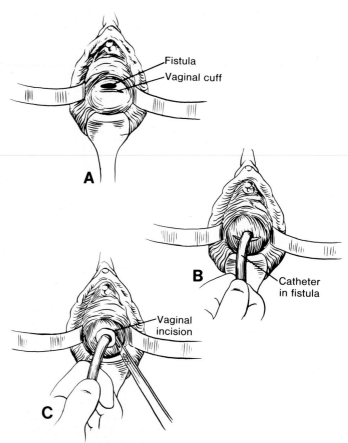

Figure 17.1. The typical location of vesicovaginal fistula is anterior to vaginal cuff (**A**). (**B**) The Foley balloon provides traction during mobilization of the fistula. (**C**) The vaginal incision circumscribes the fistulous tract. (Redrawn from *Urologic Surgery*, edited by J. F. Glenn. Harper and Row, Hagerstown, Md., 1975)

closure of the vesical and vaginal mucosa using 3-0 absorbable suture follows (Figure 17.2C). The suprapubic catheter remains in place for 7 to 10 days after the procedure.

PREOPERATIVE CORTISONE

The use of cortisone preoperatively remains controversial. The author has used this technique for 25 years. The usual dose is 100 mg of cortisone three times a day which allows repair of the fistula within 10 days to 2 weeks of injury. It is important to recognize whether or not the tissues are pliable and non-inflamed prior to surgery. Endoscopic evaluation with the urethroscope aids in this critical determination. If infection remains, at least 4 to 6 months must elapse before surgical repair.

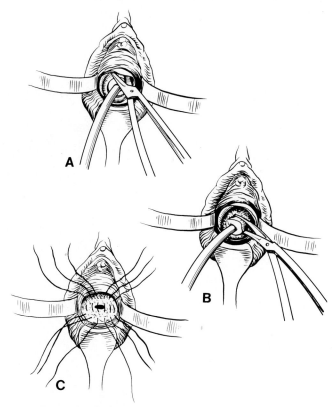

Figure 17.2 (**A**) The scissors are used to mobilize the vaginal and vesical mucosa around the fistula. (**B**) After mobilization the fistulous tract is excised, followed by closure without tension (**C**) (Redrawn from *Urologic Surgery*, edited by J. F. Glenn. Harper and Row, Hagerstown, Md., 1975.)

LATZKO PARTIAL COLPOCLEISIS PROCEDURE

The Latzko technique for vesicovaginal fistula repair by the vaginal route is a relatively new and simple surgical technique. Its success does not depend on the basic principles of fistula repair, since excision of the fistulous tract, extensive mobilization of the bladder and vagina and layered closure are not a part of the procedure.

Since there is little disturbance of the fistulous site itself and since the repair depends only upon the viability of surrounding vaginal mucosa and submucosa, the procedure lends itself to early use, thus avoiding the traditional 4- to 6-month waiting period.

Figures 17.3 and 17.4 illustrate the procedure. The typical location is just anterior to the vaginal cuff line of incision (Figure 17.3A). Prior to beginning the procedure, placement

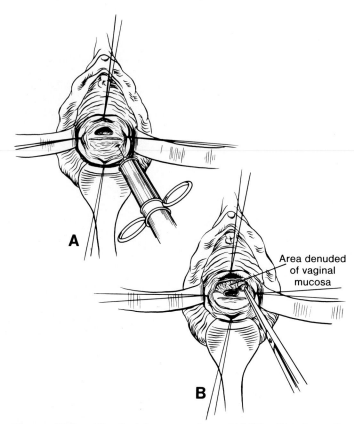

Figure 17.3. The Latzko procedure. **(A)** The fistulous site after application of four traction sutures showing typical location of fistula and the injection of a hemostatic solution. **(B)** The vaginal mucosa around the fistula is removed.

of four traction sutures and injection with a dilute epinephrine solution facilitate the dissection of the vaginal wall (Figure 17.3A). Denudation of an elliptical portion of vaginal wall at least $2\frac{1}{2}$ cm beyond the tract in all directions follows (Figure 17.3B). Closure in three layers using 3-0 absorbable suture completes the procedure (Figure 17.4A and 17.4B). The posterior vaginal wall now becomes the posterior vesical wall which eventually reepithelializes with transitional epithelium. Postoperatively a suprapubic catheter provides adequate drainage and is left in place for 7 to 10 days.

POSTOPERATIVE RESULTS

Providing the patient avoids intercourse for at least 4 months postoperatively, failures are rare with this procedure.

SUMMARY

The partial colpocleisis technique for fistula repair is easy

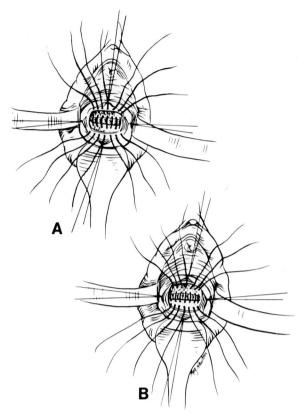

Figure 17.4. The Latzko closure. (**A**) The submucosa is closed in layers with interrupted sutures. (**B**) The vaginal wall is similarly closed.

to perform and is effective. It is applicable in patients with posthysterectomy vesicovaginal fistula and lends itself to early use, thus avoiding the traditional waiting period of 4 to 6 months.

References

1. **Collins, C.G., Pent, D., Jones, F.B.** Results of Early Repair of Vesicovaginal Fistula with Preliminary Cortisone Treatment. *Am. J. Obstet. Gynecol.* 80:1005, 1960.
2. **Diaz-Ball, F.L., Moore, C.A.** A Diagnostic Aid for Vesicovaginal fistula. *J. Urol.* 102:424–426, 1969.
3. **Glenn, J.F., Stevens, P.S.** Simplified Vesicovaginal Fistulectomy. *J. Urol.* 110:521–523, 1973.
4. **Graham, J.B.** Vaginal Fistulas Following Radiotherapy. *Surg. Gynecol. Obstet.* 120:1019–1030, 1965.
5. **Kiricuta, I., Goldstein, A.M.B.** The Repair of Extensive Vesicovaginal Fistulas With Pedicled Omentum: A Review of 27 Cases. *J. Urol.* 108:724–727, 1972.
6. **Latzko, W.** Postoperative Vesicovaginal Fistulas: Genesis and Therapy. *Am. J. Surg.* 58:211, 1942.

7. **Martius, H.** In *Martius' Gynecological Operations*, edited by M.L. McCall and K.A. Bolten. J. & A. Churchill, Ltd., London, 1957.

8. **Massee J.S., Welch, J.S., Pratt, J.H., Symmonds, R.E.** Management of Urinary-vaginal Fistula. Ten-year Survey. *J.A.M.A* 190:902–906, 1964.

9. **Moir, J.C.** *The Vesico-Vaginal Fistula*, 2nd Ed. Bailliere, Tindall & Cassell, London, 1967.

10. **O'Conor V.J.** *Suprapubic Closure of Vesicovaginal Fistula.* Charles C. Thomas, Springfield, Ill., 1957.

11. **O'Conor, V.J., Jr., Nanninga, J.B.** Surgery of Vesicovaginal Fistula. In *Current Operative Urology*, edited by E.D. Whitehead. Harper & Row, New York, 1974.

12. **Robertson, J.R.** *Genitourinary Problems in Women.* Charles C. Thomas. Springfield, Ill., 1978.

13. **Roen, P.R.** Combined Vaginal and Transvesical Approach in Successful Repair of Vesicovaginal Fistula. *Arch. Surg.*, 80: 628, 1960.

14. **Sims, J.M.** On the Treatment of of Vesico-Vaginal Fistula. *Am. J. Med. Sci.* 23:59–82, 1852.

18 Urethral Diverticula

Jack R. Robertson, M.D.

Hey described the first successful repair of a urethral diverticulum in 1805. Hunner reported three urethral diverticula in female patients and commented on the apparent rareness of the condition. In 1953, Novak stated, "This is a relatively rare condition and no gynecologist will see more than a few in a lifetime." A few years later, Davis and then Tratner developed catheters with two balloons (Figure 18.1). The two balloons effectively isolate the urethra between the intravesical balloon and a sliding or wedge shaped balloon which tamponades the external meatus. This allows the introduction of radiopaque dye into the urethra to outline urethral diverticula (Figures 18.2 and 18.3). This new diagnostic technique revealed 50 diverticula in one year, more than in the entire previous history of Johns Hopkins Hospital.

INCIDENCE

Incidence figures are infrequently reported. A recent study showed that 5% of patients in a Gynecologic Urology Clinic had diverticula, and a second study of patients prior to radiation for carcinoma of the cervix revealed a frequency of 4.7%.

CLINICAL SYMPTOMS

The clinical symptoms of urethral diverticula are common to other maladies of the lower urinary tract (Table 18.1). None are diagnostic and the classical symptoms of postmicturition dribbling and expression of pus are frequently absent. Many patients have no symptoms.

195

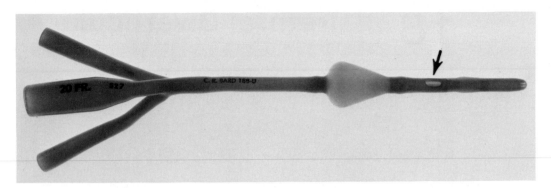

Figure 18.1. The Tratner catheter. This 3-lumen catheter has two balloons which isolate the urethra. Radiopaque dye then enters the urethra through the port indicated by the arrow.

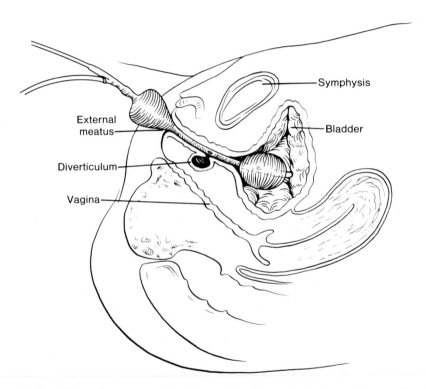

Figure 18.2. The placement of the Tratner catheter. Isolation of the urethra between the balloons allows positive pressure urethrography.

CLASSICAL PHYSICAL FINDINGS

The classical physical findings are a palpable suburethral mass and expression of pus from a tender urethra. Unfortunately, these are frequently absent and the patient may have no physical findings.

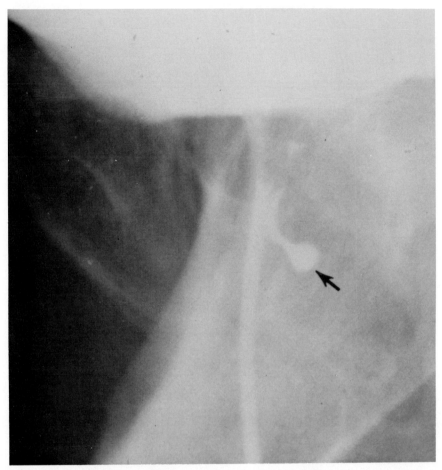

Figure 18.3. Radiographic appearance of a urethral diverticulum. The arrow indicates the diverticulum.

LOCATION OF DIVERTICULAR ORIFICES

The anatomy of the urethra includes the presence of a large number of periurethral glands entering the posterior urethra with the largest of these glands entering the posterior urethra with the largest of these glands emptying into the distal urethra (see Chapter 1). The location of urethral diverticular orifices parallels the site of entry of these glands into the urethra with more than half opening into the middle third of the urethra. Fully 50% of patients have multiple diverticula in various locations.

URETHROSCOPIC DIAGNOSTIC PROCEDURES

The technique of urethroscopy for diverticula begins with the placement of 200 cc of CO_2 in the bladder. Two fingers in the vagina push the vesical neck up against the symphysis to trap the gas in the urethra (Figure 18.4). Under direct

Table 18.1

Clinical Symptoms
Asymptomatic
Dysuria
Frequency
Urgency
Hematuria
Dyspareunia
Vaginal mass
Postmicturition dribbling
Recurrent cystitis
Pain
Incontinence
Urinary retention
Nocturia

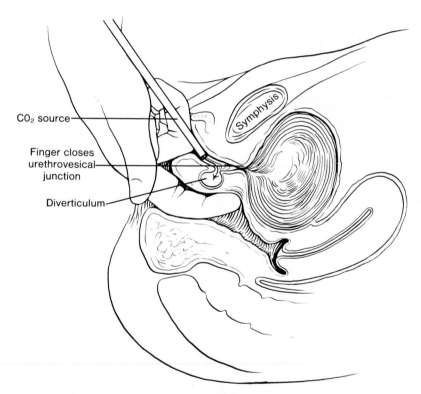

Figure 18.4.   The technique of urethral distention with CO_2. Occlusion of the urethrovesical junction with the finger allows distention of the urethra and visualization of diverticular orifices.

vision urethral massage reveals the presence of pus or urine exuding from the diverticular orifice. Visualization of stones inside the diverticulum is not uncommon.

RADIOGRAPHIC DIAGNOSTIC PROCEDURES

The two procedures in common use are voiding cystourethrography and positive pressure urethrography. The voiding radiograph depends upon the chance filling of the diverticulum during the study. Its accuracy is about 65%. Positive pressure urethrography using either the Tratner or Davis catheter is comparable to urethroscopy for accuracy (Figure 18.3). Either method diagnoses 90%.

URODYNAMIC EVALUATION

Urodynamic assessment of the urethra aids in the selection of the proper operative procedure for treatment of the diverticulum. The most important urodynamic technique is the urethral closure pressure profile and its relationship to the diverticular orifice (Figure 18.5). If the opening of the diverticulum into the urethra is distal to the peak urethral closure pressure, the Spence procedure is the operation of choice. If the diverticular orifice is proximal to the area of peak closure pressure, direct dissection of the diverticulum with closure of the urethra in layers is essential.

If a Spence procedure is done and the diverticular orifice is not distal to peak closure pressure, genuine stress incontinence is a likely result due to disruption of the muscular sphincteric mechanism of the urethra.

SURGICAL REPAIR

The standard operative approach for urethral diverticula is through the vagina. Two procedures are in use and the actual choice of the surgical method depends upon the location of the diverticular orifice in relation to the site of peak urethral closure pressure. As stated, if the orifice is proximal to this area, direct dissection of the diverticulum is necessary. Dissection is difficult due to the normal anatomical fusion of the urethra to the anterior vaginal wall,

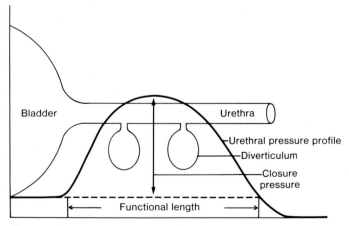

Figure 18.5. The urethral closure pressure profile with superimposed diverticular orifices proximal and distal to peak closure pressure.

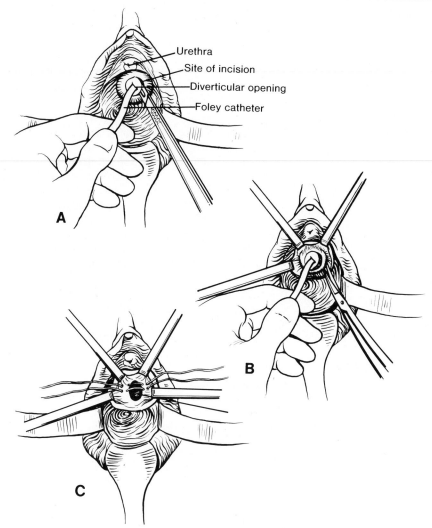

Figure 18.6. Total excision of urethral diverticulum. **(A)** The vaginal incision and exposure of the diverticulum for direct dissection with placement of a Foley catheter for traction. **(B)** Gradual dissection of the diverticulum frees it from its attachment to the urethra. **(C)** Interrupted sutures close the urethra and the base of the diverticulum. (Redrawn from *Urologic Surgery*, edited by J.F. Glenn. Harper and Row, Hagerstown, Md., 1975.)

the associated infection, the tendency of the diverticulum to partially surround the urethra or extend up under the base of the bladder. No cleavage planes exist and a tedious, time-consuming operation results. Basic principles of fistula surgery prevail with adequate dissection and closure in layers with minimal tension.

The procedure begins with the vaginal incision and exposure of the entire area occupied by the diverticulum (Figure 18.6A). At this point it is helpful to enter the diverticulum and place a Foley catheter for traction (Figure 18.6B).

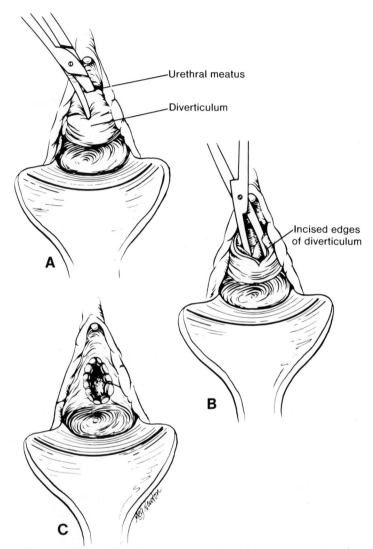

Figure 18.7. The Spence procedure for marsupialization of urethral diverticula. **(A)** The scissors enter the diverticulum and **(B)** incise the full thickness of the urethrovaginal diverticulum septum. **(C)** A running locking suture around the incised edges secures hemostasis.

Tedious sharp dissection continues until the entire diverticulum is free from all surrounding attachments and the connection to the urethra is definitively identified (Figure 18.6B). The division of the urethral attachment completes the removal of the diverticulum and closure of the urethra follows (Figure 18.6C).

An alternative technique for closure involves the creation of two vaginal flaps, one of which is denuded of its vaginal epithelial covering (Figure 18.8A). Placement of the de-

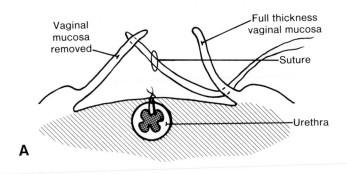

A

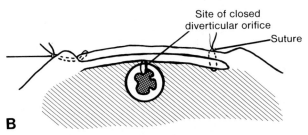

B

Figure 18.8. The vaginal flap technique for closure over the urethral defect. **(A)** After denuding one side of the freed vaginal flaps, the denuded flap is sutured underneath the intact full thickness flap **(B)**. (Redrawn from Judd and Marshall (9).)

nuded flap between the dissection site and the full thickness vaginal wall allows a layered closure without tension (Figure 18.8B).

When the diverticular ostium is distal to the peak urethral closure pressure, the Spence procedure is the operation of choice. This is an operation designed to marsupialize the diverticulum. The procedure involves placement of one blade of the scissors in the urethra and the other in the vagina (Figure 18.7A). The scissors divide the intervening septum between the floor of the urethra and the vagina to complete the marsupialization (Figure 18.7B). After trimming the edges, a running, locking suture along the edges assures hemostasis (Figure 18.7C). Catheterization is not necessary and the patients go home a few hours after the procedure. Subsequent granulation creates the appearance of a large meatotomy.

SURGICAL RESULTS

In two reported series of patients genuine stress incontinence followed the Spence procedure in one of 30 and one of 26, respectively. Both patients with failures responded to vaginal estrogen application with cure of the incontinence. Direct excision of urethral diverticula has a complication rate approaching 20%. These complications are primarily urethrovaginal fistulas and urethral strictures.

SUMMARY

Diverticular symptoms and physical findings mimic many other lower urinary tract abnormalities. Suspicion of the presence of one or more diverticula exists with every urethroscopic examination. It is helpful to combine urethroscopic, radiologic and urodynamic evaluation to select the correct operative procedure. If the diverticular orifice is distal to the area of peak urethral pressure, the Spence marsupialization operation is the procedure of choice; otherwise, direct dissection and removal is indicated.

References

1. **Andersen, M.J.F.** The Incidence of Diverticula in the Female Urethra, *J. Urol.* 98:96, 1967.
2. **Cook, E.N., Pool, T.L.** Urethral Diverticulum in the Female. *J. Urol.* 62:495–497, 1949.
3. **Davis, H.J., Cain, L.G.** Positive Pressure Urethrography: A New Diagnostic Method. *J. Urol.* 75:753, 1956.
4. **Hey, W.** *Practical Observations in Surgery.* J. Humphreys, Philadelphia, 1805.
5. **Hirschhorn, R.C.** A New Surgical Technique for Removal of Urethral Diverticula in the Female Patient. *J. Urol.* 92:206–209, 1964.
6. **Huffman, J.W.** Detailed Anatomy of the Paraurethral Ducts in Adult Human Female. *Am. J. Obstet. Gynecol.* 55:86–101, 1948.
7. **Hunner, G.L.** Calculus Formation in a Urethral Diverticulum in Women: Report of Three Cases. *Urol. Cutan. Rev.* 42:336, 1938.
8. **Hyams, J.A., Hyams, N.M.** New Operative Procedure for Treatment of Diverticulum of the Female Urethra. *Urol. Cutan. Rev.* 43:573–577, 1939.
9. **Judd, G.E., Marshall, J.R.** Repair of Urethral Diverticulum or Vesicovaginal Fistula by Vaginal Flap Technique. *Obstet. Gynecol.* 47:627–629, 1976.
10. **Lichtman, A.S., Robertson, J.R.** Suburethral Diverticula Treated by Marsupialization. *Obstet. Gynecol.* 47:203, 1976.
11. **Moore, T.D.** Diverticulum of the Female Urethra: Improved Technique of Surgical Excision. *J. Urol.* 68:611–616, 1952.
12. **Novak, R.** Editorial Comment. *Obstet. Gynecol. Surv.* 8:423, 1953.
13. **Robertson, J.R.** *Genitourinary Problems in Women.* Charles C. Thomas, Springfield, Ill., 1978.
14. **Spence, H.M., Duckett, J.W.** Diverticulum of the Female Urethra: Clinical Aspects and Presentation of a Single Operative Technique for Care. *J. Urol.* 104:432, 1970.
15. **Young, H.H.** Diverticulum of Female Urethra. *South. Med. J.* 31:1043–1047, 1938.

19 Lower Urinary Tract Infection and Its Effects on Vesical and Urethral Function

Stuart L. Stanton, F.R.C.S., M.R.C.O.G.

An acceptable definition of cystitis is an inflammation of the urinary bladder with or without bacteriuria which is usually symptomatic. The clinical diagnosis is frequently difficult because a number of women complain of recurring episodes of frequency and dysuria unassociated with an actual infecting organism. In many women these symptoms originate in the urethra without inflammatory involvement of the bladder. Yet, if one subjects the same group of patients to bladder biopsy, a surprisingly high proportion of patients have chronic inflammatory cells indicating the presence of previous urinary infection.

A significant bacteriuria requires the uncontaminated cultures of at least 10^5 organisms in three successive fresh, clean catch midstream specimens of urine. These three specimens allow a 90% confidence in the diagnosis of infection. With only two successive specimens this confidence level decreases to about 85%.

INCIDENCE

The incidence of urinary tract infection varies with age (Figure 19.1). At birth the male has a higher incidence of urinary tract infections and the incidence in the female gradually increases thereafter. Asymptomatic bacteriuria increases from an incidence in preschool children of 1% to 5% during the reproductive age groups and peaks at 10% in the postmenopausal female (4).

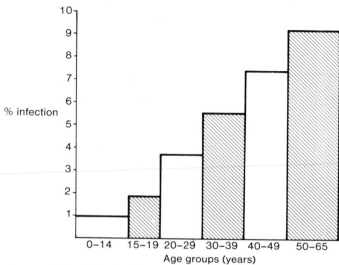

Figure 19.1. The incidence of urinary tract infection in women of various age groups.

ETIOLOGIC FACTORS

The incidence of excess urinary tract infections in the female is multifactorial in origin: the short length of the female urethra, urethral contamination by rectal pathogens, introital colonization by pathogenic bacteria (2–4, 10, 11), and the decreased resistance in the urethral epithelium as a result of the decreased levels of estrogen during the menopause (Table 19.1). In both normal women and women with recurrent urinary tract infections the short female urethra constantly harbors bacteria, especially in its outer one-third (2). In young girls bacteria pass more easily from the external meatus into the bladder which frequently accounts for infections in this age group. When the short urethra coexists with persistent meatal contamination and/or colonization with rectal pathogens, recurrent urinary tract infections frequently result. Exacerbation of this problem commonly follows the hypoestrogenism of the peri- and postmenopausal periods when the hypoestrogenic urethral and trigonal epithelium lose their resistance to contaminating pathogens. The beginning of sexual activity is an added related factor causing urethrovesical bacterial inoculation.

Additional factors include incomplete and infrequent voiding in the woman who is too busy or the little girl whose mother preaches that there are only two safe places to void: your home and the local exclusive department store (5). Voiding at any other place increases the hazard of contracting an infection from the toilet seat and, therefore, some young girls believe their mothers and during childhood develop the tendency to void infrequently, a habit which continues into adulthood. It is felt that this produces ischemic areas within the bladder mucosa, increasing the susceptibility to the ingress of bacteria to initiate and maintain this cycle of chronic urinary infection.

Table 19.1. Factors in the Etiology of Symptoms of Cystitis in Women, Including Urinary Infection[a]

A. Source of urinary pathogens
    1. Normal bowel flora (usual source)
    2. From sex partner
    3. Hematogenous via kidney
    4. Cross infection in hospital
B. Perianal accumulation of pathogens
    1. Bowel dysfunction
    2. Defective toilet hygiene
    3. Perianal disorders
        a. Fissures
        b. Hemorrhoids
        c. Abscesses
        d. Fistulas
        e. Pinworm
C. Progressive colonization by pathogens
    1. Bacterial motility
    2. Poor hygiene
    3. Sexual activity
D. Introital multiplication of urinary pathogens
    1. Infection
        a. *Trichomonas vaginalis*
        b. Monilia
        c. *Corynebacterium vaginalis*
        d. Venereal
        e. Non-specific
    2. Trauma
        a. Sexual
        b. Retained foreign body
    3. Chemical
        a. Vaginal aerosols
        b. Bath salts and oils
        c. Body lotions
        d. Antiseptics in bath
        e. Spermicidal foam
    4. Allergy
    5. Inadequate vulval ventilation
    6. Postmenopausal atrophy
E. Other causes of vaginal discharge
    1. Hormonal
    2. Chronic cervicitis
    3. IUCD
F. Increased vaginal alkalinity
G. Urinary frequency and incontinence
H. Other causes of pruritus vulvae
    1. Leukoplakia
    2. Pediculosis
I. Factors allowing pathogens access to the bladder
    1. Shortness of urethra (anatomical)
    2. Urethral sphincter weakness
        a. Urethritis
        b. Senile atrophy

(continued on p. 208)

Table 19.1—continued

3. Urethral disorders
   a. Caruncle
   b. Mucosal prolapse
   c. Diverticulum
   d. Coitus
   e. Urethrovesical reflux
   f. Turbulent urine flow
   g. Instrumentation or catheterization
   h. Pathogen virulence
   i. Diabetes mellitus
J. Defective clearance of pathogens from bladder
   1. Inadequate fluid load
   2. Infrequent voiding
   3. Incomplete voiding
      a. Obstructed
      b. Inhibited
      c. Neuropathic
   4. Reduced cellular immunity
K. Other causes or symptoms of cystitis
   1. Almost any urological condition
      a. Tumor
      b. Stone
      c. Obstruction
      d. Tuberculosis
L. Other pelvic inflammatory disease
   1. Appendicitis
   2. Salpingitis
   3. Central nervous system dysfunction
   4. Sexual and psychosexual problems
   5. Psychosomatic
   6. Anxiety

[a] Modified from Rees (8).

Additional sources of increased risk of infection include vulvovaginitis, particularly in association with poor hygiene, the menopause and the decreased resistence of the vaginal epithelium during pregnancy. All of these increase the risk of spread of infection into the bladder. Similarly, indiscriminate urethral catheterization causes unnecessary contamination. Even though clean, non-sterile catheterization appears safe, it can cause infection.

With acute or chronic pelvic inflammatory disease there is the possibility of movement of bacteria from within the inflamed pelvic organs into the bladder. Infection within urethral diverticula, changes in the urethra subsequent to repeated operations around the bladder neck area and pregnancy also predispose to cystitis. The infected diverticulum discharges its pus into the urethra which then finds its way to either the urethral meatus or to the interior of the bladder. The rigid fibrotic drainpipe urethra also provides ready access of bacteria into the bladder. Screening of pregnant patients detects those patients with asymptomatic bacteriuria who require therapy because of the greater risk of acute pyelonephritis in pregnancy in the presence of bacteriuria.

Other predisposing factors include diabetes mellitus and hemoglobinolysis. A study of 209 patients reported these associated gynecological conditions, several of which occurred in the same patient: a vaginal discharge in 66% of the patients, pruritus of the vulva in just over 33%, atrophic changes in 17%, cervical erosion in 27%, and cystocele with uterine prolapse in about 10% of patients (9).

DIAGNOSTIC PROCEDURES

Indicated investigations to make the diagnosis of cystitis include culture of midstream urine specimens, and with repeated urinary tract infections, an intravenous pyelogram, a voiding cystogram to detect reflux, urethrocystoscopy to exclude congenital and pathologic changes within the bladder and urethral mucosa which precipitate, encourage or aggravate the presence of a urinary tract infection (Table 19.2). More complex evaluation techniques include the psychometric profile (8), isotopic renography, selective ureteric catheterization and percutaneous needle nephrostomy.

In order to make the diagnosis of bladder infection various techniques are available to identify the presence of a significant bacteriuria. These include immediate culture on an agar plate or various non-specific and less accurate chemical tests. Urinalysis on a fresh urine specimen is very important to identify the presence of white blood cells and bacteria. The presence of both is usually synonymous with urinary tract infection. The presence of pyuria and the absence of bacteriuria suggests the need for cultures for acid fast organisms. This requires three early morning specimens and satisfactory culture occurs in about six weeks.

Repeated urinary infections indicate the need for an intra-

Table 19.2. Diagnostic Procedures

A. Single episode
  1. Urinalysis
  2. Urine culture
B. Multiple episodes
  1. Intravenous pyelogram
  2. Voiding cystogram
  3. Urethrocystoscopy
  4. Psychometric profile
  5. Isotopic renography
  6. Percutaneous needle nephrostomy

venous pyelogram (IVP). Patients of all ages with bacteriuria are subject to the development of chronic pyelonephritis and subsequent progressive renal deterioration. Persistent hematuria or pyuria without bacteria also require radiographic evaluation. Other causes of recurring cystitis include stone formation in the bladder, either spontaneously or on sutures from previous periurethral surgery. Urethrocystoscopy is of help in ruling out these possibilities.

URODYNAMIC FINDINGS

The urodynamic findings in urinary tract infection in one study showed outlet obstruction in only 8% of the patients (9). Twenty-five percent of patients showed evidence of bladder instability, and an additional 25% of patients had poor urine flow despite an adequate detrusor contraction and without evidence of obstruction. In many situations a vicious cycle of repeated lower urinary tract infections leads to an obstructed voiding pattern with high residual urines based solely on spasm of the external striated component of the urethral sphincteric mechanism, due either to the infection itself or secondary to the pain of the acute cystitis (Figure 19.2). This in turn leads to elevated residual urines, repeated infections and poor urinary flow rates. Because of this cycle it is important to plan therapy to eradicate or suppress the infectious process to then allow more normal control of the skeletal component of the sphincter. Based on this reasoning there is no indication for urethral dilatation or urethrotomy to control recurrent urinary tract infections. Some of these urodynamic findings may also result

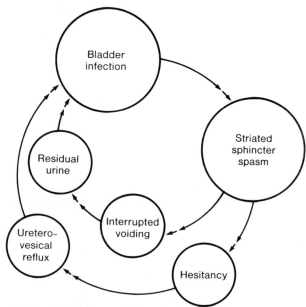

Figure 19.2. The effect of the vicious cycle of repeated urinary tract infections on urethrovesical junction.

from the recent discovery that *Escherichia coli* endotoxins cause vesical hyperactivity and urethral relaxation. Since this organism causes most lower urinary tract infections, these effects are explainable on this basis.

TREATMENT OF URINARY TRACT INFECTIONS

The management of urinary tract infections has two phases, namely prophylaxis and treatment. Therapy of acute infection requires an adequate fluid intake of $2\frac{1}{2}$ to 3 liters a day with concomitant 3 hourly voiding. Antibiotic therapy is the mainstay of treatment. Generally, cultures are of aid in the selection of antibiotics in persistent infections. The initial therapy of the acute urinary tract infection includes sulfisoxazole, nitrofurantoin, ampicillin or trimethoprim-sulfamethoxazole. All acute infections require at least one post-therapy urine culture to detect persistence of infection and to avoid the development of chronic pyelonephritis. The causes of relapse include the wrong choice of initial antibiotic therapy, inadequate duration or dosage of drug, the emergence of a resistant strain of organism and other predisposing factors, such as bladder calculi and vesicoureteric reflux.

Prophylactic screening of women with lower urinary tract infections demonstrates two groups of patients: those detected by routine screening and those with recurrent acute infections. Routine screening is usually directed to case finding in young school age girls and pregnant women. This asymptomatic bacteriuria is treated as an acute infection with close surveillance thereafter for recurrence. Many require continuous antibiotic suppression for prolonged periods of time.

Those women with recurrent acute infections require an appropriate evaluation to determine the exact etiology. Attention to vulvar and perineal hygiene and the avoidance of vaginal deodorants are very important in this group of patients. Voiding after intercourse decreases the vesical inoculum of organisms associated with sexual activity (1). Many patients relate all of their acute episodes of cystitis to intercourse. These patients benefit greatly from a single nitrofurantoin or trimethoprim-sulfamethoxazole tablet postcoitally. Many patients need chronic suppression for many years to clear their chronic cystitis along with urinary acidification. Treatment with a low dose of nitrofurantoin or trimethoprim-sulfamethoxazole usually suffices.

SUMMARY

Women are prone to urinary infections, especially before puberty and after the menopause. The main effect of infection on vesicourethral function is that 25% of the patients have uninhibited detrusor contractions with associated urethral relaxation. *E. coli* endotoxin causes these findings in many patients. In many patients urethral striated sphincteric spasm results, creating a vicious cycle of retention, obstructed voiding and repeated infection. The treatment is elimination of the infection by chemotherapeutic means. Urethral dilatation has little to offer the adult patient.

References

1. **Asscher, W.** Diseases of the Urinary System. *Br. Med. J.* 1: 1332–1335, 1977.
2. **Elkins I.B., Cox, C.E.** Perineal, Vaginal and Urethral Bacteriology of Young Women. I. Incidence of Gram Negative Colonization. *J. Urol.* 111:88, 1974.
3. **Fair, W.R., Timothy, M.M., Millar, M.A., Stamey, T.A.** Bacteriologic and Hormonal Observations of the Urethra and Vaginal Vestibule in Normal Premenopausal Women. *J. Urol.* 104:426, 1970.
4. **Lacy, S.S.** Urinary Tract Infection. In *Gynecologic and Obstetric Urology*, edited by H.J. Buchsbaum and J.D. Schmidt. W.B. Saunders, Philadelphia, 1978, pp. 301–324.
5. **Lalli, A., Lapides, J.** The Infrequent Voider. *Radiology* 92: 1177–1183, 1969.
6. **Marsh, F. P., Murray, M., Panchamia, P.** Relationship between Bacterial Cultures of Vaginal Introitus and Urinary Infection. *Br. J. Urol.* 44:368–375, 1972.
7. **Nergardh, A., Boreus, L.O., Holme, T.** The Inhibitory Effect of Coli-endotoxin on Alpha-adrenergic Receptor Functions in the Lower Urinary Tract. An in vitro Study in Cats. *Scand. J. Urol. Nephrol.* 11:219–224, 1977.
8. **Rees, D. L., Farhoumand, N.** Psychiatric Aspects of Women with Recurrent Cystitis. *Br. J. Urol.* 49:649–658, 1977.
9. **Rees, D.L.** Urinary Tract Infection. In *Clinics in Obstetrics and Gynecology-Gynecological Urology*, edited by S.L. Stanton. W.B. Saunders, London, 1978, 168–192.
10. **Stamey, T.A.** The role of introital enterobacteria in recurrent urinary infections. *J. Urol.* 109:467, 1973.
11. **Stamey, T.A., Sexton, C.C.** The Role of Vaginal Colonization with Enterobacteriaceae in Recurrent Urinary Infections. *J. Urol.* 113:214, 1975.
12. **Tanagho, E.A., Miller E.R., Lyon, H.P., Fisher, R.** Spastic Striated External Sphincter and Urinary Tract Infections in Girls. *Br. J. Urol.* 43:69, 1971.

20 The Effect of Drugs on the Lower Urinary Tract

Donald R. Ostergard, M.D.

Recent advances in the understanding of the neurology and the neuropharmacology of the lower urinary tract indicate that a multiplicity of different types of drugs influence the physiological activity of the bladder and urethra. In many instances drugs given for unrelated disease produce symptoms which bring the patient to the gynecologist. Unless the gynecologist knows the urologic effects of drugs used in medical therapy, he may overlook the possibility that the patient's symptoms may be caused by her current drug therapy. This drug awareness allows him to be more effective in dealing with the patient's lower urinary tract complaints.

This chapter provides the reader with information regarding the effect of drugs on the autonomic nervous system and their subsequent effects on the lower urinary tract. It also provides guidelines for the use of these drugs in specific urologic therapy.

PARASYMPATHETIC DRUGS

Cholinergic (Parasympathomimetic) Medications

Parasympathomimetic drugs are of three types (17, 26). Each exerts its influence by an alteration of the action of the naturally occurring neurotransmitter, acetylcholine. The first type exerts its affect through a direct stimulation of the end organ by actual substitution for the naturally occurring neurotransmitter. These drugs are chemically similar to acetylcholine. The second type prevents the destruction of acetylcholine by inactivating its degrading enzyme, acetylcholinesterase. These drugs are anticholinesterases. The

Table 20.1. Drugs Stimulating the Parasympathetic Nervous System[a]

Drug Name: Generic (Trade)	Dosage Forms	Dosage[b]
Bethanechol (Urecholine, Myocholine)	Tabs: 5, 10, 25 mg	5–30 mg
	Inj: 5 mg/ml	2.5–5 mg SQ
Neostigmine (Prostigmin)	Tabs: 15 mg	15–45 mg
	Solution: 0.25, 0.5, 1.0 mg/ml	0.5–1 mg IM or SQ

[a] See Appendix II (Table II.1) for non-urologic drugs.
[b] Dosages given are oral tid to qid unless otherwise specified.

Table 20.2. Drugs Inhibiting the Parasympathetic Nervous System[a]

Drug Name: Generic (Trade)	Dosage Forms	Dosage[b]
Dicyclomine (Bentyl)	Caps: 10 mg	10 mg
	Tabs: 20 mg	20 mg
	Syrup: 2 mg/ml	
	Solution: 10 mg/ml	
Flavoxate (Urispas)	Tabs: 100 mg	100–200 mg
Hyoscyamine (Cystospaz)	Tabs: 0.15 mg	0.15–0.3 mg
	Timed release: 0.375 mg	0.375 mg q 12 hr
Imipramine (Tofranil)	Tabs: 10, 25, 50 mg	25–50 mg
	Inj.: 25 mg/2 cc	75–200 mg/day
	Timed release: 75, 100, 125, 150 mg	
Isopropamide (Darbid)	Tabs: 5 mg	5 mg q 12 hr
Methantheline (Banthine)	Tabs: 50 mg	50–100 mg
	Powder: 50 mg/ampule	50 mg IM or IV
Oxybutynin (Ditropan)	Tabs: 5 mg	5 mg bid or tid
Oxyphencyclimine (Daricon, Viothene)	Tabs: 10 mg	5–10 mg bid
	Timed release: 10 mg	
Propantheline (Probanthine)	Tabs: 5, 7, 15 mg	7.5–15 mg + 30 mg h.s.
	Timed release: 30 mg	30 mg im or iv
	Powder: 30 mg/vial	

[a] See Appendix II (Tables II.2 and II.3) for non-urologic drugs.
[b] Dosages given are oral tid to qid unless otherwise specified.

third group directly stimulates the acetylcholine receptor sites to produce their parasympathomimetic effects; however, they are not chemically related to acetylcholine. These drugs have as their primary effect on the lower urinary tract a stimulation of detrusor contractility. They have little effect on the urethra. Table 20.1 lists those drugs which have therapeutic importance in urogynecology (10, 22, 24, 40). These drugs stimulate vesical contraction in patients with urinary retention secondary to vesical hypotonia. Appendix II (Table II.1) contains a partial list of additional parasympathomimetic drugs (1, 32, 37). Any of these may produce symptoms of urinary frequency and urgency.

ANTICHOLINERGIC (PARASYMPATHO-LYTIC) DRUGS

Medications in this group directly antagonize the effect of acetylcholine at the end organ (17, 26). Atropine is the classical prototype in this group, and its primary effect on the lower urinary tract is to relax the detrusor muscle. These drugs have little effect on the urethra. Similarly, since atropine blocks the effects of the acetylcholinomimetics and the anticholinesterases, it is also useful as an antidote for these medications. Table 20.2 lists the anticholinergic medications which are therapeutically important in urogynecology (3, 5, 7, 8, 12, 15, 18, 20, 23, 33, 35, 36, 39, 40). Appendix II (Tables II.2 and II.3) lists drugs which do not have primary therapeutic importance, but which may produce symptoms of urinary retention or difficulty in initiating or maintaining micturition (1, 32, 37).

SYMPATHETIC DRUGS

The sympathetic nervous system contains two types of receptors: alpha and beta. Various organs have one or the other type of receptor predominating (2). In the lower urinary tract the detrusor has primarily a beta-adrenergic innervation, whereas the urethra has primarily alpha-adrenergic innervation. The classification of a sympathetic drug reflects which type of receptor it stimulates predominately in a given organ. Certain medications are general adrenergic neuron stimulators or blockers and act on both alpha and beta receptor sites.

GENERAL ADRENERGIC BLOCKERS

Adrenergic blockers are of two types: ganglionic blockers and those which block the postganglionic neuron. Neither has a place in urogynecologic therapy. However, since these drugs have profound secondary effects upon the lower urinary tract, Appendix II (Table II.4 and II.5) lists these agents (1, 31, 32, 37). These agents relax the trigone and the urethral sphincteric mechanism which results in urinary incontinence.

A variety of proprietary combinations of drugs have similar effects. Appendix II (Table II.6) lists these preparations (1, 32, 37).

ALPHA ADRENERGIC BLOCKING AGENTS

The effect of alpha adrenergic stimulation is to increase the tone of the urethral sphincteric mechanism. The agent which blocks the adrenergic neuron relaxes the sphincter and causes the appearance of pseudourinary stress incontinence. However, alpha adrenergic blocking agents may also have therapeutic usefulness in the patient who has spasm of the urethral sphincteric mechanism from whatever cause.

Table 20.3. Drugs Affecting the Sympathetic Nervous System[a] Alpha Adrenergic Blocker

Drug Name: Generic (Trade)	Dosage Forms	Dosage[b]
Phenoxybenza-mine (Diben-zyline)	Caps: 10 mg	10 to 50 mg

[a] See Appendix II (Table II.7) for non-urologic drugs.
[b] Dosages are oral tid to qid unless otherwise specified.

Table 20.4. Drugs Affecting the Sympathetic Nervous System[a] Beta Adrenergic Blocker

Drug Name: Generic (Trade)	Dosage Forms	Dosage[b]
Propranolol (In-deral)	Tabs: 10, 40 mg Solution: 1 mg/ml	10 to 40 mg

[a] See Appendix II (Table II.8) for non-urologic drugs.
[b] Dosages are oral tid to qid unless otherwise specified.

Relief of this spasm will then diminish the symptoms of urgency, frequency and retention. Only one of the alpha adrenergic blocking agents (phenoxybenzamine) has clinical therapeutic usefulness for the urogynecologist (4, 19, 21, 27). It decreases the contractility of the smooth muscle component of the urethral sphincter (Table 20.3) or relaxes the surrounding vascular bed. Appendix II (Table II.7) lists other alpha adrenergic blocking agents whose specific lower urinary tract effects are unknown (1, 6, 11, 32, 37–39).

BETA ADRENERGIC BLOCKING AGENTS

A variety of agents are under investigation for their selective beta adrenergic blocking action. Only one of these drugs (propranolol) is currently available in the United States (Table 20.4) (16).

Since beta adrenergic stimulation causes relaxation of the urethral sphincter, beta blocking agents may be useful in those patients who have urinary stress incontinence of a mild degree. This blockade of the beta adrenergic neuron also allows the alpha adrenergic neuron to function more efficiently in the maintenance of continence. Appendix II (Table II.8) lists other beta adrenergic blocking agents (1, 32, 37).

GENERAL ADRENERGIC STIMULATORS

Various drugs possess general adrenergic neuron stimulating capabilities which cause contraction of the urethral sphincteric mechanism. This increased muscular tone leads to symptoms of obstruction which may be accompanied by urgency and frequency. Only one of these medications (ephedrine) has clinical usefulness in urogynecology (Table 20.5) (9). Several anecdotal reports indicate that this drug is effective in the treatment of patients with mild urinary stress incontinence. Appendix II (Table II.9) contains a list of other general adrenergic stimulators (1, 32, 37). In addition, there are a variety of proprietary medications with sympathetic stimulating effects. Appendix II (Table II.10) lists these combined preparations (1, 32, 37).

ALPHA ADRENERGIC STIMULATING AGENTS

Alpha adrenergic stimulating agents increase the tone of the urethral sphincteric mechanism. Therefore, these drugs have potential therapeutic usefulness for the treatment of urinary stress incontinence. Three drugs appear to have usefulness for the urogynecologist. (Table 20.6) (5–7, 18, 28, 34). The antidepressant medication, imipramine, may prove to be especially important since it has alpha adrenergic stimulating properties along with parasympatholytic activity. An additional group of medications has similar effects but unknown clinical application at the present time (Appendix II, Table II.11) (1, 32, 37).

BETA ADRENERGIC STIMULATING AGENTS

The large number of beta adrenergic stimulating agents benefit the asthmatic due to their potent bronchial dilating effects. Although these agents have potential use in urogynecology due to urethral relaxant effects, verification is

Table 20.5.   Drugs Affecting the Sympathetic Nervous System[a] General Adrenergic Stimulators

Drug Name: Generic (Trade)	Dosage Form	Dosage[b]
Ephedrine (Efedron, Ephetonin)	Tabs: 15, 25, 30, 50, 60 mg Syrup: 20 mg/5 ml	15 to 50 mg

[a] See Appendix II (Tables II.9 and II.10) for non-urologic drugs.
[b] Dosages are oral tid to qid unless otherwise specified.

Table 20.6.   Drugs Affecting the Sympathetic Nervous System[a] Alpha Adrenergic Stimulators

Drug Name: Generic (Trade)	Dosage Forms	Dosage[b]
Imipramine[c] (Tofranil)	Tabs: 10, 25, 50 mg Inj: 25 mg/2 cc	25 to 50 mg
	Timed Release: 75, 100, 125, 150 mg	75 to 200 mg/day
Phenylephrine	Elixir: 5 mg/5 ml	10 mg
Phenylpropanolamine (Propadrine)	Caps: 25, 50 mg Elixir: 20 mg/5 ml	25 to 50 mg

[a] See Appendix II (Table II.11) for non-urologic drugs.
[b] Dosages are oral tid to qid unless otherwise specified.
[c] Also with anticholinergic effects, see Table 20.2.

Table 20.7.   Drugs Affecting the Sympathetic Nervous System[a] Beta Adrenergic Stimulators

Drug Name: Generic (Trade)	Dosage Forms	Dosage[b]
Isoproterenol (Isuprel)	Tabs: 10, 15 mg Solution: 0.2 mg/ml	Unknown
Isoxuprine (Vasodilan)	Tabs: 10 mg Solution: 5 mg/ml	10 to 20 mg 5 to 10 mg IM
Metaproterenol (Alupent, Metaprex)	Tabs: 20 mg	20 mg

[a] See Appendix II (Table II.12) for non-urologic drugs.
[b] Dosages are oral tid to qid unless otherwise specified.

lacking at the present time. Table 20.7 lists those agents with potential therapeutic usefulness (1, 32, 37). Appendix II (Table II.12) lists other beta adrenergic stimulators (1, 32, 37).

MISCELLANEOUS DRUGS WITH EFFECTS ON THE AUTONOMIC NERVOUS SYSTEM AND THE LOWER URINARY TRACT

Several classes of medications with unrelated primary indications have secondary autonomic effects which alter the sphincteric mechanism of the urethra.

The phenothiazine derivatives constitute one group which appears to possess alpha adrenergic blocking activity and may produce urinary stress incontinence (Appendix II, Table II.13) (1, 6, 13, 25, 32, 38, 39). However, these drugs may also cause urinary retention. In a similar fashion, certain antihistamines may cause urinary retention while others in certain patients may produce incontinence (Appendix II, Tables II.13 and II.14) (1, 32, 39). Also, certain estrogenic medications in excessive amounts, phenytoin (30), as well as progestational agents (6, 24), may cause urinary stress incontinence. However, the estrogen dependent urethral sphincteric mechanism usually responds to estrogen therapy with increased muscular tone (6, 14, 40). Estrogen therapy has definite clinical usefulness for the treatment of hypoestrogenic patients with mild stress incontinence. The reason for these apparent discrepancies is not known at the present time.

An additional group of medications produces hesitancy, urgency and frequency of micturition (Appendix II, Table II.14) (1, 32, 39). The exact mechanism of symptom production is unknown.

Sulfonamides may cause mechanical urinary obstruction from crystals deposited in the urethra.

COMMENT

The multiplicity of effects of drugs on the lower urinary tract produces an aura of extreme complexity. In spite of this apparent maze, the subject lends itself to simplification in the form of several generalizations which are useful in the management of urogynecologic patients. There are four basic areas of concern which involve bladder or urethral contraction and relaxation and the ability of the physician to either stimulate or inhibit these effects.

The first of these is the pharmacologic inhibition of spontaneous bladder contractions. Anticholinergic medications in appropriate dosages accomplish this bladder restraint (Table 20.1). The second is the inability of the bladder to contract efficiently when challenged with a volume load or when the patient desires to micturate. The judicious use of cholinergic agents improves the functional activity of the bladder (Table 20.2). The third area of concern involves the urethra which either generates excessive or low intraluminal pressures or demonstrates discordant functional activity during vesical contraction. Alpha adrenergic blockade or beta stimulation produces a decrease in urethral tone in these patients (Tables 20.3 and 20.7). The fourth area involves the association of genuine stress incontinence with low intraurethral pressures. Alpha adrenergic stimulation provides a means for decreasing intraurethral pressure (Tables 20.4 to 20.6).

Some patients require both anticholinergic and alpha adrenergic stimulation when uninhibited bladder contractions are associated with low intraurethral pressures. A potentially important drug (imipramine) combines these effects and appears to have therapeutic usefulness for these patients.

The hypoestrogenic, postmenopausal patient with mild genuine stress incontinence benefits from the topical application of estrogenic creams to the vagina. The local estrogen stimulates and supports the urethral and trigonal smooth musculature and epithelium, thereby improving the physiologic function of these structures in the support of urinary continence.

In summary, it is possible to manipulate drugs in the therapy of various urethral and detrusor malfunctions. These drugs are effective and provide our patients with symptomatic and objective relief. In many instances it is possible to avoid unnecessary operative procedures for urinary stress incontinence through the application of these pharmacologic principles.

References

1. **AMA Drug Evaluations**, 2nd ed. Publishing Sciences Group, Inc., Acton, Mass., 1973.

2. **Awad, S.A., Bruce, A.W., Carro-Ciampi, G., Downie, J., Lin, M., Marks, G.S.** Distribution of α- And β- Adrenoceptors in Human Urinary Bladder. *Br. J. Pharmacol.* 50:525–529, 1974.

3. **Awad, S.A., Bryniak, S., Downie, J.W., Bruce, A.W.** The Treatment of the Uninhibited Bladder with Dicyclomine. *J. Urol.* 117:161–163, 1977.

4. **Awad, S.A., Downie, J.W.** Sympathetic Dyssynergia in the Region of the External Sphincter: A Possible Source of Lower Urinary Tract Obstruction. *J. Urol.* 118:636–640, 1977.

5. **Benson, G.S., Sarshik, S.A., Raezer, D.M., Wein, A.J.** Bladder Muscle Contractility; Comparative Effects and Mechanisms of Action of Atropine, Propantheline, Flavoxate, and Imipramine. *Urology* 9:31–35, 1977.

6. **Caine, M., Raz, S.** Some Clinical Implications of Adrenergic Receptors in the Urinary Tract. *Arch. Surg.* 110:247–250, 1975.

7. **Diokno, A.C., Hyndman, C.W., Hardy, D.A., Lapides, J.:** Comparison of Action of Imipramine (Tofranil) and Propantheline (Probanthine) on Detrusor Contraction. *J. Urol.* 107:42–43, 1972.

8. **Diokno, A.C., Lapides, J.** Oxybutynin: A New Drug with Analgesic and Anticholinergic Properties. *J. Urol.* 108:307–309, 1972.

9. **Diokno, A.C., Taub, M.** Ephedrine in Treatment of Urinary Incontinence. *Urology* 5:624–625, 1975.

10. **Diokno, A.C., Lapides, J.** Action of Oral and Parenteral Bethanechol on Decompensated Bladder. *Urology* 10:23–24, 1977.

11. **Donker, P.J., Ivanovici, F., Noach, E.L.** Analyses of the Urethral Pressure Profile by Means of Electromyography and the Administration of Drugs. *Br. J. Urol.* 44:180–193, 1972.

12. **Draper, J.W., Zorgniotti, A.W.** The Effect of Banthine and Similar Agents on the Urinary Tract. *N.Y. State J. Med.* 54:77–83, 1954.

13. **Edwards, J.G.** Unwanted Effects of Psychotropic Drugs: II. Drugs for Schizophrenia. *Practitioner* 218:696–700, 1977.

14. **Faber, P., Heidenreich, J.** Treatment of Stress Incontinence with Estrogen in Postmenopausal Women. *Urol. Int.* 32:221–223, 1977.

15. **Farrar, D.J., Osborne, J.L.** The Use of Bromocriptine in the Treatment of the Unstable Bladder. *Br. J. Urol.* 48:235–238, 1976.

16. **Gleason, D.M., Reilly, R.J., Bottaccini, M.R., Pierce, M.J.** The Urethral Continence Zone and Its Relation to Stress Incontinence. *J. Urol.* 112:81–88, 1974.

17. **Goodman, L.S., Gilman, A.** *The Pharmacological Basis of Therapeutics,* 5th ed. Macmillan Publishing Co., New York, 1975.

18. **Gregory, J.G., Wein, A.J., Schoenberg, H.W.** A Comparison of the Action of Tofranil and Pro-Banthine on the Urinary Bladder. *Invest. Urol.* 12:233–235, 1974.

19. **Khanna, O.P., Gonick, P.** Effects of Phenoxybenzamine Hydrochloride on Canine Lower Urinary Tract. Clinical Implications. *Urology* 6:323–330, 1975.

20. **Kohler, F.P., Morales, P.A.** Cystometric Evaluation of Flavoxate Hydrochloride in Normal and Neurogenic Bladders. *J. Urol.* 100:729–730, 1968.

21. **Krane, R.J., Olsson, C.A.** Phenoxybenzamine in Neurogenic Bladder Dysfunction. II. Clinical Considerations. *J. Urol.* 110: 653–656, 1973.
22. **Lapides, J., Friend, C.R., Ajemian, E.P., Reus, W.F.** A New Test for Neurogenic Bladder. *J. Urol.* 88:245–247, 1962.
23. **McGrath, W.R., Lewis, R.E., Kuhn, W.L.** The Dual Mode of the Antispasmodic Effect of Dicyclomine Hydrochloride. *J. Pharmacol. Exp. Ther.* 146:354–358, 1964.
24. **Melzer, M.** The Urecholine Test. *J. Urol* 108:728–730, 1972.
25. **Merrill, D.C., Markland, C.** Vesical Dysfunction Induced by the Major Tranquilizers. *J. Urol.* 107:769–771, 1972.
26. **Meyers, F.H., Jawetz, E., Goldfien, A.** *Review of Medical Pharmacology*, 4th ed., Lange Medical Publications, Los Altos, Calif.
27. **Mobley, D.F.** Phenoxybenzamine in the Management of Neurogenic Vesical Dysfunction. *J. Urol.* 116:737–738, 1976.
28. **Nuessle, W.F., Miller, H.E., Norman, F.C.** Urinary Retention from Ornade. *Geriatrics* 23:166–169, 1968.
29. **Raz, S., Zeigler, M., Caine, M.** The Effect of Progesterone on the Adrenergic Receptors of the Urethra. *Br. J. Urol.* 45:131–135, 1973.
30. **Raz, S., Zeigler, M., Caine, M.** The Effect of Diphenylhydantoin on the Urethra. *Invest. Urol.* 10:293–294, 1973.
31. **Raz, S. Kaufman, J.J., Ellison, G.W., Mayers, L.W.** Methyldopa in the Treatment of Neurogenic Bladder Disorders. *Urology* 9:188–190, 1977.
32. **Remington, J.P.** *Remington's Pharmaceutical Sciences*, 15th ed. Mack Publishing Co., Easton, Pa., 1975.
33. **Stanton, S.L.** A Comparison of Emepronium Bromide and Flavoxate Hydrochloride in the Treatment of Urinary Incontinence. *J. Urol.* 110:529–532, 1973.
34. **Stewart, B.H., Banowsky, L.H.W., Montague, D.K.** Stress Incontinence: Conservative Therapy with Sympathomimetic Drugs. *J. Urol.* 115:558–559, 1976.
35. **Thompson, I.M., Lauvetz, R.** Oxybutynin in Bladder Spasm, Neurogenic Bladder, and Enuresis. *Urology* 8:452–454, 1976.
36. **Ulmsten, U., Andersson, K.E.** The Effects of Emeprone on Intravesical and Intraurethral Pressures in Women with Urgency Incontinence. *Scand. J. Urol. Nephrol.* 11:103–109, 1977.
37. **Osol, A., Pratt, R., Geuraro, A.R.** *The U.S. Dispensatory*, 27th ed. J.B. Lippincott, Philadelphia, 1973.
38. **Van Putten, T., Malkin, M.D., Weiss, M.S.** Phenothiazine-Induced Stress Incontinence. *J. Urol.* 109:625–626, 1973.
39. **Whitfield, H.N., Doyle, P.T., Mayo, M.E., Poopalasingham. N.** The Effect of Adrenergic Blocking Drugs on Outflow Resistance. *Br. J. Urol.* 47:823–827, 1976.
40. **Youssef, A.F.** (Ed.) *Gynecological Urology.* Charles C. Thomas, Springfield, Ill., 1960.

21 The Differential Diagnosis of Urinary Incontinence

Thomas A.McCarthy, M.D.

In the absence of fistulas, urinary incontinence occurs when the forces of expulsion exceed the forces of retention. This requires an upset in the balance of forces such that the intravesical pressure exceeds the intraurethral pressure. Any of a variety of diverse pathological entities which affect the urethra, bladder, or the central or peripheral nervous system are potentially etiologic. Considerations in the differential diagnosis of incontinence also include a complex group of anatomical defects involving both the integrity of the lower urinary tract as a conduit and its anatomical supports. Although the actual etiology of urinary incontinence is complex, in the absence of fistulas the basic problem is always an imbalance between intravesical and intraurethral pressure. This chapter presents an outline of the causes of urinary incontinence.

ACTIVE INCREASE OF EXPULSIVE FORCES

The causes of active increases in expulsive forces include uninhibited detrusor contractions of various neurological or local etiologies and drug therapies (Table 21.1).

Uninhibited detrusor contractions result from any type of central nervous system lesion which decreases the volitional control of micturition by interference with Loop I reflex mechanisms.

Additionally, certain Loop II defects are causes for uninhibitable detrusor contractions. Increased sensory input

Table 21.1. Active Increase of Expulsive Forces

I. Uninhibited detrusor contractions
  A. Neurological causes
    1. Upper motor neuron lesions
      a. Cerebrovascular disease
      b. Multiple sclerosis
      c. Parkinson's disease
      d. Senile dementia
      e. Tumors
      f. Meningomyelocele
  B. Local causes
    1. Infections
      a. Trigone
      b. Bladder
      c. Urethra
      d. Bladder stones
      e. Bladder tumors
  C. Pharmacological
    1. Parasympathomimetics

Table 21.2. Passive Increase of Expulsive Forces (Overflow Incontinence)

I. Decreased bladder wall compliance
  A. Radiation fibrosis
  B. Intrinsic vesical disease
    1. Recurrent vesical infection
    2. Interstitial cystitis (Hunner's ulcer)
  C. Extrinsic pelvic disease
II. Bladder atony
  A. Neurological causes
    1. Lower motor neuron lesion
    2. Autonomic neuropathy
  B. Endocrine disease
    1. Hypothyroidism
  C. Local detrusor disease
    1. Recurrent vesical overdistention

along the afferent limb overfacilitates the detrusor reflex, resulting in loss of volitional control. Possible sources for increased sensory input are infection, bladder stones and bladder tumors. As with skeletal muscle, interruption of the efferent upper motor neuron pathway results in peripheral spasm and uninhibitable vesical hypertonicity.

The other category of factors causing an active increase of intravesical pressure is pharmacological, particularly with the parasympathomimetics, which stimulate detrusor muscle activity. Fortunately, patients rarely require these drugs for more than a short period of time and they don't present a major problem. These drugs are primarily used for gastrointestinal disease, such as, gastric atony after bilateral vagotomy for ulcer disease, and rarely for paroxysmal tachycardias and peripheral vascular disease, such as Raynaud's phenomenon. This possibility reinforces the need for a good drug history in evaluating the patient with incontinence.

PASSIVE INCREASE OF EXPULSIVE FORCES (OVERFLOW INCONTINENCE)

There are two general categories for passive causes of increased expulsive forces. These are: (1) decreased bladder wall compliance, and (2) bladder atony (Table 21.2). Decreased bladder wall compliance causes elevation of intravesical pressure by diminution of available bladder volume. Normally, as the bladder fills, there is little increase in pressure. With decrease in bladder wall compliance, however, volume increase is accompanied by intravesical pressure rise. Causative entities are radiation fibrosis, extrinsic pelvic disease and intrinsic bladder disease. Abnormal facilitation of central nervous system reflex activity from these disease processes may also overfacilitate detrusor activity.

Bladder atony is generally of neurogenic origin (Table 21.2) and is a form of decreased bladder wall compliance. As the bladder overfills and exceeds the limits of distensibility, this causes an intravesical pressure increase. Conditions predisposing to bladder atony are those which affect the lower motor neurons, such as diabetic peripheral neuropathy. Endocrine disease and recurrent overdistension may also play a role in the etiology of bladder atony.

DECREASED RETENTIVE FORCES

Several factors cause a decrease in intraurethral pressure. These are anatomic, iatrogenic, physiologic, pharmacologic, infectious and neurologic in origin.

Anatomic causes of lowered intraurethral pressure are several. The most important factor is the urethra which responds inadequately to the stress of increased abdominal pressure, vesical filling or position changes due to altered anatomical relationships causing decreased functional length and closure pressure. Descent of the bladder neck and the associated urethral shortening decreases resting urethral muscle tone. This is expected, since Starling's law requires an optimal stretch for efficient function of both striated and smooth muscle. The shortened muscle fibers of the urethral sphincteric mechanism in this situation respond less well to a given stimulus. This urethra is incapable of responding to neurological reflexes generated by stress to produce sufficient intraluminal pressure to prevent urine loss. Another factor is failure of intra-abdominal pressure transmission to the urethra due to anatomical displacement of the urethra outside of the abdomial cavity. Normally, intra-abdominal pressures are transmitted to the proximal urethra as well as to the bladder. If the proximal urethra descends outside the abdominal cavity, any increase in intra-abdominal pressure transmits fully to the bladder but transmission to the urethra is suboptimal and less than that received by the bladder. This results in an upset of the balance of forces and intravesical pressure now exceeds the intraurethral resistance.

Iatrogenic causes of decreased retentive forces include the scarred, rigid urethra. The most common etiology is vaginal and/or suprapubic surgery near the urethra. For this reason, the urethra is unable to compensate for the stress of increased intra-abdominal pressure by augmenting functional length and/or closure pressure urine loss. This rigid urethra causes continuous incontinence and these patients rarely demonstrate a pressure increase in the urethra in response to the hold command.

Physiologic causes of lowered intraurethral resistance to loss of urine are primarily based on hormonal effects. Many patients experience incontinence for the first time during pregnancy which usually resolves during the postpartum period. This is thought to be due, in part, to the elevated progesterone levels in pregnancy. Since progesterone acts as a beta adrenergic stimulator and since the urethra responds to beta stimulation by relaxation, a lowered intraurethral pressure is the result.

Many patients experience the onset of incontinence during the menopause. Hypoestrogenism causes decreased periurethral vascularity, mucosal atrophy and muscular hypotonia in the estrogen dependent urethra and trigone. Any or all of these mechanisms may cause incontinence beginning in the menopause.

Similarly, prescribed drug therapy causes urethral smooth muscle hypotonia through alpha blockade or beta stimulation which produces incontinence.

Acute or chronic infection of the urethra or bladder may result in urinary incontinence in women. With therapy of the infection, the incontinence usually resolves. The incontinence related to urinary infection with certain strains of *Escherichia coli* may be due to the endotoxin which inhibits the alpha adrenergic receptor function of the lower urinary tract.

Neurological lesions also cause a lowered intraurethral pressure through the effects of chronic urethral denervation. The urethras of patients with chronic bladder denervation frequently demonstrate an exaggerated pressure response to alpha adrenergic drugs. This suggests that urethral denervation is a clinical entity and behaves in accordance with

Table 21.3. Decreased Retentive Forces

I. Anatomic
    A. Urethral position
    B. Decreased length of urethra
    C. Decreased urethral closure pressure
    D. Decreased compensation in pressure or length with bladder filling or position changes
II. Iatrogenic
    A. Postoperative rigid urethra
III. Physiologic
    A. Pregnancy
    B. Menopause
    C. Pharmacologic
    D. Alpha blockers
    E. Beta stimulators
IV. Infection
    A. Alpha blockade
V. Neurologic disease
    A. Chronic urethral denervation

Table 21.4. Bypass of Continence Mechanism

Fistulas
Diverticula
Ectopic ureter

the responses described for other denervated organs. That is, the organ reacts with a supersensitivity response to its neurotransmitter after a period of denervation.

BYPASS OF CONTINENCE MECHANISMS

A rarer form of incontinence is due to bypass of the normal continence mechanisms (Table 21.3). These are non-physiologic conduits for urine, such as ureterovaginal, vesicovaginal or urethrovaginal fistulas, ectopic ureters and diverticula. Except for those with diverticula, these patients experience continuous wetness and the diagnosis is relatively easy. However, some patients present with symptoms of stress incontinence only. Similarly, the late appearance of incontinence from congenital lesions also occurs.

Characteristically, diverticula present with postmicturition dribbling, associated with virtually any combination of lower urinary tract symptoms. The postmicturition urine loss is due to the accumulation of urine in the diverticulum which empties when the patient stands up. On the same basis, the patient's history may mimic stress incontinence. Urethroscopic examination or urethral radiographic procedures substantiate the diagnosis.

SUMMARY

Urinary incontinence in women is a complex phenomenon with many etiologic factors to consider. The three main categories of increased expulsive forces, decreased retentive forces or bypass of the normal continence mechanism form a convenient categorization.

History alone is inadequate to provide a definitive diagnosis of the cause of the patient's incontinence. It is incumbent upon the physician to perform an adequate evaluation of the lower urinary tract in all incontinent patients and to rule out non-surgical diagnoses prior to a surgical procedure. Certain patients require a thorough urodynamic evaluation prior to incontinence surgery. By careful attention to the basic principles of evaluation of the lower urinary tract the physician learns to recognize which patients to refer for in depth urodynamic evaluation.

References

1. **Bradley, W.E., Timm, G.W.** Cystometry VI. Interpretation. *Urology* 7:231, 1976.
2. **Bruschini, R.S., Schmidt, R.A., Tanagho, E.A.** Effects of Urethral Stretch on Urethral Pressure Profile. *Invest. Urol.* 15:107, 1977.
3. **Diokno, A.C., Taub, M.** Ephedrine in the Treatment of Urinary Incontinence. *Urology* 5:624, 1975.
4. **Drutz, H.P., Shapiro, B.J., Mandel, F.** Do Static Cystourethrograms Have a Role in the Investigation of Female Incontinence? *Am. J. Obstet. Gynecol.* 130:516, 1978.
5. **Enhorning, G.E.** A Concept of Urinary Incontinence. *Urol. Int.* 31:3, 1976.
6. **Faber, O., Heidenzeich, J.** Treatment of Stress Incontinence With Estrogen in Postmenopausal Women. *Urol. Int.* 32:321, 1977.
7. **Hebjorn, J.T., Andersen, J.T., Walter, S., Dam, A.M.** Detrusor Hyperreflexia. *Scand. J. Urol. Nephrol.* 10:103, 1976.
8. **Nergardh, A., Boreus, L.O., Holme, T.** The Inhibitory Effect of Coli Endotoxin on Alpha Adrenergic Receptor Function in the Lower Urinary Tract. *Scand. J. Urol. Nephrol.* 11:219, 1977.
9. **Raz, S., Zeigler, M., Caine, M.** The Effect of Progesterone on the Adrenergic Receptors of the Urethra. *Br. J. Urol.* 45:131, 1973.
10. **Stewart, B.H., Banowsky, L.H.W., Montague, D.K.** Stress Incontinence: Conservative Therapy With Sympathomimetic Drugs. *J. Urol.* 115:558, 1976.

22 Evaluation and Therapy of the Unstable Bladder

Stuart L. Stanton, F.R.C.S., M.R.C.O.G.

One of the most thought provoking medical entities in the lower urinary tract is the pathophysiology of the unstable bladder. It remains a diagnostic enigma and its therapy is frequently unsatisfactory. This chapter reviews its definition, etiology, clinical presentation, treatment and those areas which remain elusive.

DEFINITION

The unstable bladder, or detrusor instability, is the occurrence of involuntary, uninhibited detrusor contractions greater than 15 cm of water or a true detrusor pressure greater than 15 cm of water in the presence of a normal bladder capacity during bladder filling (see Appendix I). When the physician suspects the presence of uninhibited contractions and they do not occur with cystometry using slow bladder filling, he employs various provocative stimuli to induce a vesical contraction, such as rapid bladder filling, coughing, standing erect with a full bladder or filling the bladder while erect.

This terminology represents an evolution of definitions occurring over many years. Urgency incontinence is an older term which describes the symptoms of the patient who complains of sudden inability to control her bladder, with resultant urine leakage. These patients usually experience a sudden desire to micturate prior to the event. The term uninhibited bladder, dyssynergic detrusor dysfunction and unstable bladder followed. All of these terms refer to uninhibited detrusor contractions as defined above.

ETIOLOGY

In many cases the etiology of the unstable bladder is unknown (Table 22.1). In some patients it is secondary to upper motor neuron disease, such as multiple sclerosis. Following retropubic surgery for incontinence, some patients develop uninhibited detrusor contractions or a steep rise in bladder pressure during the CMG (4). The exact mechanism is unknown but could be related to a partial denervation of the bladder (see Chapter 29).

In a certain number of patients psychosomatic disease is the cause, as evidenced by the fact that therapy with biofeedback or bladder drill cures a certain proportion of these patients (1). Outflow obstruction in the male produces detrusor instability; its comparable role in the female is unknown. A syndrome in the elderly caused by cerebrovascular atherosclerosis also results in an unstable bladder.

INCIDENCE

The proportion of patients with incontinence due to detrusor instability is quite significant but also quite variable. In 1963, Hodgkinson et al. gave a percentage of 8.7% in a patient population referred for evaluation of incontinence (8) and in 1975, Farrar et al. reported 63% (6), with other authors reporting intermediate results.

CLINICAL PRESENTATION

In a personal series using urodynamic techniques the author compared 100 patients with detrusor instability with 100 women with genuine stress incontinence (3). Their ages, parity and the number of previous pelvic operations were similar. In a comparison of symptoms between the two groups of patients, no particular symptom stood out to separate those with detrusor instability from those with genuine stress incontinence (Table 22.2). Thus, a good medical history is, by itself, not sufficient to make a definitive diagnosis. The only generalization possible is that a greater proportion of patients with uterovaginal prolapse had genuine stress incontinence than detrusor instability.

Urodynamic data revealed a difference in first sensation of bladder filling in the two groups. Those patients with detrusor instability had an earlier first sensation and a reduced bladder capacity. The vesical filling pressure in the supine position was just over 27 cm H_2O in those patients

Table 22.1. Etiology of the Unstable Bladder

Unknown
Upper motor neuron lesions
Psychosomatic
Incontinence surgery
Outflow obstruction
Cerebral atherosclerosis

Table 22.2. The Incidence of Symptoms Associated with Genuine Stress Incontinence and Detrusor Instability[a]

	Genuine Stress Incontinence	Detrusor Instability
Stress incontinence	89	49
Diurnal and nocturnal frequency		
Urge and stress incontinence	19	26
Urge incontinence	55	38
Present enuresis	14	13
Past enuresis	13	24
Wet on standing up	45	31
Diurnal frequency	57	79
Nocturnal frequency	38	69
Diurnal and nocturnal frequency	28	56
Difficulty voiding	6	9
Prolapse sensation	42	18

[a] Adapted from Cardozo and Stanton (3).

with detrusor instability compared to 5 cm H_1O in those patients with genuine stress incontinence. There was also a difference in the maximum voiding pressure between the two groups, with the unstable bladder group having a greater voiding pressure. The peak flow rates during micturition were similar.

A demonstration of the anatomical changes associated with genuine stress incontinence require the use of radiologic techniques. In the erect oblique position with straining, 65% of the patients with detrusor instability and 85% of those with genuine stress incontinence demonstrated descent of the urethrovesical junction.

Many authors report the usefulness of the voluntary ability of the patient to interrupt the urinary stream as a differentiating feature between stress incontinence and detrusor instability. However, in this author's series, 31% of patients with detrusor instability and 38% of patients with genuine stress incontinence lacked the ability to interrupt the urinary stream on command. During urodynamic radiological screening 85% of both groups interrupted their urinary streams.

THERAPY

There are many methods available to treat detrusor instability (Table 22.3). The use of multiple solutions to any medical problem usually indicates that the problem is poorly understood and the precise therapy is in doubt. Surgery is a last resort for the management of this condition,

Table 22.3. Treatment Methods

Drugs
Anticholinergics
Beta adrenergic stimulants
Calcium antagonists
Musculotrophics
Prostaglandin synthetase inhibitors
Bladder drill
Psychotherapy
Biofeedback
Electronic suppression
Surgery:
    Infravesical nerve resection
    Selective sacral denervation

since this is irreversible with the potential for serious side effects.

Anticholinergic drugs are the most effective, yet only produce a cure or improvement rate in the range of 50 to 60% (See Chapter 21). Banthine in a dose of 10 to 15 mg, three times a day is effective, but has the disadvantage of producing side effects such as dry mouth and retention of urine in some patients. A similar drug is propantheline. Emepromium bromide is used in Europe in a dose of 200 mg, four times a day. A main side effect is mucosal ulceration which is prevented by ingestion of the medication with a full glass of water. Beta adrenergic stimulants are potentially useful and are in the research stage. However, these have the disadvantage of producing various cardiac symptoms and the clinical results with this classification of medications are poor. Calcium antagonists increase the degree of bladder distention at which detrusor contractions occur (11). These drugs act by inhibiting the passage of calcium into the muscle and, therefore, affect its contractility. Musculotrophic drugs, especially flavoxate, in a dosage of 200 mg, four times a day, are sometimes useful but are not particularly successful. Prostaglandin synthetase inhibitors are also under investigation. Prostaglandins in the E2 and F2 series cause detrusor contractions both in vivo and in vitro. A double blind trial using the prostaglandin synthetase inhibitor, indomethacin with bromocriptine, revealed no significant differences between the two drugs using subjective response indicators (2). On the other hand, indomethacin, in a dosage of 100 mg, twice a day, increased urinary frequency but had very little effect on urgency and urge incontinence. It also caused significant side effects on the gastrointestinal tract, including nausea and indigestion, along with headaches. An objective study using cystometry with flurbiprofen, another prostaglandin synthetase inhibitor, revealed that many patients had reduced frequencies of uninhibited detrusor contractions and others had no contractions at all (5).

Bladder drill is another technique for the therapy of the unstable bladder. Patients enter the hospital for a period of ten days during which time they have their problem explained to them in detail. They learn to use a urinary diary to record voiding times and amounts, and they void at more regular and gradually increasing intervals (7).

Biofeedback is an alternative mode of bladder training used because it is thought that the bladder is no longer under cortical control (1). With a pressure line inserted into the full bladder and attached to a sound generating unit, the patient receives an audible signal when bladder pressure increases (Figure 22.1). The tone varies according to the pressure change in the bladder. By means of a mirror the patient also views the recording pen of the pressure recorder. When an uninhibited vesical contraction occurs, not only is the patient aware of the sound change but the patient also sees the pen move. Over a period of an hour long treatment session and with successive filling of the patient's bladder several times to stimulate the appearance of these contractions, the patient attempts to retain herself by means of practice with muscle relaxing exercises to

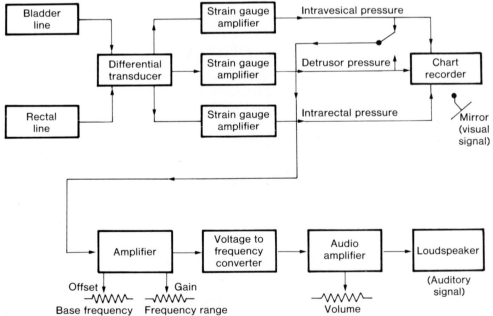

Figure 22.1.   Block diagram of the biofeedback apparatus. The transducers and amplifiers translate the pressures recorded by the bladder and rectal pressure lines to visual and auditory stimuli. (Reproduced by permission of L. Cardozo and the Editor, *British Journal of Urology* 50:521–523, 1978.)

reduce the pen deflection and the noise produced by the apparatus. After six or seven weekly treatment sessions many patients achieve satisfactory results. Failures occur in those patients with severe detrusor instability, particularly when associated with overwhelming domestic circumstances, such as marital upset. Fifty percent of patients described improvement of diurnal and nocturnal frequency as well as urgency, urge incontinence and enuresis. Using objective studies in 15 patients, including cystometry at six months, cure resulted in 6 patients, improvement in 8 and failure in 1 patient. Using the Urilos nappy test as an absolute indicator of urine loss, objective cure resulted in 7 patients, improvement in 2 and failure in 6. We conclude that the method works well and that the patient's symptoms do not always correspond to objective findings.

Surgery is the last mode of therapy. The physician reserves surgery for those patients demonstrating failure of previous conservative therapy. There are two approaches to surgery. The first is a vesical denervation procedure carried out per vaginum (10). Abolishment of uninhibited detrusor contractions by unilateral or bilateral local anesthetic blockade of the infravesical nerve precedes surgery in order to evaluate the potential effectiveness of the procedure and to determine the requirement for unilateral or bilateral resection of the nerve. The literature reports an overall cure rate of 60%.

Another surgical method of denervation is selective sacral root resection with selective sacral neurectomy at either S2, S3 or S4 (13). Fifty percent of patients noted improvement with a reduction in uninhibited detrusor contractions, an increased vesical capacity, decreased urge incontinence and a variable effect on frequency.

SUMMARY

The etiology of the primary unstable bladder is still unclear and therapy lacks specificity and consistency. Although a variety of treatment modalities exist, drug therapy is the conservative therapy of first choice, followed by a program of bladder drill or biofeedback. Surgery is the therapy of last resort.

References

1. **Cardozo, L., Abrams, P., Stanton, S., Feneley, R.** Idiopathic Bladder Instability Treated by Biofeedback. *Br. J. Urol.* 50: 521–523, 1978.
2. **Cardozo, L., Stanton, S. L.** A Comparison between Bromocriptine and Indomethacin in the Treatment of Detrusor Instability. Proceedings of the 8th International Continence Society Meeting, Manchester, England; Pergamon Press Ltd., Oxford, 1978, pp. 59–62.
3. **Cardozo, L., Stanton, S.L.** Genuine Stress Incontinence and

Detrusor Instability: A Clinical and Urodynamic Review of 200 Cases. *Br. J. Obstet Gynaecol.* 87:184, 1980.

4. **Cardozo, L., Stanton, S.L., Williams, J.E.** Detrusor Instability Following Surgery for Genuine Stress Incontinence. *Br. J. Urol.* 51:204–207, 1979.

5. **Cardozo, L., Stanton, S.L., Robinson, H., Hole, D.** Evaluation of Flurbiprofen in the Management of Detrusor Instability. Proceedings of the 9th International Continence Society Meeting, Rome, Guido Guidotti Editore, 1979, pp. 47–51.

6. **Farrar, D.J., Whiteside, G., Osborne, J., Turner-Warwick, R.** Urodynamic Analysis of Micturition Symptoms in the Female. *Surg. Gynecol. Obstet.* 141:875–881, 1975.

7. **Frewen, W.K.** An Objective Assessment of the Unstable Bladder of Psychosomatic Origin. *Br. J. Urol.* 50:246–249, 1978.

8. **Hodgkinson, C.P., Ayers, M., Drukker, B.** Dyssynergic Detrusor Dysfunction in the Apparently Normal Female. *Am. J. Obstet. Gynecol.* 87:717–730, 1963.

9. I.C.S. Definitions, Standardization of Terminology of Lower Urinary Tract Function. *Urology* 9:237–241, 1977.

10. **Ingleman-Sundberg, A.** Partial Denervation of the Bladder. *Acta Obstet. Gynecol. Scand.* 38:487–501, 1959.

11. **Rud, T., Andersson, K., Ulmsten, U.** Effects of Calcium Antagonists in Women with the Unstable Bladder. Proceedings of 8th International Continence Society Meeting, Manchester, England; Pergamon Press, Oxford, 1978, pp. 53–57.

12. **Stanton, S.L.** A Comparison of Emepronium Bromide with Flavoxate Hydrochloride in the Treatment of Urinary Incontinence. *J. Urol.* 110:529–532, 1973.

13. **Torrens, M., Griffiths, H.** Control of Uninhibited Bladder by Selective Sacral Neurectomy. *Br. J. Urol.* 46:639–644, 1974.

23 Psychiatric Aspects of Lower Urinary Tract Dysfunction*

Charles B. Stone, M.D.

Three syndromes of lower tract urinary dysfunction in women are complex phenomena with multiple contributing etiologies which may include psychogenesis. These are the urethral syndrome, urge incontinence or unstable bladder of the detrusor dyssnergia type and psychogenic retention. Primary care physicians, especially gynecologists and urologists, recognize that psychosocial factors in some patients contribute significantly to symptom production. Psychiatric evaluation of these patients contributes significantly to their care by defining underlying psychopathology and situational stresses and offers recommendations for appropriate treatment.

REVIEW OF NON-PSYCHIATRIC LITERATURE

In 1900 Bierhoff described the irritable bladder syndrome or bladder neurosis. He noted that a phlegmatic woman describes her pain as only a little discomfort while the neurasthenic type may magnify this into unbearable discomfort or "stabbing, cutting pains." He reported that of 57 patients, 4 had nervous conditions and in only 1 was there no appreciable vesical or perivesical cause.

In 1962 Smith found little in the literature about the influence of the psyche on urinary function although physicians relate such influence since ancient times. He quoted a Chinese proverb, "The bladder is the mirror of the soul."

* This work was supported by a National Institute of Mental Health Grant MH 10792-12.

Smith found that in psychosomatic cystitis the symptoms fluctuated with frequency only for a few hours each day; in psychogenic frequency there was usually an absence of nocturia, which implied normal bladder capacity despite frequent small voidings during the day; discomfort was not related to the act of urination, but was vague, poorly localized and without apparent correlations. He uniformly found sexual frustration in patients with psychosomatic cystitis. Smith condemned empirical organic therapy, including any form of manipulative or operative treatment, because it convinced the patient erroneously that there was serious organic disease. He emphasized that psychotherapy was the definitive treatment, since in addition to their urinary symptoms these patients had psychosexual difficulties with deep and basic psychological problems. The fact that a large proportion of these patients experienced relief of their vesical and other neurotic symptoms by psychotherapy was further proof of the verity of Smith's observations.

In 1963 Zufall reported that in eight years he treated 190 women with urethral syndrome, manifested by frequency, dysuria and pain in the back, flanks or abdomen. In diagnostic studies, including pyelograms and cystoscopies, he found no consistent pathological changes. With any form of treatment he noted that about one-third of his patients improved for more than 12 weeks. He also noted a history of dyspareunia in only nine patients. He regarded his patients as suffering from neuroses with hysterical somatization of emotional problems.

Bors and Comarr stated that psychic causes account for the symptom of frequency in 10% of women with this complaint. Other complaints accompanying psychogenic bladder dysfunction are also autonomic, such as headache, nausea and constipation; these women refer associated pain to the suprapubic region, lower abdomen, urethra or vagina. Psychodynamically, sexual factors are the most common cause, but other conflicts also enter the picture, such as self-punishment, fear of renal disease or grief for a friend who died of renal disease. Fear leads to frequency or "stress," as in the case of the middle-aged woman after an auto accident, who then wetted herself every time she came near a car.

In 1963 Hodgkinson et al. introduced the term dyssynergic detrusor dysfunction. They calculated the incidence of detrusor dyssynergia as 8.7% in their series of 735 patients with deficient urinary control. They commented that on the basis of medical custom the term neurogenic was as acceptable as dyssynergic. They emphasized that extreme detrusor dysfunction may develop in the apparently normal female. In their terminology "apparently normal" seems to imply the absence of positive neurologic or gynecologic findings but avoids taking psychogenic factors into account.

In responding to discussion of his paper, Hodgkinson described a patient operated upon five times for stress incontinence and apparently never cured. Finally, direct urethrocystometry yielded findings characteristic of voluntary voiding. He considered her to have psychogenic incontinence, associated with difficulties in her relationship with her husband, a chronic alcoholic, who remained sympathetic and relatively sober only so long as she had urinary difficulties. Hodgkinson then pointed out that the patient used her incontinence to keep her husband from drinking. Thus, he implicitly acknowledged a psychogenic factor, that is, the secondary gain to the patient from her symptom.

According to Green, detrusor dyssynergia is the second most common cause of urinary incontinence in women. He estimated that about 10% of all patients complaining of urinary incontinence suffer from pure detrusor dyssynergia, and that one-half of these women have this type of functional stress incontinence without abnormalities of anatomic support. He emphasized the importance of recognizing this latter group, since operations designed to correct anatomic stress incontinence fail to alleviate and usually increase the severity of the symptoms in patients with detrusor dyssynergia.

Green stated that detrusor dyssynergia is psychosomatic and functional fifty to eighty per cent of the time. He reported variability of symptoms in patients with detrusor dyssynergia, which is in keeping with its psychosomatic basis. He found that hyperirritable detrusor activity in these women, whose anatomic support mechanism is generally normal, is usually a manifestation of a readily recognizable underlying anxiety state and is often of long duration, sometimes dating back to early childhood. Thus, Green acknowledged the chronicity of the underlying psychopathology in these patients. Regarding treatment, Green reported that management of patients with detrusor dyssynergia was frequently difficult, and the results of treatment were unpredictable and often unsatisfactory. As important initial steps he advocated reassurance, with firm emphasis that no anatomic support problem existed, and an attempt to provide the patient with an understandable explanation of the mechanism involved as well as some insight into its underlying functional nature. Psychiatrically, these measures recommended by Green are quite useful. One meaning to the patient of such reassurance and explanations is that she receives positive suggestion from the physician. To the extent that these patients have underlying hysterical personality traits, which we believe is often the case, they are characteristically receptive to suggestion. That is, positive suggestion from an important person, the gynecologist, may immediately start the patient toward improvement. Green also mentioned the treatment of underlying anxiety or depression with appropriate sedatives, tranquilizers and antidepressants. The acknowledgment of psychogenic factors is a positive contribution to the literature. However, an alternative approach is probably preferable to psychopharmacologic treatment, namely, psychotherapuetic discussion with the patient about situational problems which we find almost invariably associated with chronic depression and anxiety in these patients.

Jeffcoate and Francis as well as Frewen emphasized psychosocial factors in reviewing etiology of functional types of urinary incontinence.

Marshall and Judd developed a definitive guide for the management of women with symptoms arising in the lower urinary tract. They recommend referral for psychiatric consultation when patients with urethral syndrome fail to respond to a variety of generally applicable therapies such as local applications of 5% silver nitrate, urinary antibiotics, urethral dilatation, urinary analgesics and tranquilizers. Psychiatric consultation frequently occurs in patients with incontinence who fail to respond to recognized therapy or whose incontinence fails to fit into a recognized diagnostic group. They found psychiatric consultation helpful in a number of cases in which the lower urinary tract symptoms proved to be a component of an unrecognized emotional disturbance, frequently depression.

REVIEW OF PSYCHIATRIC LITERATURE

Two types of chronic incontinence, urge incontinence and unstable bladder or detrusor dyssynergia, as well as urethral syndrome, are common psychosomatic disorders. However, there is very little in the English language psychiatric literature about them. Neither textbooks of psychiatry nor treatises on psychosomatic gynecology even mention them. The few psychiatric studies reviewed here represent nearly all available published contributions. Since we believe there are some similarities in underlying psychodynamics in patients with incontinence and those with acute psychogenic retention, we include some psychiatric studies of patients with retention. The psychoanalytic literature offers relevant formulations about psychodynamics.

In 1905 Freud wrote that children concern themselves with the problem of what sexual intercourse consists of, and they usually seek a solution to the mystery in some common activity concerned with the function of urination or defecation. Urination particularly appeals to their developing sense of logic since it is the only function of the phallus known to them. Also, Freud thought the urinary apparatus served temporarily in the place of the as yet undeveloped sexual apparatus to satisfy the child's curiosity. In 1908 Freud described the sexual instinct of man as highly complex and put together from contributions made by numerous constituents. Important contributions to sexual excitation are furnished by peripheral excitations of certain specifically designated areas of the body, including genitals, mouth, anus and urethra, which therefore deserve to be described as "erotogenic zones." Do character traits have a connection with excitation of particular erotogenic zones? Freud offered the opinion that intense burning ambition could develop in adults who earlier suffered from enuresis.

Menninger found that urination may at times express both erotic and aggressive elements of the personality. In some cases he regarded urination as having a sexual masturbatory meaning. He thought that either frequency or retention on a psychogenic basis expressed self-punitive tendencies, which in turn the individual used in attempting to atone for guilt over sexual thoughts or activities.

Wahl and Golden offered the hypothesis that urinary symptoms in adults represent an association with a wish to reexperience infantile pleasure in urination that is no longer acceptable to adults. Repression of this early infantile wish might account for the symptoms of retention. They found with remarkable regularity in patients with urinary retention that there were genital sexual conflicts of a repressed character. Genitals were considered taboo, and the individual invested the act of urination with forbidden, sensual, erotic feelings. Also, the wish for catheterization had sexual meaning, that of vicarious sexual gratification. They found their patients using their symptoms to permit avoidance of sexual relations, to provide an opportunity to be dependent, or to serve as acceptable punishment for the patient's neurotic guilt feelings.

Hollender found that women with psychogenic urinary retention struggled within themselves with the need to control angry, hostile or aggressive impulses. Aggressive impulses may take the form of a bodily symptom such as urination.

Larson et al. reported 37 cases of psychogenic urinary retention. Each patient had psychosomatic symptoms in other organ systems, predominantly headaches, low back pain and a variety of gastrointestinal symptoms. They evaluated 25 patients psychiatrically and found 17 to be neurotic and 8 psychotic. Of the 17 neurotics, they diagnosed 12 as having conversion hysteria and 3 as having

neurotic depression. Of the 8 psychotics, 5 were schizo-
phrenic and 3 psychotically depressed.

Yazmajian reported the psychoanalytic treatment of three
adult patients, all toilet trained before the age of two years
and never enuretic, in whom excessive functional urination
took the place of weeping, crying or sobbing. Each patient
went through a prolonged period in early childhood when
he or she wept, cried or sobbed bitterly because of the
mother's withdrawal of love and attention. Weeping released feelings of abandonment coupled with rage and a
sense of absolute helplessness which was the affective tone
that dominated this phase of their lives. As an adult, one
patient found that whenever she was inclined to weep, the
impulse to urinate supervened to restore emotional detach-
ment. When aware of this the patient wept briefly and while
shedding tears the impulse to urinate disappeared.

Straub, Ripley and Wolf reported an experimental psychiatric study of both men and women patients with either
urinary urgency and frequency or with retention. They
studied all their patients both urologically and neurologically and found them free of irritative or obstructive lesions
of the genitourinary tract or structural neurologic disease.
They found a commonly overt association between bladder
hyperfunction and urinary frequency with a reaction of
anxiety and resentment accompanying conflict. Bladder
hypofunction with urinary retention usually accompanied
emotional repression and a general reaction of withdrawal
and being overwhelmed. In some patients the two patterns
of disturbance alternated. In the authors' opinion such
patients dealt differently from time to time with conflict
situations. They found an association of tension, anxiety
and comparatively aggressive behavior with vesical hyperfunction, and an association of either blandness or dejection
and non-aggressive behavior with vesical hypofunction.
They concluded that recognition of psychosomatic phenomena involving the bladder depends on positive identification
of situational conflicts which correlate with bladder disturbance.

In 1962 Aboulker and Chertok reported the successful
treatment of a twenty-four year old woman with chronic
incontinence unresponsive to four pelvic and bladder-neck
operations. Psychotherapeutic interviewing followed by
hypnosis resulted in complete cessation of incontinence.
They reported follow-up of three years without recurrence
of incontinence. They failed to find a single reference in
the literature acknowledging the role of emotional factors
in diurnal incontinence.

In 1977 Chertok, Bourguignon, Guillon and Aboulker reported on both clinical aspects and the evolution of etiolog-

ical concepts of the urethral syndrome. They reviewed the literature in the German and French languages published in the past century. As early as 1859 Briquet noted the occurrence of the urethral syndrome in hysterical women. They regard Dejerine and Gauckler as having advanced etiological thought in 1911 in maintaining that disturbance of micturition and urogenital pain derived from disorders of sexuality. They state that today there is no satisfactory etiological explanation of the syndrome. They regard the psychological component in urethral syndrome as particularly important for several reasons: (1) The frequent absence of any physical lesion; even when present the lesion does not explain the severity of the symptoms. Moreover, the existence of an organic lesion in no way excludes the possibility of a coexisting psychological component. (2) The coincidence of the inception or recurrence of the disorder with a conflictual situation. (3) The presence of psychosexual disturbances in all patients. (4) The possible aggravation of the condition by local treatment or surgical operations, which leads in some cases to polysurgery. (5) The potentialities of psychotherapy. (6) The special character and expressive value of the pain. Concerning clinical aspects these authors found that about 20% of women attending a urological clinic in a Paris hospital had the urethral syndrome. The usual definition of disturbance of micturition and vesical pain may be too restrictive since frequently the pain involves not only the bladder area but the entire pelvic region as well. They studied the records of 55 women patients seen from 1952 to 1970. Eighteen of these patients suffered solely from pain, either vesical, urethral or genital; 19 patients had both dysuria and pain. Sixty-three percent complained of pain in other areas, such as headaches, heaviness of the stomach, heartburn or polysystemic complaints. In 40% there were complaints of anxiety, depression or phobias. The most significant line of inquiry was the patients' verbalization of their symptoms. In some there were thinly disguised sexual or pregnancy fantasies. The age of onset was 36 to 50 years. Most were married and many had no sexual activity. Of 23 patients who agreed to psychotherapy, 11 discontinued after two or three sessions, 9 discontinued after one to two months, and 3 continued for one to three years. They conducted follow-up interviews with eight patients. These were of three types. One group experienced no change in their symptoms. These patients gave up on any further steps to secure treatment, pretended they had never had treatment, felt angry with their physicians or felt a sense of defeat of their physicians. A second group discontinued psychotherapy but continued to make the rounds of other doctors' offices. A third group were those who recovered with psychotherapy. Some had "veritable therapeutic miracle cure" after one interview. These authors recommend that most patients not consult psychiatrists, since the patient derives the greatest benefit from a sustained relationship with her own physician—a professional relationship based upon the patient's trust and the doctor's readiness and availability to "listen" and to understand.

In 1977 Hafner, Stanton and Guy reported a psychiatric study of women with urgency and urgency incontinence in the absence of organic structural bladder and urethral abnormality. They wished to determine the extent to which these symptoms yield to psychological and behavioral treatments. Those patients who appeared most disturbed had symptoms that were often bizarre or atypical, with pain in areas other than the bladder as a common feature. Most had grossly disturbed interpersonal relationships, had recently lost a close relative, or had a history of repeated bereavement. In four patients whose husbands had serious accidents, the urinary symptoms appeared related to this and to the stress of coping with the consequent disablement and loss of earnings and status. These patients reluctantly acknowledged any emotional or interpersonal problems; they tended to suffer more from incontinence than frequency. These authors found that treatment by group and individual psychotherapy benefited one-third of the patients considerably; one-third refused treatment or ceased therapy prematurely and one-third improved slightly or not at all.

PRESENT STUDY

Twenty patients with chronic urinary incontinence were referred from the Gynecological Urology Clinic to the Gynecological Psychiatry Clinic at the Harbor-UCLA Medical Center. Before referral these patients received thorough urogynecologic examinations and treatment as described recently by Marshall and Judd. During these examinations various "challenges" were directed at the bladder. These included jolt, cough, straining or bearing down, and at times the use of cold or bethanechol injection to provoke the detrusor to contract independently. Patients unable to stop or interrupt the stream while voiding usually had an unstable bladder which could be related to the dynamics of psychosomatic symptom production. Patients who failed to respond to treatment, including anticholinergic drugs, received psychiatric evaluation and treatment. Sixteen of the 20 patients were in the 40- to 60-year age group, which is generally the time when patients seek treatment for such incontinence. Fifteen of these patients in the 40 to 60 age range were multiparous and 12 had previous hysterectomies. Of the entire group of 20 patients, only 3 gave a history of childhood enuresis. A fourth patient had had urge incontinence since the age of 12 years.

In this study the author used psychotherapeutic interviewing as the exclusive method of psychiatric evaluation. This chapter contains a detailed description of this method which

Chertok et al., Friederich, and Stone and Judd strongly advocate. There were three major psychiatric findings. First, in all 20 patients there were severe prolonged life situational stresses, that is, serious problems in the environment of the patient, especially in significant relationships. All of the patients except the three oldest, aged 59, 63 and 75 years, had available sex partners, but all of these patients regarded themselves as suffering too much from their incontinence to be able to participate in sex. The second prominent finding in 19 patients was chronic depression, which was, with one exception, associated mainly with situational problems rather than with biological factors, and therefore, not amenable to treatment with antidepressant drugs. The one exception was a 59-year-old woman with involutional depression and both urgency incontinence and detrusor dyssynergia. Treatment with a combination of imipramine, thioridazine and psychotherapy resulted in relief of both her depression and her urinary incontinence.

The third major psychiatric finding in 12 patients was functional symptomatology in other organ systems, i.e., polysystemic somatization of anxiety characteristic of hysterical personalities. The most frequent functional symptoms in these patients were the same as those previously reported in association with acute urinary retention by Larson et al, namely, headaches, backaches and gastrointestinal symptoms.

A few patients with urethral syndrome were referred for psychiatric evaluation. Tentatively, it appears that these patients have similar psychiatric findings, with chronic depression, hysterical personality traits and severe prolonged life situational problems in all patients. Our findings so far are in accord with those reported by Chertok et al. One patient was successfully treated for urge incontinence and detrusor dyssynergia and then developed painful urethral syndrome.

Three patients with psychogenic urinary retention received evaluation and therapy in the Gynecological Psychiatry Clinic. A detailed description of them and a patient with the urethral syndrome follow.

CASE REPORTS

Case 1. This 39-year-old separated unemployed black woman, mother of four teen-age children, had had a vaginal hysterectomy and anteroposterior vaginal repair four years previously. For two years she received treatment in the Gynecological Urology Clinic for detrusor dyssynergia and urge incontinence. For several months she complained of "bladder pain" not always associated with urination. She was considered to have chronic pelvic pain and was referred to the Gynecological Psychiatry Clinic. During the initial psychotherapeutic interview she complained of severe bladder pain for many months. She related the onset of her depression to the time that her husband left her five years earlier for a younger woman. She said she did not want any other man and still loved her husband, although he did not want to see her or have anything to do with her. Her depression intensified in recent years due to the deaths of close relatives, which she felt as further abandonments. Her husband refused to see two of their children, which evidently deeply pained her. Three weeks later on the second visit, she was symptom-free and reported she had had no pain since her first interview. On two months follow-up she remained asymptomatic.

It was, of course, unpredictable that the interpretation of her deep pain as related to her husband's attitude was helpful to her. Perhaps this was a psychosomatic version of a "transference cure," in which there are special positive meanings to a patient, usually not consciously known by the patient, as a result of the meeting with the psychotherapist. Chertok et al. also reported remarkable relief of chronic pain with one psychotherapeutic interview with similar patients.

Case 2. This 49-year-old white married woman had had a total abdominal hysterectomy ten years earlier and a Marshall-Marchetti procedure four years earlier, since which time she had been under treatment in the Gynecological Urology Clinic for urge incontinence and unstable bladder syndrome. The onset of depression caused her referral to the Gynecological Psychiatry Clinic. She walked with a marked limp and had limited use of her withered right arm due, she said, to a birth injury and cerebral palsy. Her disabled husband was unemployable. She spoke at length about her frustrations in attempting to deal with social agencies upon which she depended for a meager disability pension. She was chronically depressed, tearful and felt trapped in a difficult life situation. At first she challenged the interviewer and showed disrespectful behavior, but with gradual rapport she expressed appreciation for the interest shown in her. Considering the difficult life situation and chronic depression, the goal of psychotherapy was to encourage her to take increasing doses of imipramine to treat her incontinence. She required six months of biweekly psychotherapy before she agreed to take 100 mg of imipramine each night. Two weeks later she reported that she did not like the side effect of dry mouth, but that her incontinence was no longer a problem when she took the imipramine for several nights consecutively.

This case illustrates the formidable psychological resistance in some patients to accepting a regimen of pharmacological treatment. Rather than regarding this as a problem in compliance, it is preferable to conceptualize the problem as that of establishing a treatment alliance between the physician and the patient. In this case it was first essential that the physician not be put off by the patient's defensive and unpleasant attitude. Secondly, the patient had to develop some feeling of trust and a sense of true interest on the part of the physician.

Case 3. This 26-year-old white single woman had been unable to urinate except by self-catheterization for three years following a Marshall-Marchetti procedure to correct overflow incontinence. She developed a vesicocutaneous fistula requiring several surgical procedures. On admission to Harbor-UCLA Medical Center for treatment of suprapubic skin breakdown, surgeons removed a 5×4 cm mass containing a sinus tract and inflammatory tissue. Postoperatively, she continued to be unable to urinate except by self-catheterization. She continually pleaded for "shots" for severe lower abdominal pain. Injections of normal saline solution completely relieved her pain. Repeated cystoscopic and urethrocystometric pressure studies revealed no anatomical or physiological explanation for her inability to urinate. Psychiatric examination disclosed a moderately mentally retarded young woman with hysterical personality traits who was chronically under emotional stress in her home situation. Her anxious and protective parents kept her from being sexually involved with a young man with cerebral palsy who wanted to date her. She and her parents reluctantly accepted transfer from the Urology Service to the Psychiatric In-Patient Unit. Upon reaching the psychiatric unit and for the ten days she remained there, she willingly gave up her catheter and urinated almost every hour during the day by running warm water over her pelvic area to initiate urination. She did not urinate at night. She received no psychotrophic drugs. She was quite happy with this result but on return home she soon reverted to self-catheterization. Her parents refused to bring her for psychiatric follow-up, insisting upon the need for further urological procedures.

Case 4. This 43-year-old white married woman required referral from the Gynecological Urology Clinic to the Gynecological Psychiatric Clinic for evaluation of her unusual behavior. She had required an indwelling Foley catheter for three months following a Burch procedure and posterior repair for treatment of genuine stress incontinence. This necessitated hospitalization on the Gynecological Service three times for a total of five weeks to treat her urinary retention, which remained refractory to treatment. On psychiatric examination she was grossly hypomanic and restless and had pressured speech. Psychiatric hospitalization followed for six weeks. At age 20 she married a taxi driver who supported her well. There were three sons, 19, 15 and 11 years of age. Severe marital problems resulted in the absence of sexual relations for the two years prior to her referral. According to her husband, for years she frequently had gone to hospital emergency rooms and doctors' offices complaining of multiple insignificant bodily symptoms. Also, prolonged bouts of depression alternated with hyperactive behavior for several years. During psychiatric hospitalization treatment consisted of milieu therapy and a total dose of thioridazine of 100 mg daily. Shortly after admission to the psychiatric unit, she began to improve and within three weeks both her hyperactive behavior and her urinary symptoms subsided. The final psychiatric diagnosis was cyclothymic personality, a benign mild variant of manic depressive illness. She continued treatment with thioridazine for a few months after hospitalization. Brief psychotherapy visits in the Gynecological Psychiatric Clinic continued for four years. During that time she remained free of both hyperactive behavior and urinary symptoms.

Psychodynamically, both patients in Cases 3 and 4 hesitated to express resentment or angry feelings, felt trapped in difficult life situations from which they felt unable to extricate themselves, and had sexual inhibitions. Both probably gained substitutive sexual gratification from catheterization.

**PSYCHO-
THERAPEUTIC
INTERVIEW**

Green observed that management of patients with detrusor dyssynergia was frequently difficult, and the results of treatment were unpredictable and often unsatisfactory. This statement is equally applicable to some patients with urethral syndrome, especially when the symptomatology is significantly psychosomatic or functional. Nevertheless, patients generally expect the primary physician to provide all necessary treatment and do not wish to be referred to psychiatrists. In order for treatment to be most effective the physician is responsible for developing a "working alliance" with the patient. Greenson suggested the concept of working alliance. This concept describes the patient's regard for the physician as an ally in a mutual working relationship rather than as a formidable, frightening authority figure. Development of a satisfactory working alliance enhances the patient's motivation to overcome her illness and sense of helplessness, stimulates her conscious and rational willingness to cooperate, and maximizes her potential ability to follow the physician's instructions. According to Greenson the psychological process that makes this possible is the patient's identification with the physician's approach to understanding the patient. That is, the patient needs to realize the physician's interest in her as a person who is ill, rather than as a case of a disease.

What can the physician do to develop the working alliance? The primary care physician provides the necessary psychotherapeutic intervention as an integral aspect of treatment. The best means to accomplish this is the psychotherapeutic interview, which has the practical advantage of being both a diagnostic and therapeutic process at the same time. The diagnostic aspect consists of talking with the patient to find out whether she has significant life situational problems, whether she is chronically depressed and whether she has functional symptoms in other organ systems characteristic of hysterical personality trends. With experience, such an interview need not take more than 10 or 15 minutes.

An inquiry about life situational stresses uses certain specific questions. Does she get satisfaction from everyday activities? Are there difficulties in her closest relationships, such as with husband, immediate family members, relatives, co-workers or employers? The focus is on present life situations. It is not necessary to delve deeply into the past or development history, except for one question about childhood enuresis. Specifically, this line of inquiry is aimed at finding out how well the patient coped with situational problems just preceding the onset of urinary symptoms. To the patient her distress in her current life is real and as much a source of disability as the "real" genitourinary pathology for which the physician searches in order to explain her symptoms. When treating a patient with chronic complicated situational problems, the physician obviously need not expect himself to solve all the patient's life problems. It is a valuable service to the patient to offer a sympathetic ear plus a little useful objective advice about any part of the problem.

Chronic depression is readily recognizable, even though the patient may maintain a facade of smiling cheerfulness on certain important occasions, such as a visit to her physician. The so-called "smiling depression" is chronic. The chronic patient cannot remember specifically when the depression began nor can she spontaneously connect it with any happening in her life. She usually relates abandonment of whatever her life goals may have been. An ominous but useful finding in psychiatric history-taking is that the patient as a girl did not have any life goals or ambition for her future. Such history usually indicates a patient who had severe traumatization of her self-image in early childhood. As an adult she tends to welcome invalidism. Usually she feels herself miserably trapped with no hope of extricating herself. Often these include her home and marriage, and she sadly accepts her fate, but in ill health. Patients with chronic incontinence tend to feel too indisposed to participate in sex. In our experience those with urethral syndrome say they tend to avoid sex, but not as consistently as the patients with chronic incontinence. The chronically depressed patient feels like crying, but embarrassment prevents it. She prefers to be alone to cry, and when she cries she isn't sure of just exactly what she is crying about, and characteristically does not get much relief from crying.

The third area of inquiry in the brief psychotherapeutic interview regards functional symptoms in other organ systems. To elicit these symptoms it is often useful to ask the patient if she ever feels nervous in any part of her body. Often the physician discovers that the patient never before attempted to verbalize her bodily feelings. The process of verbalization is in itself psychotherapeutic, since the patient immediately changes perceptions of vague physical uneasiness into secondary process, that is, logical language. This process may in itself reduce anxiety and lead to prevention of anxiety through understanding of the emotional significance of physical sensations or symptoms. The usual alternative of prescribing minor tranquilizing drugs tends to perpetuate the patient's fear of helplessness in preventing symptom recurrence.

PSYCHIATRY AND THE URETHRAL SYNDROME

Pain is a prominent clinical feature in many women patients with urethral syndrome. The reports of Bierhoff, Smith, Zufall, and Bors and Comarr all discuss the symptoms of pain. In recent psychiatric studies reviewed above, Hafner et al. found pain in some patients while Chertok et al. placed major emphasis upon it. In studying women with chronic pelvic pain Friederich found that some also had dysuria, urgency or frequency. Chertok et al. discuss their patients' sexually symbolic fantasies associated with descriptions of pain, its chronicity and tenacity, refractoriness to treatment, and the tendency to invalidism.

Friederich states that it is possible for pain to be completely a psychic experience based on unconscious memories or fantasies, that is, a patient describing a pain as sharp and sticking like a knife, probably never actually had a knife plunging into her body. This is a fantasy that may be unlike someone else's fantasy. In discussing psychodynamics, Friederich explained that early life or recent rejection probably evoked great anger, but the patient suppressed her anger via guilt feelings. When she evokes forbidden angry feelings, a woman may develop pain as a way of coping. In the sexual sphere, if as a child a patient felt guilty about expressed sexual feelings, in situations of sexual arousal as a woman, she may develop pain. Another setting for pain is loss, actual, threatened, or fantasied. Identifying with the lost person through pain is an unconsciously determined way of continuing a relationship in the patient's mind and of emotionally holding on to the lost person. Pain is more likely if the patient had ambivalent feelings with strong anger and guilt feelings about the lost person. The pain in this sense keeps the lost one present inside the patient and helps diminish the intense grief that may threaten to overwhelm the patient.

We concur completely with these clinical observations and psychodynamic formulations presented by both Chertok et al. and by Friederich. These findings are similar to our own unpublished findings in a group of over 40 women patients with chronic pelvic pain whom we studied psychiatrically. Referral to the Gynecological Psychiatry Clinic at Harbor-UCLA Medical Center occurred after extensive gynecological evaluation and treatment both for the pelvic pain and for the urethral syndrome. Tentatively we regard women patients with painful urethral syndrome as psychiatrically similar to those with chronic pelvic pain. Our opinion that painful urethral syndrome is a clinical variant or subgroup of chronic pelvic pain is supported by the opinion of Chertok et al. that the present nomenclature is too restrictive, insofar as the patient expresses pain not only in the vesical area, but frequently also in the pelvic regions as well.

DRUG THERAPY

The use of minor tranquilizing or antidepressant drugs involves serious therapeutic dilemmas in these patients. Minor tranquilizers, such as diazepam or chlordiazepoxide, assist in the management of mild anxiety or depression only if used sporadically. This specifically contraindicates daily uninterrupted use for weeks or months. Such prolonged use leads to loss of the initial benefit and results in habituation to the drug. The patients under consideration here all have chronic subjective distress associated with chronic situational problems and are not likely to be satisfied with only a few days' use of minor tranquilizers. The likelihood of becoming habituated to these drugs correlates with personality traits of dependency, either clearly evident passive-dependency or more subtle unsatisfied dependency needs in seemingly active, vigorous people. Recent studies of pharmacology of minor tranquilizers suggest that these drugs in therapeutic doses impair mental acuity and that this is more of a problem in older patients. Imipramine, a tricyclic antidepressant, does not cause drug dependence, but has other limitations. When treating a depressed patient, the physician must rule out suicidal tendency, since overdoses with imipramine are difficult to treat and are likely to be fatal due to production of heart block and ventricular arrhythmias. The therapeutic dosage range is narrow. The usual minimum therapeutic dose is 50 to 75 mg daily, while the generally accepted maximum dose is 300 mg daily, at which level patients usually do not tolerate the distressing side effects. Imipramine relieves chronic urinary incontinence in some patients, such as the patient in the second case report above. The mechanism of action is not clearly understood and may not be adequately explained as due either to the anticholinergic effect, the alpha stimulating effect or the central antidepressant effect or some combination of effects. Nevertheless, imipramine is an appropriate empirical therapy for some patients with chronic urinary incontinence.

URINARY RETENTION

Compared with urethral syndrome or incontinence, it is a relatively rare psychosomatic disease, but definitely does occur, as evidenced by two cases from one teaching hospital. The psychopathology in patients with psychogenic retention tends to be so severe that the primary care physician must involve a psychiatric consultant in management of the case. This contrasts with the main thrust of this presentation, which encourages the primary care physician to provide all necessary care, including psychotherapeutic intervention.

CONCLUSIONS

The clinical experience described here, together with reports by Chertok et al., Hafner et al., and Stone and Judd and others, suggests that there are significant psychosocial etiological factors in some women patients with two common psychosomatic disorders of lower tract urinary dysfunction, urethral syndrome and chronic incontinence of the urgency type or detrusor dyssynergia. Three major psychiatric findings in a group of 20 patients with incontinence reported here are prolonged severe life situational stresses, chronic depression and hysterical personality traits. These findings are similar to those reported by others in patients with urethral syndrome, as well as in patients with incontinence. Further psychiatric studies of such patients are needed to determine whether these findings apply to larger numbers of patients. Treatment of these patients by the primary care physician includes psychotherapeutic interviewing in order to allow recognition and treatment of significant psychosocial problems.

References

1. **Aboulker, P., Chertok, L.** Emotional Factors in Stress Incontinence. *Psychosom. Med.* 24:507, 1962.
2. **Bierhoff, F.** On the so-called "Irritable Bladder" in the Female. *Am. J. Med. Sci.* 120:670, 1900.
3. **Bors, E., Comarr, A. E.** *Neurological Urology.* University Park Press, Baltimore, 1971, pp. 120–121.
4. **Chertok, L., Bourguignon, O., Guillon, F., Aboulker, P.** Urethral Syndrome in the Female (Irritable Bladder): The Expression of Fantasies about the Urogenital Area. *Psychosom. Med.* 39:1, 1977.
5. **Freud, S.** Character and Anal Erotism. In *Standard Edition of the Complete Psychological Works of Sigmund Freud*, Vol. 9. Hogarth Press, London, 1959.
6. **Freud, S.** Three Essays on the Theory of Sexuality. In *Standard Edition of the Complete Psychological Works of Sigmund Freud*, Vol. 7. Hogarth Press, London, 1963.
7. **Frewen, W. K.** Urgency Incontinence. *J. Obstet. Gynaecol. Br. Commonw.* 79:77, 1972.
8. **Friederich, M. A.** Psychological Aspects of Chronic Pelvic Pain. *Clin. Obstet. Gynecol.* 19:399, 1976.
9. **Green, T. H., Jr.** Urinary Stress Incontinence: Differential Diagnosis, Pathophysiology, and Management. *Am. J. Obstet. Gynecol.* 122:368, 1975.
10. **Greenson, R. R.** The Working Alliance and Transference Neurosis. *Psychoanal. Q.* 34:155, 1965.

11. **Greenson, R. R.** *The Technique and Practice of Psychoanalysis.* International Universities Press, New York, 1967, pp. 192–193.
12. **Hafner, R. J., Stanton, S. L., Guy, J.** A Psychiatric Study of Women with Urgency and Urgency Incontinence. *Br. J. Urol.* 49:211, 1977.
13. **Hodgkinson, C. P., Ayers, M. A., Drukker, B. H.** Dyssynergic Detrusor Dysfunction in the Apparently Normal Female. *Am. J. Obstet. Gynecol.* 87:717, 1963.
14. **Jeffcoate, T. N. A., Francis, W. J. A.** Urgency Incontinence in the Female. *Am. J. Obstet. Gynecol.* 94:604, 1966.
15. **Larson, J. W., Swenson, W. M., Utz, D. C., Steinhilber, R. M.** Psychogenic Urinary Retention in Women. *J.A.M.A.* 184:697, 1963.
16. **Marshall, J. R., Judd, G. E.** Guide for the Management of Women with Symptoms Arising in the Lower Urinary Tract. *Clin. Obstet. Gynecol.* 19:247, 1976.
17. **Menninger, K. A.** Some Observations on the Psychological Factors in Urination and Genitourinary Affections. *Psychoanal. Rev.* 28:117, 1941.
18. **Nesbitt, R. E., Jr., Hollender, M. H., Feldman, P. M., Glazer, J. A., Hayes, R. C., Ferro, P. L.** Psychogenic Urinary Retention. *Int. Psychiatry Clin.* 2:561, 1965.
19. **Smith, D. R.** Psychosomatic 'Cystitis.' *J. Urol.* 87:359, 1962.
20. **Stone, C. B., and Judd, G. E.** Psychogenic Aspects of Urinary Incontinence in Women. *Clin. Obstet. Gynecol.* 21:807, 1978.
21. **Straub, L. R., Ripley, H. S., Wolf, S.** Disturbances of Bladder Function Associated with Emotional States. *J.A.M.A.* 141:1139, 1949.
22. **Wahl, C. W., Golden, J. S.** Psychogenic Urinary Retention. In *New Dimensions in Psychosomatic Medicine*, edited by C. W. Wahl. Little Brown, Boston, 1964, pp. 313–335.
23. **Yazmajian, R. V.** Pathological Urination and Weeping. *Psychoanal. Q.* 35:40, 1966.
24. **Zufall, R.** Treatment of the Urethral Syndrome in Women. *J.A.M.A.* 184:138, 1963.

24 Functional Electrical Stimulation

Thomas A. McCarthy, M.D.

Nearly two decades ago, investigators began to use electrical stimulation of the pelvic floor for the treatment of various voiding disorders. It provides effective therapy for urinary incontinence due to sphincter weakness and uninhibited bladder contractions in certain patients (4, 10, 11). Electrical bladder stimulation may reestablish detrusor contractions in patients with atonic, areflexic bladders as well (21). Due primarily to the lack of knowledge of basic detrusor urethral neurophysiology and to the neuromuscular complexity of voiding disorders, progress in this area continues to be slow. However, it holds sufficient promise to consider it as potential therapy for the relief of incontinence in selected patients.

MECHANISM OF ACTION

The basic functions of the lower urinary tract are storage and emptying. The muscles of the pelvic and genitourinary diaphragms, bladder wall and the intrinsic and extrinsic muscles of the urethra control these functions. Balanced nervous system reflexes and voluntary nervous system control orchestrate the coordinated activity of these different muscles. The central and peripheral nervous systems constitute a complex network which initiates and transports minute electrical impulses from one point to another. Alteration of these impulses, or creation of new impulses, enhances or inhibits the function of the urethral and vesical end organs. In various disease states or anatomical conditions, the preexisting normal neural control over these end

255

organs is insufficient for proper control and maintenance of continence. Functional electrical stimulation improves that control by applying external electrical impulses to the neural regulatory system (17, 18).

MECHANICS

Functional electrical stimulation (FES) stimulates the pelvic floor or inhibits the bladder by means of several different delivery methods. The first attempts to supply external electric current to the pelvic floor involved surgically implanted devices for the control of stress incontinence (4). Through a retropubic approach the investigators applied permanent electrodes directly to the pelvic floor musculature. With stimulation, tetanic contraction of the pelvic floor resulted and some patients became continent. In spite of initial success, implanted devices often broke or the electrodes migrated from their original placement sites, rendering the device functionless. This required repeat operation (2). Because of these disadvantages, the second generation of FES stimulators included removable external devices (Figures 24.1 and 24.2).

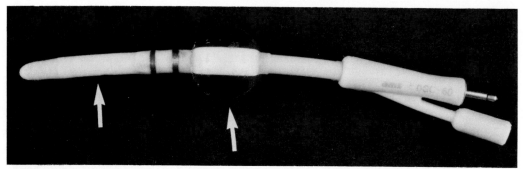

Figure 24.1. The intra-anal FES stimulating electrode. The two balloons (arrows) assure retention in the anal sphincter. (American Medical Systems, Minneapolis, Minn.)

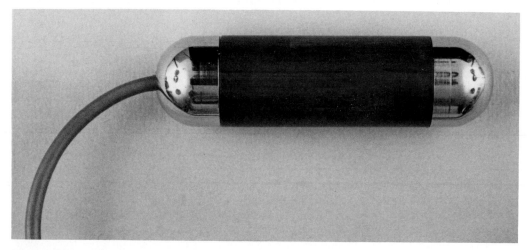

Figure 24.2. The intravaginal FES stimulating electrode. (Brown Corp, Santa Barbara, Calif.)

The first such external device was an anal plug electrode (15), which delivered a constant tetanizing current. Some patients with stress urinary incontinence achieved fair results. At about the same time a vaginal pessary appeared which delivered electrical current through the vagina in an effort to achieve the same effects (1, 3, 5). Because of various technical difficulties with these devices, the next few years saw alterations in their electromechanics. The introduction of biphasic currents stopped electrode blackening, tissue injury, and resulting poor function (16, 17). The results of trials of different pulse widths, frequencies and voltage ranges improved results and helped to determine the mode of action of the devices.

Initially, the effect of electrical stimulation was thought to be on the basis of direct stimulation to the levator muscles, which, upon contraction, kept the patient continent. An added benefit was that the patients slowly reeducated those muscles which were important in continence control and this facilitated their pelvic floor exercise programs (9, 20). As the electrophysiology developed further, it became apparent that a major mode of action of FES was via reflex pathways activating the pudendal nerve (22). Further study implicated other reflex pathways which caused inhibition of vesical contractility. This discovery increased the potential usefulness of FES (12, 13, 19).

Most recently several elegant studies using both animal and human subjects further elucidated the mode of action of FES, as well as determined its applicability to various clinical conditions (8). Using vaginal plug electrodes these investigators demonstrated several major characteristics of FES. Most importantly, they showed that the pudendal nerve mediates the effect of electrical stimulation, via both its afferent and efferent limbs (Figure 24.3). Efferent pudendal nerve stimulation mediated the increase in urethral closure pressure required for effective control of stress incontinence. Blocking the neuromuscular junction with succinyl choline abolished the effect of FES on the urethra (8). There was no evidence that spinal reflex mechanisms are important in augmenting urethral closure pressure. It required only an intact pudendal motor innervation. Their studies also indicated that precise placement of the active electrode within a narrow range of 1.0 cm is critical to maximize results. Since such electrode placement is specific for each patient, the urethral closure pressure profile best determined the site of optimal placement.

Two reflex arcs mediate bladder inhibition during FES (Figure 24.3). The afferent limb of the pudendal nerve initiates both reflex arcs. At low intravesical pressures the hypogastric (sympathetic) efferents mediate bladder inhibition. At high pressures, inhibition of the pelvic (parasym-

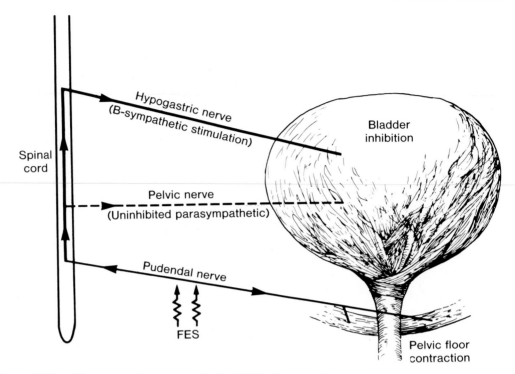

Figure 24.3.   Nervous pathways mediating FES. Direct stimulation of the pudendal nerve stimulates pelvic muscle contraction and inhibits detrusor contraction by inhibition of the pelvic nerve (parasympathetic) and stimulation of the hypogastric nerve (beta stimulation).

pathetic) efferents completes the reflexogenic bladder inhibition. Whether this occurs through a spinal mechanism which selects one pathway over the other dependent upon bladder volume or whether both reflex pathways are always active concurrently is open to question. In any case, detrusor inhibition occurs.

For both urethral closure and bladder inhibition the pudendal nerve is the initial pathway mediating FES (Figure 24.3). Since the desired results are unique and the portion of the pudendal nerve to be stimulated differs for each organ, a maximal response with minimal energy consumption requires two types of electrical characteristics. For urethral closure, a stimulation frequency of 50 Hz, a pulse duration of 1 to 2 msec using alternating pulses and intermittent stimulation is the most efficient. Intermittent, rather than constant, stimulation circumvents the problem of muscle fatigue without sacrificing effectiveness. Bladder inhibition, on the other hand, responds best to a stimulation frequency of 10 Hz with a pulse duration of 2 msec. The patient's individual needs and the urodynamic findings determine the specific frequency and pulse duration. Individual adjustment of voltage from 2 to 12 volts improves efficacy and patient tolerance. For those patients with mixed urge and stress incontinence, pulse characteristics similar to those for urge incontinence are the most effective.

Currently the removable anal and vaginal FES devices are the most popular. Patient acceptance and the ability to retain the device are the major determinants of which device to employ. The vaginal plug is more versatile because its placement can be changed to coincide with maximally efficient stimulation positions (8).

CLINICAL USEFULNESS

The important question to be answered with FES involves its ultimate clinical usefulness. Early reports were quite optimistic. However, more recent reports indicate that FES is most applicable to patients with stress incontinence who are also the best operative candidates (6, 7, 14). This includes the younger age groups and patients without prior incontinence surgery. Since surgery with adequate preoperative evaluation is successful in 80 to 95% of cases of genuine stress incontinence, others suggest that FES is a second line of defense for women who are poor operative risks or refuse surgery (19).

It seems that FES has a major potential clinical usefulness in the treatment of patients with uninhibited detrusor contractions where medical therapy has limited usefulness. If investigators develop FES technically as a specific inhibitor of reflex bladder contractions, it will become a major clinical therapeutic modality.

SUMMARY

The use of functional electrical stimulation of the pelvic floor for voiding disorders spans approximately 20 years. Since its development, investigators directed extensive efforts in an attempt to make it clinically useful. Because of initial technical difficulties and because of the existence of other treatment modalities which work as well, if not better, FES is not overly popular. Recently, insight into the mechanism of action of FES, particularly in detrusor reflex inhibition, makes this a promising future therapy of this condition. In addition, FES may become an important therapy for genuine stress incontinence for those patients who are not surgical candidates.

References

1. **Alexander, S., Rowan, D.** An Electric Pessary for Stress Incontinence. *Lancet* 1:728, 1968.
2. **Alexander, S., Rowan, D.** Electrical Control of Urinary Incontinence. A Clinical Appraisal. *Br. J. Surg.* 57:766, 1970.
3. **Alexander, S., Rowan, D., Millar, W. et al.** Treatment of Urinary Incontinence by Electric Pessary. *Br. J. Urol.* 42:184, 1970.
4. **Caldwell, K.P.S., Cook, P.J., Flack, F.C. et al.** Stress Incon-

tinence in Females: Report on 31 Patients Treated by Electrical Implant. *J. Obstet. Gynaec. Br. Commonw.* 75:777, 1968.

5. **De Soldenhoff, R., McDonnell, H.** New Device for Control of Female Urinary Incontinence. *Br. Med. J.* 4:230, 1969.

6. **Edwards, L., Malvern, J.** Electronic Control of Incontinence: A Critical Review of the Present Situation. *Br. J. Urol.* 44: 467, 1972.

7. **Edwards, L. E.** The Investigation and Management of Incontinence of Urine in Women. *Ann. R. Coll. Surg. Engl.* 52:69, 1973.

8. **Erlandson, B.E., Fall, M.** Intravaginal Electrical Stimulation in Urinary Incontinence. An Experimental and Clinical Study. *Scand. J. Urol. Nephrol.* Suppl. 44, 1977.

9. **Glen, E.S.** Effective and Safe Control of Incontinence by the Intra-anal Plug Electrode. *Br. J. Surg.* 58:249, 1971.

10. **Godec, C., Cass, A.C., Ayala, G.F.** Bladder Inhibition with Functional Electrical Stimulation. *Urology* 6:663, 1975.

11. **Godec, C., Cass, A.C.** Electrical Stimulation for Incontinence. Technique, Selection and Results. *Urology* 7:388, 1976.

12. **Godec, C., Cass, A.C.** Electrical Stimulation for Incontinence in Myelomeningocele. *J. Urol.* 120:729, 1978.

13. **Godec, C., Cass, A.C.** Electrical Stimulation for Voiding Dysfunction After Spinal Cord Injury. *J. Urol.* 121:73, 1979.

14. **Harrison, M.B., Paterson, P.J.** Urinary Incontinence in Women Treated by an Electronic Pessary. *Br. J. Urol.* 42:481, 1970.

15. **Hopkinson, B.R., Lightwood, R.** Electrical Treatment of Incontinence. *Br. J. Surg.* 54:802, 1967.

16. **Hopkinson, B.R.** Electrical Treatment of Incontinence Using an External Stimulator with Intra-anal Electrodes. *Ann. R. Coll. Surg. Engl.* 50:92, 1972.

17. **McNeal, D.R.** Peripheral Nerve Stimulation—Superficial and Implanted. In Neural Organization (and its Relevance to Prosthetics) Symposia Specialists, Miami, Fla., 1973.

18. **McNeal, D.R., Reswick, J.B.** Control of Skeletal Muscle by Electrical Stimulation. *Adv. Biomed. Eng.* 6:209, 1976.

19. **Merrill, D.C., Conway, C., DeWolf, W.** Urinary Incontinence. Treatment with Electrical Stimulation of the Pelvic Floor. *Urology* 5:67, 1975.

20. **Sotiropoulos, A.** Urinary Incontinence. Management with Electronic Stimulation of Muscles of Pelvic Floor. *Urology* 6: 312, 1975.

21. **Timm, G.W., Bradley, W.E.** Electrostimulation of the Urinary Detrusor to Effect Contraction and Evacuation. *Invest. Urol.* 6:562, 1969.

22. **Tontelj, J.V., Janko, M., Godec, C. et al.** Electrical Stimulation for Urinary Incontinence. A Neurophysiologic Study. *Urol. Int.* 29:213, 1974.

25 Triage of Patients with Lower Urinary Tract Symptoms

Donald R. Ostergard, M.D.

Since a variety of lower urinary tract pathological states manifest similar symptomatology, in most instances it is not possible to rely upon medical history alone to provide a satisfactory triage for patients with lower urinary tract complaints. Triage of these patients requires initial screening procedures which may progress to in-depth urodynamic, pharmacologic and electrophysiologic evaluation. Initial screening procedures eliminate the need for further testing in nearly 90% of patients, since these evaluations provide an adequate preliminary diagnosis which allows the institution of treatment. Less than 10% of patients with lower urinary tract symptoms require in-depth urodynamic evaluation. This preliminary triage schema is subject to modification as new knowledge accumulates in this rapidly advancing area of medicine (Figure 25.1).

PHASE I TRIAGE

The initial triage of patients with lower urinary tract symptoms begins with an adequate urine culture obtained by catheterization or suprapubic aspiration. Those patients with documented infection need routine follow-up cultures at the conclusion of therapy. This identifies resistant organisms and continued infection which commonly results in damage to the upper urinary tracts with resultant progressive deterioration of renal function. Any patient with documented recurrent urinary tract infections requires an evaluation of the upper tracts by intravenous pyelogram and other procedures as needed.

261

PHASE II TRIAGE

Those patients with negative cultures enter the next phase of the triage schema, which includes a complete urogynecologic history and physical examination (see Chapter 4), along with a urologically oriented screening neurological examination (see Chapter 5). Indicated procedures include urethroscopy, uroflowmetry and CO_2 cystometry. CO_2 cystometry, when negative, obviates the need for water cystometry. Due to a high percentage of false positive indications of uninhibited bladder contractions with CO_2 cystometry, water cystometry is always necessary when this occurs. Many patients have posterior periurethral glandular exudate and/or obstructed uroflow patterns which generally respond to serial urethral dilatations, especially when performed under bladder pillar block anesthesia to a maximum of 38F (see Chapter 16). This evaluation also detects fistulas and diverticula.

Cystoscopy frequently enters the triage schema when symptoms other than those of stress incontinence persist. When only stress incontinence symptoms remain, it is appropriate to perform a primary retropubic incontinence procedure without further testing.

PHASE III TRIAGE

A small proportion of patients (less than 10%) enter the final major triage level for major urodynamic studies, which include water cystometry, urethral closure pressure profiles, cough profiles, studies of urethrovesical pressure dynamics, and vesical contraction inhibition (see Chapters 7 to 10). The results of these studies dictate the next step in the evaluative process. Certain tests and therapies are common to many of these diagnoses. These include the universal need for vaginal estrogens in hypoestrogenic patients, and the frequent imposition of bladder training and psychiatric evaluation in the the triage schema. Although some patients have positive results in several areas, clinical judgment indicates which pathology deserves priority. Surgical procedures for genuine stress incontinence, unless this is the patient's only complaint, rarely fall into the limited priority category.

Hypotonic Bladder

If the patient demonstrates a large capacity bladder which lacks voluntary or involuntary contractile ability, a determination of its etiology follows. In this context vesical denervation sensitivity testing (see Chapter 14) and glucose tolerance testing for diabetes mellitus are necessary. Specific therapy depends upon component results of several procedures, especially the results of urethral pressure testing. This emphasizes the interdependence of these evaluative procedures.

Uninhibited Detrusor Contractions

If the patient demonstrates intrinsic vesical activity which she cannot inhibit, this diagnosis prevails (see Chapter 22). Pharmacologic testing helps to confirm the diagnosis and also provides an indication of future therapeutic respon-

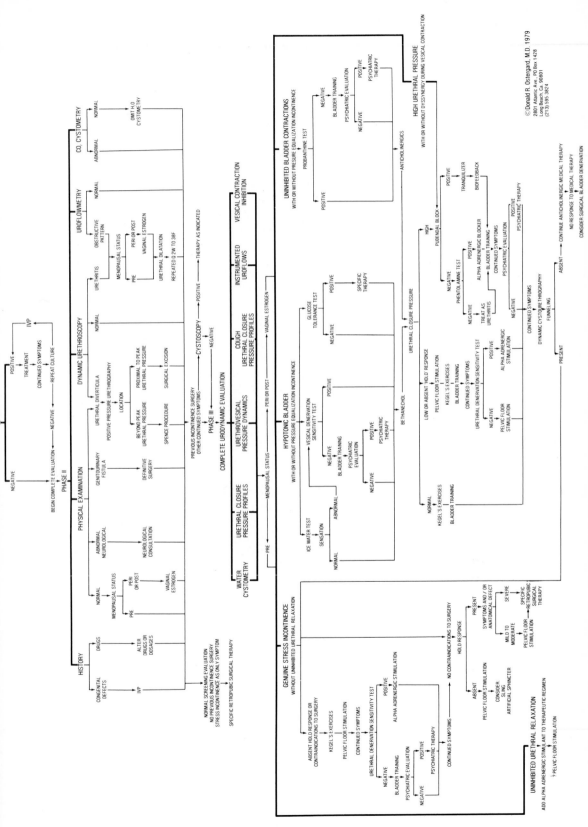

Figure 25.1. Triage of patients with lower urinary tract symptomatology.

263

siveness (see Chapter 15). Again, therapy interrelates with other testing results and other therapeutic needs.

Uninhibited Urethral Relaxation

This diagnostic entity has a specific therapy for use in conjunction with other coincidental diagnoses (see Chapter 10).

Genuine Stress Incontinence

This is the classical genuine stress incontinence which characteristically reveals a negative closure pressure during stress, particularly in the erect position with a full bladder. Retropubic surgical repair is the procedure of choice for the management of these patients, taking care not to damage the delicate urethral sphincteric mechanism during the procedure (see Chapters 7, 10, 28).

Hyperactive Urethral Sphincter

The overactive spastic urethral sphincter reveals itself by generating excessively high intraurethral pressures. Local anesthesia and pharmacologic means distinguish between the relative contributions of the smooth and striated sphincteric components (see Chapter 7). Specific therapy corrects the effect of the predominating contributing element.

Psychiatric Evaluation

Concurrent with or in place of any other objectively demonstrable urologic diagnosis may reside an underlying or predominating psychiatric disturbance (see Chapter 23). Inclusion of psychiatric evaluation is important from both the diagnostic and therapeutic standpoints.

SUMMARY

This algorithm or triage schema (Figure 25.1) for the evaluation and management of patients with lower urinary tract complaints includes many areas where present knowledge is fragmentary at best. Future investigations and clinical evaluations continually provide additional information which serve to modify this system with time. Its true test will be in the years to come.

IV SURGICAL TREATMENT OF GENUINE STRESS INCONTINENCE

26 Retropubic Procedures for the Surgical Repair of Genuine Stress Incontinence*

Donald R. Ostergard, M.D.
C. Paul Hodgkinson, M.D.

Since 1914, when Goebell-Stoeckel-Frangenheim introduced their retropubic surgical procedures for anatomic incontinence, various attempts at improving results and decreasing complications produced several major changes in the operative technique. In the original operation the authors tunneled beneath the urethra and placed a strip of rectus fascia through this tunnel and attached it to the contralateral rectus fascia. Major complications of this operation included urethral injury and subsequent urethrovaginal fistula. Millen and Read slightly modified this procedure. Aldridge described a combined approach utilizing an initial anterior vaginal wall dissection of the urethra followed by the suprapubic component of the operation. This modification decreased the frequency of serious complications. The use of this operation continued until Marshall, Marchetti and Krantz introduced their procedure in 1949 which changed the existing concepts for the use of retropubic urethropexies. Unfortunately, a small percentage of patients developed osteitis pubis due to the periosteal placement of suture material. In order to minimize the possibility of this complication, future modifications avoided the periosteum as the site of suspension. Since the upper suture at the urethrovesical junction is the most important in the evaluation of this anatomical area, movement of its attachment site appeared advantageous. Burch's

---

* See Preface for origin of this chapter.

and Hodgkinson's modifications utilized elevation of the paravaginal fascia for attachment to Cooper's ligament bilaterally. The use of the more substantial vaginal fascia provides a more secure urethral supporting mechanism.

PLACE OF HYSTERECTOMY

In the treatment of anatomic (genuine) stress incontinence, certain patients benefit from combining retropubic urethropexy with abdominal hysterectomy. The preoperative metallic bead chain cystourethrographs of this multiparous woman disclose the specific indications for combining these procedures (Figure 26.1). Because radiographic details photograph poorly, artist's tracings demonstrate the specific changes in urethrovesical pubic relationships. With the patient erect, the anteroposterior radiographs show the lowest bladder level to be midpubic. With straining, it descends to the inferior border of the symphysis. The upper half of the bladder shadow shows three unusual features. First, the shape is very irregular. Second, two lateral ears

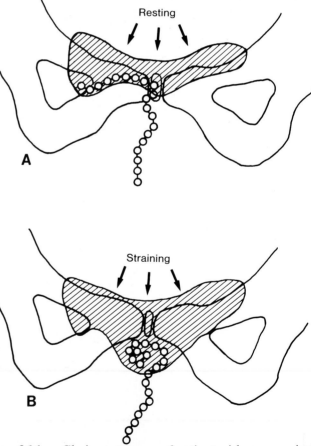

Figure 26.1.   Chain cystogram of patient with supravesical mass. **(A)** Resting and **(B)** straining. The descent below the symphysis indicates a significant cystocele.

project upwards. Third, there is a lack of uniformity of the density, and shadow lines extend transversely. These distorted changes suggest the presence of a supravesical mass pressing inward on the bladder dome. The lateral radiograph obtained during straining shows the urethrovesical junction depressed to the lowest bladder level with minimal rotation of the bladder posterior to the urethrovesical junction. These findings on the lateral x-ray are characteristic of genuine stress incontinence. Downward pressure from an extravesical mass distorts the superior surface of the bladder shadow which also pushes on a segment of bladder far anterior to the symphysis. Clinical examination confirmed the mass to be the enlarged uterine fundus.

Patients who have large pelvic tumors and those with a history of multiple pelvic operations frequently demonstrate these radiographic characteristics. The objectives of combining retropubic urethropexy and abdominal hysterectomy are, first, to relieve supravesical pressure to permit uniform bladder distention; second, to facilitate downward rotation of the bladder posterior to the urethrovesical junction; and third, to correct the forward suprapubic bladder displacement.

RETROPUBIC VAGINAL SUSPENSION OPERATION

The patient is on the operating table in a supine position with thighs abducted and knees flexed over rolled blankets (Figure 26.2A). Appropriate arrangement of the drapes permits access to the vagina from above. The physician incises the skin and anterior rectus sheath transversely. After division of their tendonous insertions into the pubic rami, entry into the retropubic space allows visualization of the bladder which is gently displaced downwards and medially to the level of the pelvic floor (Figure 26.2B). The middle finger of the right hand in the vagina strongly lifts the anterior vaginal wall upwards into the retropubic space (Figure 26.2C). This produces an upward pressure cone of vaginal wall at the level of urethrovesical junction. Medial displacement of the bladder from over the peak of the pressure cone is the first step, followed by blunt dissection and separation of the muscles and fascia of the pelvic floor to the level of the paravaginal fascia. This separation allows the shiny white fibers of the perivaginal fascia to protrude. Two sutures encompass the entire thickness of the vaginal wall and continue through Cooper's ligament at the pelvic brim using 2-0 non-absorbable material (Figure 26.3A). The surgeon delays tying the sutures until after the completion of the procedure on the opposite side. After tying the sutures, the vaginal walls bilaterally approximate Cooper's ligament (Figure 26.3B). This forms a strong vaginal wall sling to support the urethra and the urethrovesical junction. The bladder is free to rotate backwards and downwards.

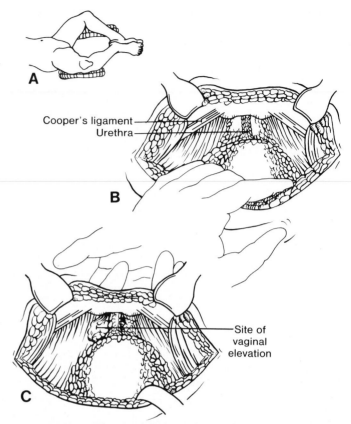

Figure 26.2. The position of the patient for retropubic surgery **(A)**. The retropubic space with the bladder reflected downwards and medially **(B)**. The vaginal finger raising anterior vaginal wall **(C)**.

ROUND LIGAMENT PROCEDURE

Hodgkinson described the round ligament technique for retropubic urethropexy in 1957 for use in patients with recurrent intractible genuine stress incontinence. The round ligaments act as a suburethral sling. Barns in England described this same procedure in 1950. The procedure has certain advantages in that the round ligaments serve as whole organ transplants and their muscular composition produces a softer sling material which is less traumatic than rectus muscle fascia. In an experience of over 125 patients, pressure necrosis of the urethra is conspicuous by its absence. Patients with recurrent genuine stress incontinence, particularly when the anterior vaginal wall is thick and scarred, are the best candidates for a combined round ligament vaginal and retropubic approach, since retropubic urethropexy by vaginal wall suspension is impractical due to short vaginal length.

The vaginal portion of the operation begins with injection of dilute epinephrine solution to achieve hemostasis. After

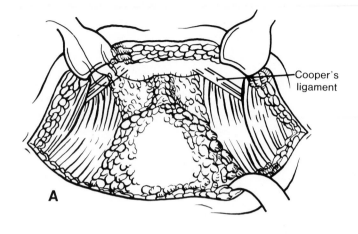

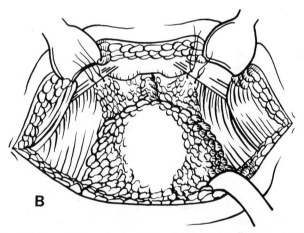

Figure 26.3.   The placement of the suture through the perivaginal fascia and Cooper's ligament (**A**). The sutures tied and the operation completed (**B**).

the longitudinal vaginal incision the mucosal dissection extends laterally to the level of the inferior symphysis (Figure 26.4A). By blunt finger and occasional sharp dissection, the surgeon enters the inferior retropubic space and places two strands of suture material beneath the urethra and packs the ends into the retropubic spaces (Figure 26.4B). These sutures will be attached to the round ligaments to pull them beneath the urethra.

After closure of the vaginal wall incision, a lower paramedian skin incision follows with dissection through the trans-

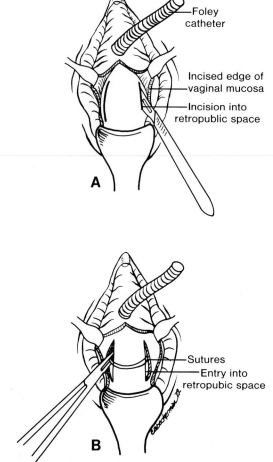

Figure 26.4.   The vaginal incision of the round ligament procedure with bilateral entry into the retropubic space **(A)**. The placement of the suburethral sutures into the retropubic space **(B)**.

versalis fascia to the space of Retzius and then to the site of the ends of the previously placed suture strands on each side of the urethra. Palpation of the retroperitoneal space locates the round ligament as it ascends to enter the internal inguinal ring. It is a white shiny cord of tissue, and by palpation it feels like the ureter. Cutting the adjacent peritoneum with about 0.5 cm of peritoneum attached to each side of the round ligament improves its strength and conserves the blood supply (Figure 26.5A).

In the patient with a previous hysterectomy, the end of the round ligament extends to the vaginal vault and must be identified by palpation. After proper identification, division

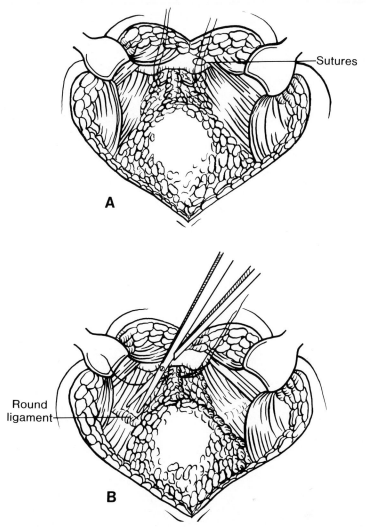

Figure 26.5. The recovery of the suburethral sutures (**A**). The freeing and division of the round ligaments (**B**).

of the round ligament between clamps follows (Figure 26.5B). Suture ligatures on each end achieve hemostasis. The suture arms are left long for use later to aid in pulling the round ligament beneath the urethra. After peritoneal closure to-and-fro traction on the suburethral suture ends identifies the respective suburethral suture strands. The surgeon appropriates and ties the suburethral suture strands to the ligatures attached to ends of the round ligaments and then pulls the round ligaments beneath the urethra by gentle traction (Figure 26.6A).

Sufficient traction shortens the round ligaments to elevate

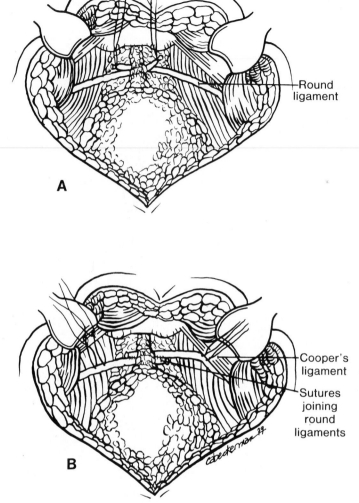

Figure 26.6. Placement of the round ligaments beneath the urethra **(A)**. Suturing of the round ligaments to Cooper's ligaments **(B)**.

the urethrovesical junction to a high retropubic level. While maintaining appropriate traction, interrupted sutures of 4-0 non-absorbable plastic sutures unite the two round ligaments with fine bites of tissue. It is important to avoid encirclement of the ligaments by the sutures for fear of interrupting blood supply. When joined in this way, the round ligaments serve as whole organ transplants and provide broad suburethral support. Being composed of smooth muscle and fibrous tissue, the round ligaments are less incisive to the urethra than are fascial strips. After the round ligaments are securely joined, the surgeon fixes the

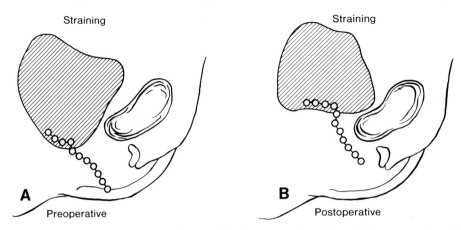

Figure 26.7. Straining cystourethrographs. Preoperative **(A)** and Postoperative **(B)**.

round ligaments to Cooper's ligaments at the pelvic brim using two sutures on each side; this procedure provides additional elevation and stability to the urethrovesical junction (Figure 26.6B).

SURGICAL RESULTS OF ROUND LIGAMENT PROCEDURE

As compared to the preoperative radiograph on the left of Figure 26.7, the postoperative metallic bead chain cystourethrograph on the right demonstrates high elevation of the urethrovesical junction. During straining, the urethrovesical junction maintains this position and the bladder tends to rotate downward and backwards. These are favorable urethrovesical relationships which are characteristic of all types of successful retropubic urethropexy operations. This technique generates few complications. In this series of over 125 patients, one developed a retropubic infection and another, a severe diabetic, developed osteitis pubis. Cure rates are 95% at two years and 94% at five years.

SUMMARY

Retropubic surgical procedures in patients with recurrent anatomic (genuine) stress incontinence require accurate placement of the urethrovesical junction in a high retropubic position. Either suspension of the anterior vaginal wall directly to Cooper's ligament or a round ligament suspension procedure accomplishes this purpose. Proper preoperative selection of the appropriate surgical procedure results in successful correction of most cases of recurrent genuine stress incontinence.

References

1. **Arnold, E.P.** Proceedings: Cystometry—Postural Effects in Incontinent Women. *Urol. Int.* 29:185, 1974.
2. **Barns, H.H.F.** Round Ligament Sling Operation for Stress Incontinence. *J. Obstet. Gynaecol. Br. Emp.* 57:404, 1950.

3. **Bayer, H.** Urinary Incontinence in Women and Pregnancy. *Zentralbl. Gynaekol.* 85:732, 1963.

4. **Berkow, S.G.** Paraurethral Fixation: A New Operation for the Cure of Relative Incontinence of Urine in Women. *Am. J. Obstet. Gynecol.* 41:1051, 1941.

5. **Drukker, B.H., Miller, D.W., Jr.** Retropubic Urethropexy by Vaginal Wall Technique in Stress Incontinence. *Clin. Obstet. Gynecol.* 21:775, 1978.

6. **Drutz, H.P., Shapiro, B.J., Mandel, F.** Do Static Cysto-Urethrograms Have a Role in the Investigation of Female Incontinence? *Am. J. Obstet. Gynecol.* 130:516, 1978.

7. **Francis, W.J.** Disturbances of Bladder Function in Relation to Pregnancy. *J. Obstet. Gynaecol. Br. Emp.* 67:353, 1960.

8. **Gould, D.W., Hsieh, A.C.L., Tinckler, R.F.** Effect of Posture on Bladder Pressure. *J. Physiol.* 129:448, 1955.

9. **Hodari, A.A., Hodgkinson, C.P.** Iatrogenic Bacteriuria and Gynecologic Surgery. *Am. J. Obstet. Gynecol.* 95:153, 1966.

10. **Hodgkinson, C.P., Cobert, N.** Direct Urethrocystometry. *Am. J. Obstet. Gynecol.* 79:648, 1960.

11. **Hodgkinson, C.P., Kelly, W.T.** Stress Urinary Incontinence in the Female—III, Round Ligament Technique for Retropubic Suspension of the Urethra. *Obstet. Gynecol.* 10:493, 1957.

12. **Ingelman-Sundberg, A.** Orthostatic Urinary Incontinence in Women. *Gynecol. Prat.* 11:561, 1960.

13. **Keith, A.** Man's Posture: Its Evolution and Disorders. *Br. Med. J.* 1:451–454, 499–502, 545–548, 587–590, 624–626, 669–672, 1923.

14. **Keller, R.J.** Certain Problems of Micturition in the Female. *Proc. R. Soc. Lond.* 49:657, 1956.

15. **Knobel, J.** Stress Incontinence in the Black Female. *S. Afr. Med. J.* 49:430, 1975.

16. **Marcel, J.E.** On Stress Incontinence. *Gynecol. Prat.* 4:445, 1960.

17. **Marshall, V.F., Marchetti, A.A., Krantz, K.E.** The Correction of Stress Incontinence by Simple Vesicourethral Suspension. *Surg. Gynecol. Obstet.* 88:509, 1949.

18. **Nemis, A., Middleton, R.P.** Stress Incontinence in Young Nulliparous Women; A Statistical Study. *Am. J. Obstet. Gynecol.* 68:1166, 1954.

19. **Read, C.D.** Stress Incontinence of Urine. With Special Reference to Failure of Cure Following Vaginal Operative Procedure. *Am. J. Obstet. Gynecol.* 59:8, 1950.

20. **Stanton, S.L., Williams, J.E., Ritchie, D.** The Colposuspension Operation for Urinary Incontinence. *Br. J. Obstet. Gynaecol.* 83:890, 1976.

21. **Warrell, D.W., Clow, W.M.** Proceedings: Critical Appraisal of Cystometry in Evaluation of Bladder Function. *Urol. Int.* 9:187, 1974.

22. **Zacharin, R.F.** A Chinese Anatomy—The Pelvic Supporting Tissues of the Chinese and Occidental Female Compared and Contrasted. *Aust. N. Z. J. Obstet. Gynaecol.* 17:1, 1977.

27 Incontinence Surgery After Previous Operative Failures*

Donald R. Ostergard, M.D.
C. Paul Hodgkinson, M.D.

It is important to recognize that the critical operation for anatomical (genuine) stress incontinence is the first one, and that the cure rate declines more or less proportionately to the number of subsequent operations performed. Many authors discuss "recurrent stress urinary incontinence," which implies that an operation achieved temporary success and then incontinence recurred. Unfortunately, many of these postoperative patients were neither cured nor improved and sometimes incontinence actually worsened.

PATIENT GROUPS

This series includes 198 patients operated upon 205 times from 1961 through 1976. All of these patients had the usual urodynamic and radiographic studies, including chain cystograms and electronic cystometrics. Of the original group of patients, 163 of them had an anatomic basis for their incontinence, with surgery expected to cure or substantially improve all of these patients.

An additional group of 42 patients had compromised anatomical (genuine) stress incontinence. These individuals had some other condition which preoperatively compromised the expected surgical results.

Of the entire group, 83 actually had total urinary inconti-

---

* See Preface for origin of this chapter.

nence requiring heavy pads with social incapacitation by their condition. The remaining 122 patients had severe incontinence requiring pads nearly all the time.

PREVIOUS SURGICAL PROCEDURES

These patients had 314 previous operations for an average of 1.58 operations per patient. The most common previous operations were vaginal procedures with anterior colporrhaphy being the most common.

Forty-nine patients had primary vaginal surgery based on the adage "Do a vaginal operaton first; if this fails go above." These patients had an anterior and posterior vaginal repair of some type first and then had a retropubic urethropexy. Fifteen had multiple vaginal operations and multiple retropubic urethropexy procedures almost too numerable to count.

REASONS FOR PREVIOUS SURGICAL FAILURES

It was possible to identify six major categories of operative failures (Table 27.1): the philosophic, the pragmatic, the subjective, the psychologic, compromise from preexisting conditions and compensation causes.

PHILOSOPHIC CAUSES

The philosophic causes of failure result from adherence to the antequated adage of "Do a vaginoplastic operation first, and if this fails go above." Failures result from inadequate investigation of urethrovesical physiology, subsequent employment of the wrong operative technique and failure to perform a hysterectomy when indicated.

Table 27.1. Reasons for Operative Failure

PHILOSOPHIC
   "Do a vaginoplastic procedure first, if this fails go above."
     Failure to adequately evaluate preoperatively
     Failure to do correct procedure
     Failure to do hysterectomy when indicated
PRAGMATIC
   Inadequate retropubic healing
   Inadequate suture material
SUBJECTIVE
   Inadequate pelvic fascia
   Congenital or acquired neuromuscular deficiencies
   Extensive pelvic irradiation
PSYCHOLOGIC
   Generally preexistent
PREOPERATIVE COMPROMISE
   Fistulas
     Vesicovaginal
     Urethrovaginal
   Pelvic irradiation
   Extensive trauma
   Detrusor dyssynergia
     Type I
     Type II

Figure 27.1 shows a diagrammatic example of an inadequately investigated patient. The urethrovesical junction is at a very high level preoperatively, therefore, a vaginoplastic operation cannot raise it to a significantly higher position or allow posterior rotation of the bladder (Figure 27.1B). In this case the choice of surgical procedure resulted from adherence to the philosophy of, "Do a vaginoplastic procedure first, if this fails go above." This antequated philosophical approach is no longer valid.

Misconceptions of the objectives of incontinence operations are common and result in performance of incorrect procedures. Unfortunately, the Marshall-Marchetti procedure became known as a "bladder lifting," "elevating," or "suspending" operation. Many of these procedures resulted in minimal elevation of the urethrovesical junction with the anterior bladder wall simply sutured to the periosteum of the symphysis. The postoperative chain cystogram of a patient who had a bladder lifting procedure reveals that the bladder, in close apposition with the posterior symphysis, moves minimally on straining (Figure 27.2). This postoperative failure resulted from a basic misconception of the objective of the incontinence operation. To be successful, the retropubic procedure must elevate the urethrovesical junction and allow the bladder free posterior rotation.

The chain cystogram also aids the preoperative evaluation through identification of concurrent pelvic pathology requiring hysterectomy (Figure 27.3). In this example an obvious impression on the bladder indicates the presence of a uterine myoma. Even though the urethrovesical junction elevation is excellent, the failure of the surgeon to ade-

Non-straining

Straining

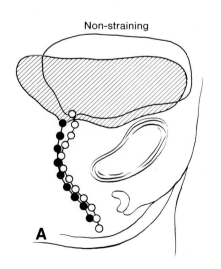
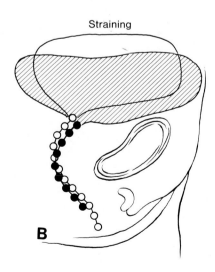

Fig. 27.1. Preoperative (solid black beads) and postoperative (clear beads) chain cystogram with urethrovesical junction high behind symphysis.

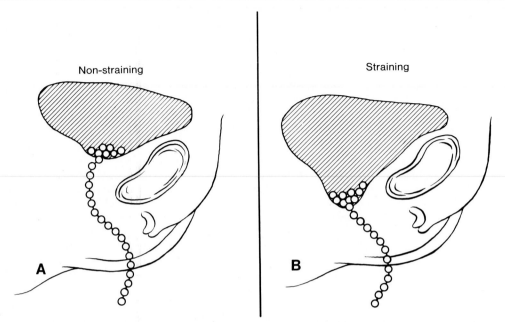

Fig. 27.2. Chain cystogram post-Marshall-Marchetti procedure. A comparison of the non-straining **(A)** and the straining **(B)** views demonstrates an immobile bladder and poorly suspended urethrovesical junction.

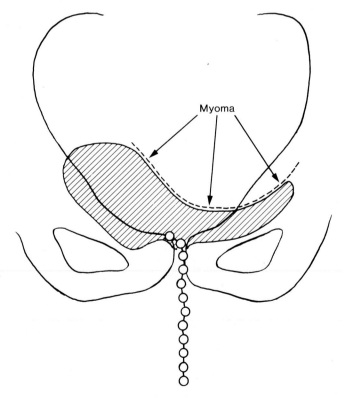

Fig. 27.3. Chain cystogram demonstrating bladder compression by a uterine myoma.

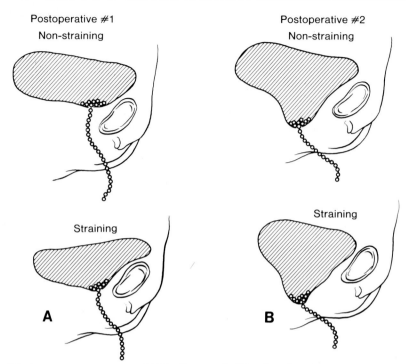

Postoperative #1
Non-straining

Postoperative #2
Non-straining

Straining

Straining

A

B

Fig. 27.4. Chain cystometrogram **(A)** before and **(B)** after breakage of suture postoperatively.

quately evaluate the patient preoperatively resulted in failure to also perform a hysterectomy.

PRAGMATIC CAUSES

The pragmatic causes of failure include the existence of inadequate tissue healing or faulty suture material. Figure 27.4 illustrates a patient who had a normal chain cystogram postoperatively and a clinical cure of her incontinence. She remained continent until she developed a severe respiratory infection. The severe coughing resulted in sufficient stress on the operative site to cause the suspended urethrovesical junction to separate from the retropubis with resulting incontinence.

SUBJECTIVE CAUSES

The multiple subjective causes for failure include inadequate pelvic fascia, congenital or acquired neuromuscular deficiencies, and previous extensive pelvic irradiation. Characteristically, an apparent cure of the incontinence gradually gives way with eventual return of the incontinence.

PSYCHOLOGICAL CAUSES

The psychological causes for surgical failure are difficult to evaluate and diagnose. Unfortunately, most of these causes are present preoperatively and indicates the importance of always including the possibility of a psychologic cause for incontinence in the preoperative differential (see Chapter 23).

Table 27.2. Techniques Used for Previous Operative Failures

	No. of Patients	Failures
Round ligament	125	1
Vaginal suspension	62	1
Marlex mesh sling	11	0
Martius fat pad transplant	6	0
Rectus fascial sling	1	0

Table 27.3. Surgical Results

	No. of Patients	Lost to Follow-up	Cure Rates	
			Partial	Complete
Genuine stress Incontinence	163	6	92%	5%
Compensation cases	5	0	25%	
Compromised	41			
Round ligament, Marlex Sling or fat pad technique	29		46%	11%
Vaginal wall	9		66%	

PREOPERATIVE CAUSES OF SURGICAL COMPROMISE

A group of 42 patients had various reasons to suggest preoperative compromise of expected surgical results (Table 27.4). These causes include vesicovaginal or urethrovaginal fistulas, previous pelvic irradiation, generalized body trauma, especially effecting the pelvis, and detrusor dyssynergia of both Type I and II varieties.

COMPENSATION CAUSES

An additional group of patients includes those seeking compensation because of incontinence. Usually, these patients have total urinary incontinence with many previous operations. Frequently, in the immediate postoperative period, these patients ask for a letter stating total disability due to total incontinence. Objective evaluation of these patients is impossible. They refuse to admit that they are continent, yet they demonstrate good anatomic support and good anatomical relationships after operation.

SURGICAL PROCEDURE

The operative treatment for previous surgical failures has one important objective: to elevate the urethrovesical junction to a high retropubic position. Table 27.2 shows the procedures used in these patients. The vaginal wall suspension and round ligament techniques are very reliable and differ little from the technique used as a primary procedure (see Chapter 26). The former technique is applicable if the vaginal wall is sufficiently relaxed so that adequate vaginal elevation is possible; the latter technique is most useful when the scarred vaginal vault is too short for adequate suspension.

Table 27.4. Preoperative Causes of Surgical Compromise

	No. of Patients	Cured	Improved	Failed
Fistulas:				
Vesicovaginal: (closed)	7	7	—	0
Urethrovaginal: (open)	6	3	2	1
Pelvic irradiation	6	3	0	3
Posttraumatic	3	2	1	0
Detrusor dyssynergia Type I	5	5	0	0
Detrusor dyssynergia Type II	14	2	0	12
Totals	41	17	6	16
		(41%)	(7%)	(39%)

CLINICAL RESULTS

In the group of patients with anatomical reasons for incontinence, 92% no longer had to wear pads and lost no urine if they coughed or sneezed (Table 27.3). An additional 5% reported improvement with occasional urine loss not requiring pads. There were two failures, one with the vaginal wall technique and one with the round ligament technique. Subsequent operation cured one of them, producing a 3% ultimate failure rate.

In the preoperatively compromised group of patients, the results were not good (Table 27.4). Twenty-nine of the patients had round ligament, Marlex or labial fat pad techniques performed. Only 46% reported cure and 11% reported improvement. The vaginal wall technique cured 6% of the patients.

However, the surgical procedure cured all 7 patients in the closed fistula group. Of the 6 with open fistulas there were three cures, 1 improvement and 1 failure. In the 6 irradiated patients half experienced cure. Of 14 patients with detrusor dyssynergia, Type II, cure resulted in only 2 of these and then only when combined with infravesical nerve resection. The presence of any type of uninhibited vesical contractions remains as a nearly absolute contraindication to a surgical procedure. The patients in the trauma group had previous life threatening accidents which seriously damaged bladder and urethral function. These included lacerations of bladder and urethra and traumatic evulsion of these structures from pelvic attachments.

POSTOPERATIVE COMPLICATIONS

These complications included one osteitis pubis in a patient with severe diabetes, two retropubic hematomas and one retropubic infection. Uneventful laceration of the bladder occurred 20 times with no subsequent fistulas.

Delayed voiding occurred in several patients with 12 requiring drainage for 30 days, 4 for 60 days, and 1 for 215 days. Three patients required internal urethrotomy. Except for two patients in the compensation group, all of the patients in the delayed voiding group experienced cure of their incontinence.

SUMMARY

The most important considerations in the problem of recurrent genuine stress incontinence are in the preoperative evaluation of the patient in order to select those patients who will benefit from surgery and the proper choice of operative technique. The preoperative identification of detrusor dyssynergia is essential to this evaluation process. Recent studies indicate that a large number of patients have unstable bladders, as demonstrated particularly with CO_2 cystometry. Unfortunately, many unstable bladders are really stable and represent an artificiality of the method. This is an important consideration, particularly when the surgeon plans to withhold surgery based on CO_2 cystometry. The appropriate selection and interpretation of available urodynamic techniques remains critical for the patient with recurrent genuine stress incontinence.

REFERENCES

1. **Beck, R.P., Grove, D., Arnesch, D., Harvey, J.** Recurrent Urinary Incontinence—treated by the Fascia Lata Sling Procedure. *Am. J. Obstet. Gynecol.* 120:613,1974.
2. **Hodgkinson, C.P.** Relationships of the Female Urethra and Bladder in Urinary Stress Incontinence. *Am. J. Obstet. Gynecol.* 65:560, 1953.
3. **Hodgkinson, C.P.** Urinary Stress Incontinence in the Female—A Program of Preoperative Investigation. *Clin. Obstet. Gynecol.* 6:154, 1963.
4. **Hodgkinson, C.P., Kelly, W.** Urinary Stress Incontinence in the Female. III. Round-ligament Technique for Retropubic Suspension of the Urethra. *Obstet. Gynecol.* 10:493, 1957.
5. **Lee, R.A., Symmonds, R.E.** Repeat Marshall-Marchetti Procedure for Recurrent Stress Urinary Incontinence. *Am. J. Obstet. Gynecol.* 122:219, 1975.
6. **Marshall, V.F., Marchetti, A.A., Krantz, K.E.** Correction of Stress Incontinence by Simple Vesicourethral Suspension. *Surg. Gynecol. Obstet.* 88:509,1949.
7. **Mohr, J.C.** The Gauze-Hammock Operation. *J. Obstet. Gynaecol. Br. Commonw.* 75:1, 1968.
8. **Morgan, J.E.** A Sling Operation Using Marlex Polypropylene Mesh for Treatment of Recurrent Stress Incontinence. *Am. J. Obstet. Gynecol.* 106:369, 1970.
9. **Nichols, D.H.** The Mersilene Mesh Gauze-Hammock for Severe Urinary Stress Incontinence. *Obstet. Gynecol.* 41:88, 1973.
10. **Ridley, J.H.** Discussion of Beck, R.P., Grove, D., Arnusch, D., Harvey, J. Recurrent Urinary Stress Incontinence Treated by the Fascia Lata Sling Procedure. *Am J. Obstet. Gynecol.* 120:613, 1974.
11. **Zacharin, R.F.** Abdominoperineal Urethral Suspension—A Ten Year Experience in the Management of Recurrent Stress Incontinence of Urine. *Obstet. Gynecol.* 50:1, 1977.

28 Genuine Stress Incontinence, the Retropubic Procedure: A Physiologic Approach to Repair

Emil A. Tanagho, M.D.

Modern understanding of the pathophysiology of genuine stress incontinence discourages the vaginal approach to surgical repair. Proper urethral function requires the establishment of good anatomical support with an adequate urethral suspension, a surgical result which the anterior vaginal repair does not provide. Instead of trying to push the urethrovesical junction into a retropubic position from below, the preferred route is through the retropubic space, which allows the placement of the urethra and urethrovesical junction in a secure, stable and normal anatomical position. The retropubic approach limits interference with the physiological function of the urethra, an important principle which requires emphasis.

Fortunately, recent advances in the understanding of the pathophysiology of genuine stress incontinence allow us to discard any procedure which fails to correct the existing pathophysiology. Prior to any repair for genuine stress incontinence it is important to eliminate all other causes of incontinence. Another important point is that the posterior urethrovesical angle is no longer of any basic importance. Modern physiological studies reveal that this angle and the axis of inclination of the urethra are of minor significance. The displacement of the urethra from its normal position and the loss of normal support of the urethra are the primary disturbances and actually cause the changes in the posterior urethrovesical angle and the urethral axis, and also produce excessive urethral mobility. Therefore, the most studied modality of genuine stress incontinence, the posterior urethrovesical angle, is really the result of the basic problem of loss of normal urethral position and normal anatomical support.

Modern surgical therapy restores urethrovesical anatomical relationships and, hopefully, also restores physiological function. It is important to realize that, in genuine stress incontinence, there is nothing wrong whatsoever with the urethral muscular sphincteric mechanism. The intrinsic structure of the muscular sphincter is totally intact, yet functionally it is very weak. Its functional weakness is due to the disadvantage at which the sphincteric units must function as a result of displacement from normal position through loss of normal support; it is not a result of loss of the integrity of muscular sphincteric elements. If surgical therapy restores normal urethral anatomy and support, normal functional ability returns. With the possible exception of lack of estrogenic support, any loss of urethral function after restoration of normal position and normal support is due to iatrogenic damage to the sphincter during the surgical procedure.

The variations in the urethral closure pressure profile with different positions emphasize the above findings. Frequently the UCPP is normal with the bladder relatively empty and with the patient supine or sitting. The closure efficiency diminishes significantly when the patient resumes the upright position. The intrinsic sphincteric mechanism is intact in the sitting or supine position with an empty bladder because of its relatively normal anatomy. With urethral displacement and loss of support from change of position, it becomes inefficient due to further loss of normal position.

The goal of surgery is nothing more and nothing less than restoration of normal anatomy in order to achieve normal muscular sphincteric function.

NORMAL URETHROVESICAL ANATOMY

By using a lateral cystogram with a soft, red Robinson catheter made opaque by the dye traversing it, definition of the relationship of the urethra to the base of the bladder, as well as its relation to the pubic bone, is made possible. In a normal patient without genuine stress incontinence and in a normal resting position, the urethrovesical junction is always opposite the lower third of the pubic bone (Figure 28.1). It assumes a more superior location in children. This radiographic study also measures the extent of urethral mobility in order to judge the intactness of its anatomical support. In those patients in whom the urethrovesical junction is not in the normal position and shows excessive mobility, these findings do not invariably indicate genuine

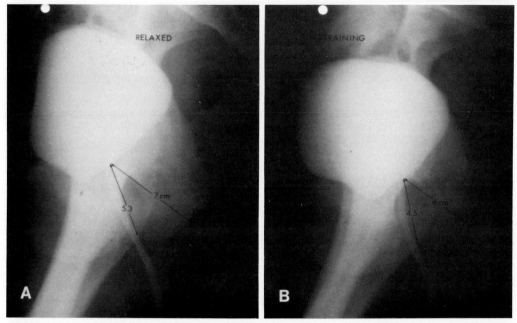

Figure 28.1. Radiographic location of the normal urethrovesical junction. **(A)** Resting. **(B)** Straining. Straining produces minimal downward movement.

stress incontinence (Figure 28.2). This radiographic procedure evaluates the presence or absence of abnormal urethrovesical position or mobility. If the patient has genuine stress incontinence and exhibits excessive mobility or abnormal position, this finding becomes significant.

If the patient is incontinent and the lateral cystograph reveals a normal position with normal mobility, the diagnosis of anatomic incontinence in 99% of cases is not tenable. The further evaluation of this patient usually shows that she has some other cause for her incontinence.

SURGICAL PROCEDURE

Position of the Patient

Since the physician must have access to the vagina during the procedure, place the patient in either the frog leg position or with the legs supported in the abducted position. A urethral catheter allows identification of the urethra and vesical neck during surgery.

Incision

The low transverse abdominal incision with separation of the rectus muscles allows adequate exposure of the retropubic space.

Dissection of the Retropubic Space

Several important points deserve emphasis regarding the dissection of the retropubic space: (1) No dissection occurs near the urethra and for 2 cm lateral on each side; (2) the procedure requires removal of all fatty tissue lateral to this midline area in order to stimulate fibrosis and fixation to the retropubis; (3) the urethra must have adequate support

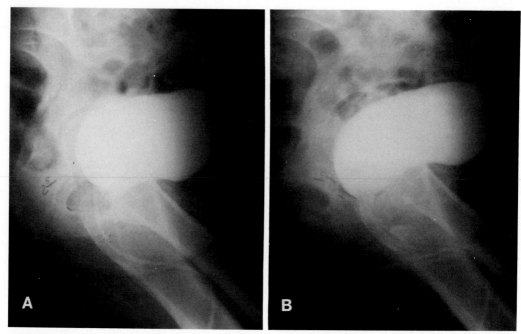

Figure 28.2.   The urethrovesical junction in a normal patient. **(A)** Nonstraining. **(B)** Straining. Even though support is lost, this patient is continent.

without kinking or strangulation; (4) tying proceeds without undue tension to avoid necrosis and breakdown at the suture placement site.

The retropubic dissection begins with mobilization of the lateral parts of the retropubic space down to the endopelvic fascia and continues with mobilization of the bladder upwards and medially on both sides, avoiding the area within 2 cm of the midline (Figure 28.3A). It is important to clear the entire retropubic space of all fatty tissue, since this allows a more durable and long-lasting firm fixation of the paracolpos to the retropubis. If fatty tissue remains in place, fixation is less durable and permits recurrence of abnormal anatomical relationships with application of sufficient force.

Suture Placement

Two sutures on either side support the urethra with the lower one at the midurethra (Figure 28.3B). The upper one is exactly at the vesicourethral junction and both are 2 cm away from the midline. Finger placement in the lateral vagina facilitates exposure and brings the paracolpos further into the operative field. Cooper's ligament is the superior site for suture placement. Tying of sutures proceeds from below upwards with the intravaginal fingers lifting up the paracolpium to facilitate approximation. In some patients vaginal walls may not reach all the way up to Cooper's ligament. Since the vaginal wall is still in contact with the lateral pelvic wall and the back of the pubis, subsequent fibrosis provides sufficient permanent adherence.

At the end of the properly performed procedure, it is possible to place two or three fingers behind the pubic bone in front of the urethra (Figure 28.4). This assures the surgeon that no kinking or compression of the urethra exists.

Suture Material

The avoidance of future complications from suture material necessitates the use of absorbable material, such as number 1 Dexon. The major complication of non-absorbable sutures is the migration into the bladder or urethra, even with suture placement far lateral to either organ. It is important to recognize that the suture material does not suspend the vaginal wall permanently, only long enough for fibrosis and

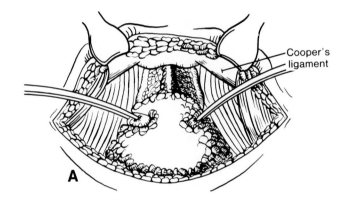

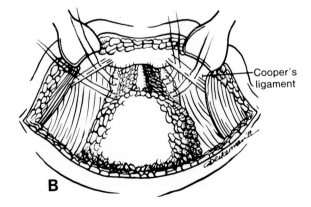

Figure 28.3. The surgical procedure. **(A)** The bladder is mobilized medially and the fat removed starting from 2 cm lateral to the urethra. **(B)** Two sutures are placed on each side from the paravaginal fascia to Cooper's ligament.

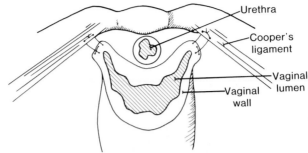

Figure 28.4. The retropubic space is free after tying of sutures without urethral compression. (Redrawn from (8).)

scarring to produce permanent adherence between the retropubis and pelvic sidewall.

Intraoperative Complications

Intraoperative bleeding from retropubic blood vessels is common. Usually packing and the tying of sutures eliminates this cause of blood loss.

Long Term Complications

Long term complications relate to various compromises in urethral function created by the procedure itself. These include urethral obstruction by compression, angulation or stimulation of scar tissue formation around the urethra. The surgeon avoids this complication by not grasping the urethra with Allis clamps or any other device and leaves the midline free from any operative insult. The muscular fibers of the urethra are delicate and fragile. Any maneuvering which causes injury or subsequent scar tissue formation is detrimental to their inherent integrity and to their function. Remember that their functional muscular elements are intact and surgical plication or other operative interference cannot improve upon this. Their preservation is critical and the purpose of the operative procedure is to reestablish proper anatomical support. Above all, the surgical procedure must not compromise urethral function.

URETHRAL STRETCH RESPONSES

The intrinsic structure of the urethra is normal in genuine stress incontinence. Restoration of normal urethral anatomical support allows full recovery of its physiological functions.

Testing of urethral stretch responses validates this concept (Figure 28.5). The functional length increases as does the closure pressure. Maximum improvement comes in the proximal smooth muscle segment of the urethra which is the most essential component of the muscular sphincteric mechanism to insure continence.

In surgery, the restoration of normal anatomical position of the urethra in humans improves the pressure profile. With

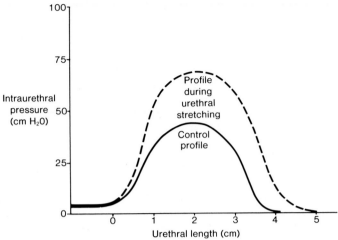

Figure 28.5. The pressure response of the urethra to stretch. Closure pressure increases in response to urethral stretching.

complete anesthesia and curarization and with the abdomen open, there is no intra-abdominal pressure effect and no effect of the voluntary sphincteric component. With traction on the dome of the bladder and without even touching the vesicourethral segment, the vaginal wall or the retropubic space, improvement in the pressure response and functional length of the proximal segment of the urethra results. After tying of sutures additional improvement also results.

It is difficult to reconcile this obvious functional urethral improvement with reports stating that no change occurs in urethral pressure profiles after surgery for genuine stress incontinence.

SUMMARY

The intrinsic mechanism of the muscular sphincter of the urethra is intact in patients with genuine stress incontinence. Any surgical procedure must restore its normal anatomical position and support while avoiding any trauma or other detrimental manipulation. Iatrogenic urethral trauma stimulates scar tissue formation which ultimately compromises urethral function. With restoration of normal anatomy and support, normal physiological function of the muscular sphincteric mechanism is the expected result.

References

1. **Burch, J.C.** Urethrovaginal Fixation to Cooper's Ligament for Correction of Stress Incontinence, Cystocele, and Prolapse. *Am. J. Obstet. Gynecol.* 81:281, 1961.
2. **Burch, J.C.** Urethrovaginal Fixation to Cooper's Ligament in the Treatment of Cystocele and Stress Incontinence. *Prog. Gynecol.* 4:591, 1963.

3. **Murnaghan, G.F.** Colposuspension in the Management of Stress Incontinence. *Br. J. Urol.* 47:236, 1975.
4. **Tanagho, E.A., Smith, D.R.** Mechanism of Urinary Continence. I. Embryologic, Anatomic and Pathologic Considerations. *J. Urol.* 100:640, 1968.
5. **Tanagho, E.A., Miller, E.R.** Functional Considerations of Urethral Sphincteric Dynamics. *J. Urol.* 109:273, 1973.
6. **Tanagho, E.A.** Simplified Cystography in Stress Urinary Incontinence. *Br. J. Urol.* 46:295, 1974.
7. **Tanagho, E.A.** Anatomy and Physiology of the Urethra. In *Urinary Incontinence,* edited by K.P.S. Caldwell. Sector Publishing Co., London, 1975.
8. **Tanagho, E.A.** Colpocystourethropexy: The Way We Do It. *J. Urol.* 116:751, 1976.

29 The Effect of Hysterectomy and Periurethral Surgery on Urethrovesical Function

Emil A. Tanagho, M.D.

Physicians treating the lower urinary tract frequently encounter patients whose urologic symptoms began after hysterectomy. Similarly, many patients relate worsening of their urinary incontinence or the onset of urologic symptoms to an anterior vaginal operation. Frequently, the purpose of vaginal operation is to remedy stress incontinence, but, unfortunately, the intervention only aggravates it.

Although no study definitely links hysterectomy and anterior vaginal operations to subsequent vesical and urethral dysfunction, it is difficult not to incriminate these procedures, because of the chronological relationship of the former to the latter. In consequence, it is imperative that the surgeon be aware of the neuroanatomy of the bladder and urethra, including their vascular supply, in order to respect these delicate structures during operation. Nevertheless, it is not possible to operate within the paravesical area without causing some damage to the parasympathetic and sympathetic nerve supply to the bladder. The result is partial denervation of the detrusor and urethra, with concomitant detrusor hyperactivity or complete urethral relaxation, and their clinical manifestations—urge incontinence or uninhibited bladder contractions.

For ten years the author has evaluated many patients with various urologic complaints with complete urodynamic studies. Many of these patients subsequently had an anterior vaginal operation, then developed uninhibited detrusor contractions, due either to detrusor overactivity or to neuropathic dysfunction of the urethra. None of them had any other abnormality. The conclusion is that a neuropathic dysfunction of the urethra, or the bladder, or both, was iatrogenically induced. Unfortunately, the actual incidence of troubles resulting from anterior vaginal surgery and hysterectomy is unknown, since there is no prospective study addressing this issue. However, in the experience of the author, the magnitude of this problem is such that one has to conclude that certain types of periurethral and perivesical operations must be avoided if at all possible.

FUNCTIONAL CONSEQUENCES OF HYSTERECTOMY AND ANTERIOR VAGINAL REPAIR

In a large personal series of women with urinary incontinence, all patients had one striking feature in common: they had had anterior vaginal operations at some time in the past. No other common factor was found. Evaluation with modern urodynamic techniques performed on all patients left no explanation for the incontinence aside from previous anterior vaginal surgery.

Anterior vaginal repair, including plication of both the urethovesical junction and the urethra, is the time-honored gynecologic method for the treatment of genuine stress incontinence. Unfortunately, many surgeons approach this procedure with the idea that it is not permanent and frequently needs to be repeated. This attitude is borne out by many studies indicating that the rate of immediate postsurgical failure is about 15%. This percentage increases dramatically after one or two years with approximately half the patients having recurrent stress incontinence. This rate of failure is unacceptably high and indicates that anterior vaginal repair has no place in the treatment of genuine stress incontinence.

STRESS INCONTINENCE

Since altered anatomy with descent of the urethrovesical junction and inadequate urethral support is the major etiologic factor in genuine stress incontinence, it must be recognized that the surgeon cannot adequately correct this anatomical defect by performing vaginal surgery. Although the symptoms may improve for a while, they generally recur. In addition, damage to the delicate smooth muscular component of the intrinsic urethral sphincteric mechanism frequently complicates these recurrences. Such sphincteric damage results from periurethral fibrosis and scarring as a direct consequence of the surgical procedure. This is a permanent defect, for which no treatment is known. Thus, it is most important to consider the possibility of sphincteric damage when contemplating vaginal surgery as a primary treatment.

A problem often encountered after vaginal anterior repair is mechanical urethral obstruction. This secondarily obstructed urethra is rigid and fibrotic from end to end. It has normal anatomical support. The result of surgery is lack of proper suspension of the urethra combined with intrinsic damage to its delicate muscular network. In such cases, these patients have no voluntary muscular activity in the urethra, even though they did have normal function before the operation.

The urethral pressure profiles of a patient before and after vaginal operation for primary repair of stress incontinence are seen in Figures 29.1 to 29.3. The postsurgical curve shows a sharp increase in pressure and a sharp decrease, with a sustained plateau between the two (Figure 29.2). However, this pressure is not due to intrinsic muscular activity of the urethra, but results from periurethral scarring. The urethra is now a rigid tube (Figure 29.3). Even though absolute intraurethral pressures appear adequate, these pressures are insufficient to maintain continence under stress because no external pressure is transmitted to the urethra. An increase in intra-abdominal force due to cough-

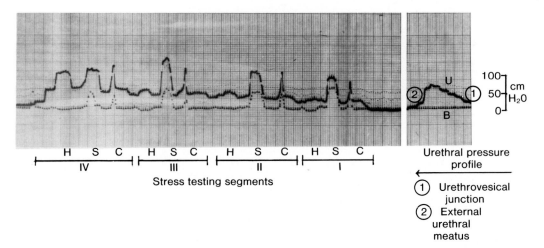

Figure 29.1. Urethral pressure profile and stress testing of a patient with a mild degree of urinary stress incontinence. The tracing reads from right to left with the heavier darker line representing the urethral pressure (**U**) and the lighter dashed line recording the intravesical pressure (**B**). The urethral closure pressure profile is on the right and the stresses of coughing (**C**) and straining (**S**) and the response to the hold command (**H**) on the left. Pressure is in centimeters of H_2O. Each segment represents the effect of these maneuvers on the urethral pressure in that part of the urethra. Segment I is closest to the urethrovesical junction and Segment IV is in the area of peak urethral pressure. On the right, note overall low closure pressure, more apparent in the proximal half of the functional length of the urethra. The effect of stress on the various segments of functional length are not markedly abnormal (left). Observe the strong response to the hold maneuver in the distal part (Section IV) of the urethral functional length (compare to Figure 29.2).

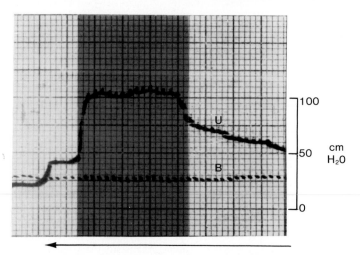

Figure 29.2. Urethral pressure profile of the same patient after vaginal repair. There is no improvement in proximal urethral pressure. However, a sharp increase in pressure reaches a plateau in the distal (shaded) half of the urethra (compare to Figure 29.3).

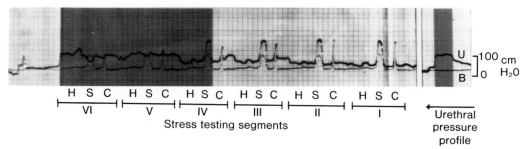

Figure 29.3. Same patient postoperatively. The right hand side of the graph repeats the pressure profile of Figure. 29.2. The left side shows the responses to stress in various urethral segments. There is no change in first half of the urethra when compared to the preoperative tracing in Figure 29.1. However, the segment with the high pressure rise and plateau shows no increase in pressure from coughing or straining because of marked fibrosis and rigidity due to scarring from vaginal repair. Despite high pressure, this portion of the urethra is not responsive to stress. Note that there is only minimal pressure increase from the hold maneuver.

ing or straining is not reflected in the external urethral walls and the urethra fails to generate sufficient intrinsic luminal pressure to negate the effect of a simultaneous and equal pressure increase within the detrusor (Figure 29.3). Pressure is equalized between the bladder and the urethra, with incontinence as the result. In addition, before surgery, the patient responded to the "hold" command with a good intraurethral pressure increase; after surgery this response is absent. The patient has a rigid, fibrotic and responsive urethra. This damage is permanent. There is no way to correct it except with an artificial sphincter.

**TRUE URGE
INCONTINENCE**

The second major problem which may occur after anterior vaginal wall surgery or hysterectomy is the phenomenon of true urge incontinence (uninhibited detrusor contractions). Urodynamic evaluation of patients with urge incontinence reveals perfectly normal urethrovesical pressure dynamics, good responses to "hold" and normal responses to stress within the urethra. However, the irritable bladder contracts freely, without volitional control from the patient. The functional length of the urethra is normal. Responses of closure pressure to bladder filling and stress are normal (Figure 29.4). However, during filling there appears to be a normal spontaneous micturition act (flow in Figure 29.5) because there is a preliminary decrease in urethral pressure followed by an increase in true detrusor pressure. This type of micturition is nevertheless abnormal inasmuch as it occurs at a very low bladder volume and the patient cannot stop urine from escaping. Urinary incontinence occurs before the patient has enough sensation to realize it. She voids incompletely, losing urine in small spurts. This phenomenon usually repeats itself as bladder filling continues, often with no change in sphincter pressure.

Thus, classic urge incontinence consists of bladder contractions that the patient cannot inhibit (uninhibited vesical activity), and of urethral sphincter activity fighting to prevent urine loss. In some patients, increased intra-abdominal pressure triggers irrepressible vesical contractions and may be the cause of incontinence.

**UNINHIBITED
SPHINCTER
RELAXATION**

Another type of postsurgical incontinence results from uninhibited sphincter relaxation. In this situation, urine loss occurs through a different mechanism, consisting of irrepressible urethral sphincter relaxation allowing pressure

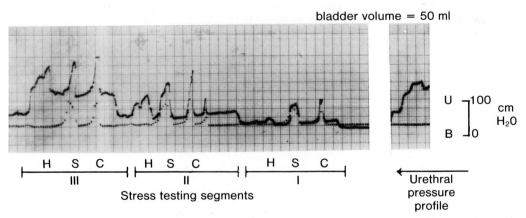

Figure 29.4. Urethral pressure profile and stress testing of a patient with urge incontinence. There is adequate closure pressure throughout the entire functional urethral length (right). Response to stress is normal throughout; again, observe the pressure increase from the hold maneuver in the distal half of urethra (Segments III and IV).

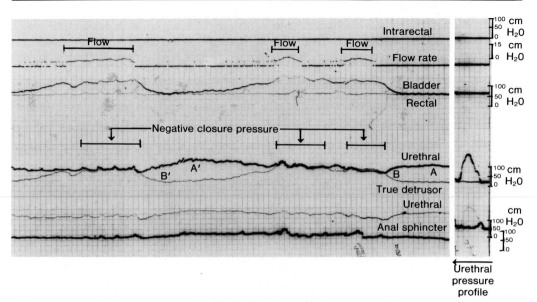

Figure 29.5.   Urethral pressure profile and cystometry of a patient with urge incontinence. This urodynamic tracing includes a record of the following parameters from top to bottom: intrarectal pressure, flow rate, intravesical and intrarectal together, urethral and true detrusor pressure together, urethral pressure and anal sphincter pressure. Urethral closure pressure is adequate or even above normal in the pressure profile (UCPP on the right). During a repeat profile, there is urethral and bladder activity associated with urinary leakage. At points A and A′ there are gradual decreases in urethral resistance which become accentuated as the true detrusor pressure increases (B and B′). Urine flow is apparent during periods of negative closure pressure. The anal sphincter is inactive.

equalization (Figure 29.6). Usually, this takes place in the absence of a bladder contraction. Sphincter relaxation is so complete that intravesical pressure exceeds intraurethral pressure with resultant urine loss. The patient's perception is basically the same as in pure urge incontinence (uninhibitable bladder contractions). For this reason, anticholinergic agents are of no benefit; the patient needs a type of medication allowing her more control of the urethral sphincteric mechanism. Frequently, an alpha-adrenergic stimulating agent is of value.

Sometimes, the sphincter relaxes before a detrusor contraction, as in a normal voiding act. In such a situation it is difficult to make the distinction between detrusor instability and urethral instability (Figure 29.5). To separate the normal voiding act from either detrusor overactivity or sphincter relaxation it must be remembered that the latter generally occurs at low intravesical volumes. This clue is useful in diagnosing the patient's problem.

SUMMARY

Periurethral surgery often results in intrinsic damage to the urethral sphincteric mechanism and concomitant vesical or urethral instability (Table 29.1). Although a definitive study showing the proportion of patients having undergone anterior vaginal repair who develop this particular problem is unavailable, it is frequently encountered. It is common

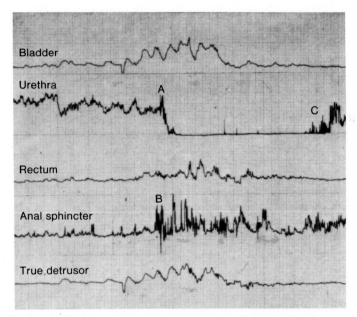

Figure 29.6. A urodynamic recording of uninhibited urethral relaxation. This tracing reads from left to right. At point A, the high urethral pressure drops precipitously. The patient's urethral sphincteric control is lost and she cannot prevent urine leakage. Beginning at point B, there is an increase in anal sphincter contractions. Some increase in intra-abdominal pressure is reflected on both bladder and rectal recordings. At point C, the patient finally recovers sphincteric control and terminates voiding.

Table 29.1. Consequences of Anterior Vaginal Surgery

Pathology	Clinical Manifestation
Partial detrusor denervation	Uninhibitable detrusor contractions
Partial urethral denervation	Uninhibitable urethral relaxation
Insufficient anatomic support	Recurrence of incontinence
Stimulation of periurethral fibrosis	Unresponsive, fibrotic rigid urethra
	Mechanical urethral obstruction

enough to make it imperative that the gynecologist be cognizant of this important postoperative complication and wisely select his patients for anterior vaginal wall repair. Many authorities state that anterior vaginal surgery is not the procedure of choice for primary surgical treatment of genuine stress incontinence. The retropubic procedure provides a better restoration of normal urethrovesical anatomical relationships. The urodynamic studies quoted in this chapter support this contention and delineate the various types of urologic problems resulting from anterior vaginal operations.

30 A Comparison of Anterior Vaginal Repair and Retropubic Colposuspension in the Treatment of Genuine Stress Incontinence

Stuart L. Stanton, F.R.C.S., M.R.C.O.G.

The standard gynecological approach to the cure of stress incontinence is by surgical repair of the anterior vaginal wall, frequently in conjunction with vaginal hysterectomy for uterine prolapse. The literature contains many reports which cast doubt on the long term effectiveness of this procedure and suggest that suprapubic operations are superior (1, 4–6). The disadvantages of these series include the absence of objective pre- and postoperative urodynamic assessment, and the lack of comparative data since each report deals with only one procedure.

This chapter describes the author's personal investigation of the effects of the anterior vaginal repair and the modified colposuspension operation on unselected patients who complained of stress incontinence with or without prolapse. In each patient the urodynamic investigation demonstrated incontinence due to urethral sphincter incompetence.

The preoperative investigation consisted of the procedures outlined in Chapter 6 and included a clinical history, physical examination and objective urodynamic assessment consisting of urine peak flow rate measurement, cystoscopy and videocystourethrography with provocative tests to exclude detrusor instability. Twenty-five patients underwent the colposuspension operation which was a modification of Burch's original procedure (2) with more extensive dissection of the bladder base and the final placement of four pair of sutures (8). Eight of these had an abdominal hysterectomy; their mean age was 46.8 years and mean parity was 2.3. Eleven of these had previous operations for incontinence. Twenty-five patients underwent a traditional anterior vaginal repair using Kelly-type plicating sutures of the urethra and vesical neck. In addition, ten had a vaginal hysterectomy and two had an amputation of the cervix and a posterior repair. Their mean age was 54.8 years and mean parity was 2.1. Three of these patients had previous operations for incontinence.

Preoperative symptoms of stress incontinence, urge incontinence, frequency and nocturia were similar between the two groups (Table 30.1). Postoperatively, all were similar except that fewer patients complained of stress incontinence in the colposuspension group. Figure 30.1 indicates the pre- and postoperative signs.

Patients in both groups had similar preoperative urodynamic data in terms of first sensation of vesical filling, total vesical capacity, maximum voiding pressure, peak flow rate and degree of anatomical descent of the bladder neck. Postoperatively, both groups had similar urodynamic findings, including elevated maximum voiding pressures and decreased peak urine flow. The latter indicates an increase in outlet resistance subsequent to both procedures.

Contrary to findings by other authors (3) the anterior repair did not predispose to the postoperative symptoms of urgency and frequency in the first six months postoperatively (Table 30.1). Table 30.2 shows the objectively determined cure rates after each procedure at this same time period. An obvious loss of contrast into the urethra during videocystourethrography on the first cough, defined marked incontinence and less obvious leakage on the second or third cough defined slight incontinence.

At six months following anterior repair, 16 of the 25 patients (64%) demonstrated incontinence on videocystourethrography; 3 of these same patients had a positive Urilos test. Following retropubic suspension only 4 of 25 patients dem-

Table 30.1 Pre- and Postoperative Urinary Symptoms in the Anterior Repair and Colposuspension Groups

Symptoms	Preoperative		Postoperative	
	Anterior repair	Colposuspension	Anterior repair	Colposuspension
Stress incontinence	100%	100%	36%	12%
Urge incontinence	52%	44%	24%	20%
Frequency	52%	72%	40%	36%
Nocturia	44%	44%	28%	20%

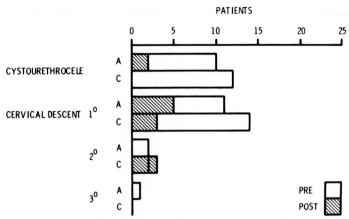

Figure 30.1. The preoperative and postoperative vaginal findings of patients who had undergone an anterior repair **(A)** or a colposuspension operation **(C)**. (Reproduced with the permission of the *British Journal of Urology*.)

Table 30.2 Objectively Determined Cure Rates by Anterior Vaginal Repair and Colposuspension Operations

	Anterior Repair	Colposuspension
Videocystourethrography		
Marked leakage	4	0
Slight leakage	12	1
Urilos positive	3[a]	3
Objective cure	9 (36%)	21 (84%)

[a] All incontinent on VCU.

onstrated incontinence, for a failure rate of only 16%. This resulted in an objective cure rate of only 36% for the anterior repair compared to 84% for the colposuspension procedure.

It is important to recognize that the individual patient's history of urinary incontinence is frequently at variance with objective assessment of the conditions under which urine loss occurs. Videocystourethrography and the Urilos test constitute objective methods of assessing incontinence and are necessary to confirm or refute the patient's history and to demonstrate why the operation failed. The former reveals whether or not the urine enters the proximal urethra during stress even though it may not be clinically evident. The Urilos test objectively indicates minute quantities of actual urine loss under the stresses of walking, running, jumping, coughing and straining. They usually produce a lower success rate than subjective evidence alone.

Although these preliminary comparative results refer only to a six-month follow-up, ongoing data collection for the colposuspension procedure indicates that cure rates of genuine stress incontinence remain at 85% at two years of follow-up.

References

1. **Bailey, K.V.** A Clinical Investigation into Uterine Prolapse with Stress Incontinence Treated by Modified Manchester Colporrhaphy. Part 1. *J. Obstet. Gynaecol. Br. Emp.* 61:291–301, 1954.
2. **Burch, J.C.** Urethrovaginal Fixation to Cooper's Ligament for Correction of Stress Incontinence, Cystocele and Prolapse. *Am. J. Obstet. Gynecol.* 81:281–290, 1961.
3. **Delaere, K.P.J., Moonen, W.A., Debruyne, F.M.J., Michiels, H.G.E., Renders, G.A.M.** Anterior Vaginal Repair, Cause of Troublesome Voiding Disorders? *Eur. Urol.* 5:190–194, 1979.
4. **Hodgkinson, C.P.** Stress Urinary Incontinence. *Am. J. Obstet. Gynecol.* 108:1141–1168, 1979.
5. **Jeffcoate, T.N.A.** Principles of Gynaecology. 3rd ed. Butterworth, London, 1967, p. 840.
6. **Morgan, J.E.** The Suprapubic Approach to Primary Stress Urinary Incontinence. *Am. J. Obstet. Gynecol.* 115:316–320, 1973.
7. **Stanton, S.L., Ritchie, D.** Urilos: Practical Detection of Urine Loss. *Am. J. Obstet. Gynecol.* 124:461–463, 1977.
8. **Stanton, S.L., Cardozo, L.** Results of the Colposuspension Operation for Incontinence and Prolapse. *Br. J. Obstet. Gynecol.* 86:693–697, 1979.

APPENDICES

I Definitions Relating to Urodynamics

All terminology used in this text is standard and conforms to that published by the International Continence Society. Reproduced below are those terms which are of importance to the understanding of the material in this text. This material is quoted and/or paraphrased from the *British Journal of Urology* 48: 39–42, 1976, and 49: 207–210, 1977; the *Scandinavian Journal of Urology and Nephrology* 12: 191–193, 1978; and as discussed at the International Continence Society Annual Meeting, Rome, Italy, October 4–6, 1979.

URINARY INCONTINENCE

Incontinence is a condition where involuntary loss of urine is a social or hygienic problem and is objectively demonstrable. Loss of urine through channels other than the urethra is extraurethral incontinence.

Stress incontinence denotes: (1) a symptom; (2) a sign; and (3) a condition = genuine stress incontinence.

The *symptom* "stress incontinence" indicates the patient's statement of involuntary loss of urine when exercising physically.

The *sign* "stress incontinence" denotes the observation of involuntary loss of urine from the urethra immediately upon an increase in abdominal pressure.

The *condition* "genuine stress incontinence" is involuntary loss of urine when the intravesical pressure exceeds the maximum urethral pressure in the absence of detrusor activity.

Urge incontinence is involuntary loss of urine associated with a strong desire to void. Urge incontinence may be subdivided into motor urge incontinence, which is associated with uninhibited detrusor contractions, and sensory urge incontinence which is not due to uninhibited detrusor contractions.

Reflex incontinence is voluntary loss of urine due to abnormal reflex activity in the spinal cord in the absence of the sensation usually associated with the desire to micturate.

Overflow incontinence is involuntary loss of urine when the intravesical pressure exceeds the maximum urethral pressure due to an elevation of intravesical pressure associated

306

with bladder distension but in the absence of detrusor activity.

CYSTOMETRY

The presence of contractions exceeding 15 cm H_2O clearly indicates an uninhibited detrusor contraction if the patient cannot suppress it. Pressure elevations smaller than 15 cm H_2O indicate the need for clinical judgment. Record when the patient indicates the first desire to void.

Maximum cystometric capacity is the volume at which the patient has a strong desire to void.

Effective cystometric capacity is the maximum cystometric capacity minus the residual urine.

Compliance indicates the change in volume for a change in pressure.

URETHRAL CLOSURE PRESSURE PROFILE

The pressure profile denotes the intraluminal pressure along the length of the urethra with the bladder at rest. Zero reference for pressure is the level of the superior edge of the symphysis pubis. To be meaningful, measure bladder pressure simultaneously.

Maximum urethral pressure is the maximum pressure of the measured profile.

Maximum urethral closure pressure is the difference between the simultaneously measured maximum urethral pressure and the bladder pressure.

Functional profile length is the length of the urethra along which the urethral pressure exceeds the bladder pressure.

Total profile length is the functional length of the urethra plus the additional length to reach zero pressure.

UROFLOWMETRY

Flow rate is the volume of fluid expelled via the urethra per unit time expressed in milliliters per second.

Flow time is the time over which measurable flow actually occurs.

Time to maximum flow is the elapsed time from onset of flow to maximum flow.

Maximum flow rate is the maximum measured value of the flow rate.

Voided volume is the total volume expelled via the urethra.

Average flow rate is voided volume divided by flow time.

Intermittent flow or continuous flow with substantial terminal dribbling applies the same parameters measuring flow time as defined above, i.e., disregard time intervals between flow episodes and the duration of very low terminal flow.

Voiding time is total duration of micturition, i.e., includes interruptions. In continuous flow situations, voiding time is equal to flow time.

PRESSURE MEASUREMENTS DURING MICTURITION

Zero reference for all pressure measurements is the level of the superior edge of the symphysis pubis. Pressures are expressed in centimeters of H_2O.

Intravesical pressure is the pressure within the bladder.

Abdominal pressure is taken to be the pressure surrounding the bladder through estimation from rectal, gastric or intra-peritoneal pressure.

Detrusor pressure is that component of intravesical pressure created by forces in the bladder wall (passive and active). It is estimated by subtracting abdominal pressure from intravesical pressure.

Opening time is the elapsed time from initial rise in detrusor pressure to onset of flow.

Premicturition pressure is the pressure recorded immediately before initial isovolumetric contraction.

Opening pressure is the pressure recorded at the onset of measured flow.

Maximum pressure is the maximum value of the measured pressure.

Pressure at maximum flow is the pressure recorded at maximum measured flow rate.

Contraction pressure at maximum flow is the difference between pressure at maximum flow and premicturition pressure.

PRESSURE FLOW RELATIONSHIPS

Driving pressure is the pressure within the bladder which accomplishes micturition. Its origin is a detrusor contraction, abdominal pressure (valsalva) or a combination of the two. The combination of these pressure flow characteristics determines the flow rate. The specific interaction of the detrusor contraction and the abdominal pressure contribution is quite variable from individual to individual and from micturition to micturition.

Obstructed flow has a low flow rate in combination with high detrusor pressure.

Normal flow rate has an associated low detrusor pressure.

Detrusor motor impairment has an intermittent flow rate, produced by abdominal wall contraction in the absence of detrusor activity.

Interrupted flow rate with an increase in true detrusor pressure and the absence of abdominal straining indicates intermittent contraction of the urethrosphincteric mechanism.

Residual urine is the volume of fluid remaining in the bladder immediately following micturition. It originates from detrusor insufficiency, urethral obstruction or psychological inhibition. It may also originate from ureteral reflux or bladder diverticula which allow urine to reenter the bladder following micturition.

NEUROMUSCULAR DYSFUNCTION OF THE LOWER URINARY TRACT

Detrusor function is either normal, overactive or underactive. The classification may change between the filling and voiding phases.

Detrusor function is normal when no significant rise in pressure occurs during the filling phase and no involuntary contractions occur.

Voiding is normal when a voluntarily initiated detrusor contraction occurs which is of sufficient duration to completely empty the bladder. The patient suppresses this contraction at will.

Overactive detrusor function occurs when the filling phase demonstrates spontaneous or provoked voluntary or involuntary contractions that the woman cannot suppress. Provocations include rapid filling, alterations of posture, coughing, walking, jumping and other triggering procedures.

Other terms also describe various aspects of detrusor function. The *unstable bladder* contracts spontaneously or on provocation during filling while the patient attempts to inhibit micturition. *Detrusor hyperreflexia* results from disturbances of the nervous control mechanisms. *A stable detrusor* demonstrates only voluntary inhibitable contractions. An *unstable detrusor* is simply one not stable on filling.

Underactive detrusor function describes the bladder without demonstrable contractions during filling. During voiding the contraction is either absent or inadequately sustained.

Detrusor areflexia exists where underactivity is due to an abnormality of nervous control with complete absence of central coordination.

URETHRAL FUNCTION   The urethral closure mechanism is either normal, overactive or incompetent. The *normal urethral closure mechanism* maintains a positive urethral closure pressure during filling even in the presence of increased abdominal pressure. Occasionally detrusor overactivity overcomes this pressure. During micturition the normal closure pressure decreases to allow flow. The normal closure mechanism has the capability of interrupting urination voluntarily.

An *overactive urethral closure mechanism* contracts involuntarily against a detrusor contraction or fails to relax during attempted micturition.

Synchronous detrusor and urethral smooth and/or striated muscle contraction is *detrusor/urethral dyssynergia* which has two subdivisions. The term *detrusor/sphincter dyssynergia* describes a detrusor contraction concurrent with contraction of the urethral and/or periurethral striated muscle. The term *detrusor/bladder neck dyssynergia* denotes a detrusor contraction concurrent with an objectively demonstrated defect of bladder neck opening.

An *incompetent urethral closure mechanism* allows leakage of urine due to several causes. The negative urethral closure pressure is persistent (continuous leakage), or due to sharp increases in abdominal pressure (genuine stress incontinence) or an involuntary fall in intraurethral pressure in the absence of detrusor activity (*unstable urethra*). Detrusor overactivity also causes leakage if there is an involuntary decrease in urethral pressure.

Sensation is either normal, hypersensitive or hyposensitive.

Pharmacology of the Lower Urinary Tract

Table II.1. Drugs Stimulating the Parasympathetic Nervous System

Generic Name	Trade Name
Ambenonium	Mytelase
Carbachol	Carcholin, Isopto-carbachol
Echothiophate	Phospholine
Edrophonium	Tensilon
Demecarium	Humorsol
Isoflurophate	Floropryl
Methacholine	Mecholyl
Pilocarpine	Pilocar
Pralidoxime	Protopam
Pyridostigmine	Mestinon

Table II.2. Drugs Inhibiting the Parasympathetic Nervous System

Generic Name	Trade Name
Adiphenine	Trasentine
Alverine	Profenil, Spacolin
Anisotropine	Valpin
Atropine	—
Belladonna extract	—
Carbofluorene	Pavatrine
Clidinium	Quarzan, Librax
Cyclopentolate	Cyclogyl
Diphemanil	Prantal
Ethaverine	Neopavrin
Eucatropine	Euphthalmine
Glycopyrrolate	Robinul
Hexocyclium	Tral
Homatropine hydrobromide	—
Homatropine methylbromide	Mesopin, Homapin, Novatrin, Malcotran
Hyoscyamine sulfate	Levsin
Isometheptene	Octin, Isometene
Mepenzolate	Cantil
Methixene	Trest
Methscopolamine bromide	Pamine
Methylatropine nitrate (Atropine methylnitrate)	Metropine
Oxyphenonium	Antrenyl
Papaverine	Cerespan, Ethaquine, Laverin, Neopavrin, Pap-Kaps, Pavabid, Pavacap, Pavacen, Pavarine, Pavatest, Paveril, Vasal, Vasospan
Pentapiperium	Antrenyl; Quilene
Penthienate	Monodral
Pipenzolate	Piptal
Piperidolate	Dactil
Poldine	Nacton
Scopolamine	—
Thihexinol	Sorboquel
Thiphenamil	Trocinate
Tincture of belladonna	—
Tricyclamol	Elorine
Tridihexethyl	Pathilon
Tropicamide	Mydriacyl
Valethamate	Murel

Table II.3. Drugs Inhibiting the Parasympathetic Nervous System: Combined Preparations

Belbarb	Kolantyl
Belladenal	Levsin with Phenobarbital
Bellergal	Milpath
Bentyl with phenobarbital	Nolamine
Butibel	Pamine
Cantil with phenobarbital	Pathibamate
Chardonna	Pathilon with Phenobarbital
Combid	Phenobarbital and Belladonna
Daricon-PB	Pro-Banthine with Dartal
Donnalate	Pro-Banthine with Phenobarbital
Donnatal	Prydonnal
Donphen	Robinul-PH
Enarax	Sidonna
Histalet	Valpin-PB
Hybephen	Trasentine-Phenobarbital
Kinesed	

Table II.4. Drugs Affecting the Sympathetic and Parasympathetic Nervous System: Ganglionic Blockers

Generic Name	Trade Name
Azamethonium	Pendiomide
Chlorisondamine	Ecolid
Hexamethonium	—
Mecamylamine	Inversine
Pentolinium	Ansolysen
Sparteine	Spartocin, Tocosamine
Trimethaphan	Arfonad
Trimethidinium	Ostensin

Table II. 5. Drugs Inhibiting the Sympathetic Nervous System: Adrenergic Neuron Blockers

Generic Name	Trade Name
Alseroxylon	Rauwiloid, Rautensin
Bethanidine	Esbatal
Bretylium	Darenthin
Debrisoquin	Declinax
Deserpidine	Harmonyl
Guanadrel	—
Guanethidine	Ismelin
Guanoclor	Vatensol
Guanoxan	Envacar
Hydralazine	Apresoline
Methyldopa	Aldomet
Methyldopate	Aldomet Ester
Nialamide	—
Pargyline	Eutonyl
Rauwolfia	Hyperloid, Raudixin, Rauja, Raulfin, Rautina, Rauval, Venibar
Rescinnamine	Cinatabs, Moderil
Reserpine	Lemiserp, Rau-Sed, Resercen, Reserpoid, Rolserp, Sandril, Serpasil, Sertina, Vio-Serpine
Syrosingopine	Singoserp
Tranylcypromine	—
Veratrum alkaloids	Unitensen, Veralba, Veriloid, Vertavis

Table II.6. Drugs Inhibiting the Sympathetic Nervous System: Combined Preparations

Aldoclor	Nyomin
Aldoril	Oreticyl
Besertal	Pentoxyglon
Butiserpazide	Protalba-R
Butiserpine	Rauvera
Diupres	Rautrax
Diutensen	Rauzide
Enduronyl	Rauwiloid with Veriloid
Esimil	Regroton
Eutron	Ruhexatal with Reserpine
Exna-R	Renese-R
Hydromox-R	Salutensin
Hydropres	Sandril with Pyronil
Maxitate with Rauwolfia	Serpasil-Esidrix
	Singoserp-Esidrix
Metatensin	Theobarb-R
Naquival	Theominal RS
Nembu-Serpin	Vertavis-Phen
Neo-Slowten	Vertina

Table II.7. Drugs Affecting the Sympathetic Nervous System: Alpha Adrenergic Blockers

Generic Name	Trade Name
Azapetine	Ilidar
Dihydroergotoxine	Hydergine
Ergot alkaloids	—
Phenothiazines	(Various, See Table II.13)
Phentolamine	Regitine
Piperoxan	Benodaine
Tolazoline	Priscoline

Table II.8. Drugs Affecting the Sympathetic Nervous System: Beta Adrenergic Blockers[a]

Generic Name	Trade Name
Alprenolol	—
Butidrine	—
Butoxamine	—
Dichloroisoproterenol	Alderlin, Nethalide, Pronethalol
Isopropylmethoxamine	—
Ko592	—
LB-46	Prinodolol
M 1999	Sotalol
Oxprenolol	—
Practolol	Eraldin

[a] None are available in the United States.

Table II.9. Drugs Affecting the Sympathetic Nervous System: General Adrenergic Stimulators

Generic Name	Trade Name
Adrenalone	Kephrine
Aminorex[a]	—
—	Aranthol
Benzphetamine	Didrex
Chlorphentermine	Pre-Sate
Clortermine	Voranil
Cyclopentamine	Clopane
Deoxyepinephrine	Epinine
Dextroamphetamine	Dexedrine
Diethylpropion	Tenuate, Tepanil
Epinephrine	—
Ethylnorepinephrine	Bronkephrine
Fenfluramine	Pondimin
Hydroxyamphetamine	Paredrine
H1032[a]	—
Isometheptene	Octin
Levamphetamine	Ad-Nil, Amodril, Cydril, Maigret
Mazindol	Sanorex
Methamphetamine	Desoxyn
Mephentermine	Wyamine
Methylaminoheptane	Oenethyl
Methylhexamine	Forthane
Naphazoline	Privine
Oxymetazoline	Afrin
Phedrazine[a]	—
Phendimetrazine	Dietrol, Plegine
Phenmetrazine	Preludin
Phentermine	Ionamin, Wilpowr
Pholedrine	Paredrinol
Propylhexedrine	Benzedrex
Pseudoephredrine	Sudafed, Ro-Fedrin
Racephedrine	—
Synephrine[a]	—
Tenaphtoxaline[a]	—
Tetrahydrozoline	Tyzine
Tramazoline	—
Tuaminoheptane	Tuamine
Tymazoline[a]	Pernazene
Xylometazoline	Otrivin

[a] Not available in the United States.

Table II.10. Drugs Affecting the Sympathetic Nervous System: Combined Preparations

Actifed-C Expectorant
Acutuss
Acutuss Expectorant with Codeine
Aerolone Compound
Amesec
Amodrine
Asbron
Ayrcap
Ayr Liquid
Bihisdin
Brondilate
Bronkometer
Bronkosol
Bronkotabs
Calcidrine Syrup
Cerose Expectorant
Chlor-Trimeton Expectorant with Codeine
Citra
Colrex Compound
Copavin
Copavin Compound
Coricidin Nasal Mist
Co-Xan
Dainite
Dainite-KI
Deltasmyl
Duo-Medihaler
Duovent
Dylephrine
Ephed-Organidin
Ephedrine and Chlorcyclizine
Ephedrine and Nembutal
Ephedrine and Secondal Sodium
Ephoxamine
Glynazan/EP
Hyadrine
Hydryllin with Racephedrine Hydrochloride
Iso-Tabs
Isuprel Compound
Luasmin
Luftodil
Lufyllin-EP
Marax
Nasocon
Nebair
Neospect
Neo-Vadrin
Norisodrine with Calcium Iodide
Novalene
Numal
NTZ
Orthoxine and Aminophylline
Phyldrox
ProDecadron
Pyracort
Pyraphed
Quadrinal
Synophedal
Tedral
Tedral-25
Tedral Anti-H
Thalfed
Triaminicin
Tri-Isohalant
Ulogesic
Ulominic
Verequad

Table II.11. Drugs Affecting the Sympathetic Nervous System: Alpha Adrenergic Stimulators

Generic Name	Trade Name
Amidephrine[a]	—
Cyclopentamine	Clopane
Dopamine[a]	Intropin
Etafedrine[a]	—
Ethylphenylephrine[a]	Effortil
Hydroxyamphetamine	Paredrine
Metaraminol	Aramine
Methamphetamine	Desoxyn, Efroxine, Methedrine, Norodin, Synodrox
Methoxamine	Vasoxyl
Methylhexaneamine	Forthane
Nordefrin[a]	Cobefrin
Norepinephrine	Levarterenol
Novadral[a]	—
Phenylephrine	Neo-Synephrine, Isophrin, Synasal, Alcon-Efrin, Biomydrin, Isohalant Improved
Phenylpropylmethylamine	Vonedrine
Propylhexedrine	Benzedrex
Tyramine[a]	—

[a] Not available in the United States.

Table II.12. Drugs Affecting the Sympathetic Nervous System: Beta Adrenergic Stimulators

Generic Name	Trade Name
Albuterol[a]	—
Bamethan[a]	—
Chlorprenaline	—
Dioxethedrine	—
Etafedrine	—
Ethylnorepinephrine[a]	Bronkephrine
Hydroxyephedrine[a]	—
Isoetharine	—
Isoproterenol	Aludrine, Isuprel, Norisodrine
Methoxyphenamine	Orthoxine
Nylidrin	Arlidin
Protokylol	Caytine
Salbutamol[a]	—
Soterenol[a]	—
Terbutaline	Bricanyl

[a] Not available in the United States.

Table II.13. Drugs Affecting the Autonomic Nervous System: Drugs Causing Retention

Generic Name	Trade Name
Acetophenazine	Tindal
Amitriptyline	Elavil
Amphotericin B	Fungizone
Benztropine	Cogentin
Biperiden	Akineton
Bromodiphenhydramine	Ambodryl
Brompheniramine	Dimetane
Butaperazine	Repoise
Carbinoxamine	Clistin
Carphenazine	Proketazine
Chlorpheniramine	Chlor-Trimeton, Hista-span, Teldrin
Chlorphenoxamine	Systral, Phenoxene
Chlorpromazine	Thorazine
Chlorprothixene	Taractan
Cycrimine	Pagitane
Deanol	Deaner
Desipramine	Norpramin, Pertofrane
Dexbrompheniramine	Disomer
Dexchlorpheniramine	Polaramine
Dimethindene	Forhistal, Triten
Diphenhydramine	Benadryl
Diphenylpyraline	Diafen, Hispril
Doxepin	Adapin, Sinequan
Doxylamine	Decapryn
Droperidol	Inapsine
Ethopropazine	Parsidol
Fluphenazine	Prolixin, Permitil
Haloperidol	Haldol
Imipramine	Tofranil, Presamine
Isocarboxazid	Marplan
Mesoridazine	Serentil
Mepazine	—
Metaxalone	Skelaxin
Methapyrilene	Histadyl
Methdilazine	Tacaryl

(continued on p. 317)

Table II.13—continued

Generic Name	Trade Name
Methylphenidate	Ritalin
Methysergide	Sansert
Molindone	Moban
Nortriptyline	Aventyl
Orphenadrine	Norflex
Perphenazine	Trilafon
Phenelzine	Nardil
Phenindamine	Thephorin
Piperacetazine	Quide
Pipradrol	Meratran
Prochlorperazine	Compazine
Procyclidine	Kemadrin
Promazine	Sparine
Promethazine	Phenergan
Protriptyline	Vivactil
Pyrilamine	—
Rotoxamine	Twiston
Thiopropazate	Dartal
Thioridazine	Melleril
Thiothixene	Navane
Tranylcypromine	Parnate
Trifluoperazine	Stelazine
Triflupromazine	Vesprin
Trihexyphenidyl	Artane, Pipanol, Tremin
Trimeprazine	Temaril
Tripelennamine	Pyribenzamine
Triprolidine	Actidil

Table II.14. Drugs Affecting the Autonomic Nervous System: Drugs Causing Miscellaneous Urologic Symptoms

Generic Name	Trade Name	Mixtures
FREQUENCY		
Iron Sorbitex	Jectofer	Etrafon
Dantrolene	Dantrium	Triavil
INCONTINENCE		
Estrogens		
Hydroxystilbamidine		
URGENCY		
Disodium Edetate	Endrate	
FREQUENCY, RETENTION and INCONTINENCE		
Levodopa	Bendopa, Dopar, Larodopa, Levodopa	
Levopropoxyphene	Novrad	

III   Data Recording Forms for Gynecologic Urology

URG-DATA BASE SYSTEM
URODYNAMICS AND GYNECOLOGIC UROLOGY
HISTORY

DONALD R. OSTERGARD, M.D.
WOMEN'S HOSPITAL
MEMORIAL HOSPITAL MEDICAL CENTER
UNIVERSITY OF CALIFORNIA IRVINE
2801 ATLANTIC AVENUE, P.O. BOX 1428
LONG BEACH, CA 90801 (213) 595-3824

FORM 1A
Page 1

DATE _____
CHART NO. _____
PATIENT NO. _____

NAME _____   _____
                    Last   First

INSTRUCTIONS TO PATIENT: Check the box if your answer is "YES"

1. Have you had treatment for urinary tract disease, such as: (Please check) stones ☐, kidney disease ☐, infections ☐, tumors ☐, injuries ☐?

2. Have you ever had paralysis ☐, polio ☐, multiple sclerosis ☐, a stroke ☐, back pain ☐, syphilis ☐, diabetes ☐, pernicious anemia ☐? (If yes, check proper ones).

3. Have you had an operation on your spine ☐, brain ☐, or bladder ☐?

4. Have you had a bladder infection during the last year? ☐

5. If yes, did it occur more than twice during the last year? ☐

6. Did the bladder infection follow intercourse at any time? ☐

7. Is your urine ever bloody? ☐

8. Have you ever been treated by urethral dilatation? ☐

9. If yes: when? _____ How many times? _____

10. Did urethral dilatation help you? ☐

11. Did you have trouble holding urine as a child? ☐

12. As a child, did you wet the bed? ☐

13. If yes, at what age did you stop? _____

14. Do you wet the bed now? ☐

15. What is the volume of urine you usually pass? (Please check) Large ☐, medium ☐, small ☐, very small ☐

16. Do you notice any dribbling of urine when you stand after passing urine? ☐

17. Do you lose urine by spurts during severe coughing ☐, sneezing ☐, or vomiting ☐?

18. If yes, in which position(s) does it occur? (Please check) Standing ☐, sitting ☐, laying down ☐

19. Do you lose urine without coughing, sneezing or vomiting? ☐

20. If yes, when does it occur? (Please check) walking ☐, running ☐, straining ☐, laying down ☐, any change of position ☐, after intercourse ☐, during intercourse ☐?

21. When you are passing urine, can you usually stop the flow? ☐

22. Did your urine difficulty start during pregnancy ☐, or after delivery of an infant ☐? (If yes, check proper one).

23. Did it follow an operation? ☐

24. If yes, check the type of operation:
☐ Hysterectomy (removal of womb), through the abdomen. Radical ☐
☐ Hysterectomy (removal of womb), through the vagina.
☐ Removal of a tumor through the abdomen.
☐ Vaginal repair operation.
☐ Suspension of the uterus or bladder.
☐ Cesarean section.
☐ Other (describe) _____

25. Did it follow X-ray treatment? ☐

26. If your menstrual periods have stopped, did the menopause make your condition worse? ☐

27. Do you lose control and pass a large amount of urine when you cough ☐, sneeze ☐, laugh ☐, lift ☐, strain ☐, vomit ☐, during intercourse ☐, after intercourse ☐?

28. Do you have difficulty holding urine if you suddenly stand up after sitting or lying down? ☐

29. Do you find it necessary to wear protection because you get wet from the urine you lose? ☐

30. If yes, at what age did you start using this protection? _____

31. When do you wear protection? (Please check) occasionally ☐, all the time ☐, only during the day ☐, only at night ☐.

32. Is your urinary problem bad enough that you would request surgery to fix it? ☐

33. List all medications you are now taking and duration of use of each medication (include contraceptives):

CODE	MEDICATION	DURATION OF USE

34. When you lose your urine accidentally, are you ever unaware that it is passing? ☐

35. Do you always have an uncomfortably strong need to pass urine before you empty your bladder? ☐

36. Do you lose urine before reaching the toilet? ☐

37. If yes, is this urine loss painful? ☐

38. Do you have to hurry to the toilet or can you take your time? (Please check) hurry ☐, take time ☐.

39. Can you overcome the uncomfortably strong need to pass urine? (Please check) usually ☐, occasionally ☐, rarely ☐.

40. Do you have an uncomfortably strong need to pass urine with a full bladder? ☐

Form 1A, Page 1.   History (English).

A6

URG-DATA BASE SYSTEM
URODYNAMICS AND GYNECOLOGIC UROLOGY
HISTORY

DONALD R. OSTERGARD, M.D.
WOMEN'S HOSPITAL
MEMORIAL HOSPITAL MEDICAL CENTER
2801 ATLANTIC AVENUE, P.O. BOX 1428
LONG BEACH, CA 90801 (213) 595-3824

Form 1A
Page 2

DATE _____
CHART NO. _____
PATIENT NO. _____

NAME _____ _____
         Last   First

INSTRUCTIONS TO PATIENT: Please check the box if your answer is "YES"

41. Do you have an uncomfortably strong need to pass urine without a full bladder? ☐

42. How many times do you void during the night after going to bed? _____

43. How many times do you void during the first hour after going to bed? _____

44. Does an uncomfortably strong need to pass urine wake you up? ☐

45. Are you usually awake and simply pass urine while up? ☐

46. After passing urine, can you usually go back to sleep? ☐

47. How much fluid do you usually drink before going to bed? _____ cups.

48. Do you have discomfort in the area above or to the side of your bladder? ☐

49. Do you have pain while you pass your urine? ☐

50. Is it painful during the entire time you pass urine? ☐

51. Is it painful only at the end of passing urine? ☐

52. Do you always feel that your bladder is empty after passing urine? ☐

53. Do you usually have painful passing of urine after intercourse? ☐

54. Do you need to pass urine more frequently after intercourse? ☐

55. Does your bladder discomfort stop completely after passing urine? ☐

56. How often do you pass urine during the day? Every _____ hours.

57. Is it necessary for you to pass urine frequently? ☐

58. Does the sound, the sight, or the feel of running water cause you to lose urine? ☐

59. Do you need to pass urine more frequently when riding in a car? ☐

60. Is your clothing slightly damp ☐, wet ☐, soaking wet ☐, or do you leave puddles on the floor ☐?

61. Is your loss of urine a continual drip so that you are constantly wet? ☐

62. Are you ever suddenly aware that you are losing or are about to lose control of your urine? ☐

63. How often does this occur? _____ / Day _____ / Week

64. Do you usually have difficulty starting your urine stream? ☐

65. Do you find it frequently necessary to have your urine removed by means of a catheter because you are unable to pass it? ☐

FAMILY UROLOGY HISTORY

Does (did) your natural mother, sister, aunt or grandmother have problems with urine loss as a child or an adult? ☐

	Mother	Sister	Aunt	GrandMother
Did she have surgery to correct this problem?	☐	☐	☐	☐
Did she wear a pad to protect against urine loss?	☐	☐	☐	☐
At what age did her problem start?	_____	_____	_____	_____
How old were you when her problem started?	_____	_____	_____	_____
Did she wet the bed as a child?	☐	☐	☐	☐
At what age did she stop?	_____	_____	_____	_____

SUMMARY:

In the space below please summarize your urine problem(s) as briefly as possible:

A7

Form 1A, Page 2. History (English).

DATOS BASICOS DEL SISTEMA
GINECO-UROLOGICO
HISTORIA GINECOUROLOGICA

DONALD R. OSTERGARD, M.D.
WOMEN'S HOSPITAL
MEMORIAL HOSPITAL MEDICAL CENTER
UNIVERSITY OF CALIFORNIA IRVINE
2801 ATLANTIC AVENUE, P.O. BOX 1428
LONG BEACH, CA 90801 (213) 595-3824

Form 1B
Pagina 1

FECHA_____
CHART NO. _____
PATIENT NO. _____

NOMBRE _____   _____

ULTIMO   PRIMERO

INSTRUCCIONES A LA PACIENTE: Favor de chequear (marcar) el cuadro si contesta sí.

1. ¿ Ha tenido usted tratamiento para enfermedades de las vías urinarias, como: piedras ☐, enfermedad de los riñones ☐, infecciones ☐, tumores ☐, lesiones ☐? (favor de marcar donde corresponda).

2. ¿ Ha tenido usted alguna vez parálisis ☐, polio ☐, multiple sclerosis ☐, serias lesiones en la espalda ☐, embolia ☐, sífilis ☐, diabetes ☐, anemia perniciosa ☐ (favor de marcar donde corresponda).

3. ¿ Ha tenido un operación en la espina ☐, el cerebro ☐, la vejiga ☐? (Favor de marcar donde corresponda).

4. ¿ Ha tenido usted infección en la vejiga durante el año pasado? ☐

5. ¿ Si contesta sí, occurrió ésto mas de dos veces durante el año pasado? ☐

6. ¿ La infección de la vejiga ocurrió después de tener relaciones íntimas en alguna ocasión? ☐

7. ¿ Tiene usted sangre en la orina a veces? ☐

8. ¿ Ha recibido usted tratamiento de dilatación de la uretra? ☐

9. ¿ Si contesta sí, cuando? _____
¿ cuantas veces? _____

10. ¿ Le ayudó la dilatación de la uretra? ☐

11. ¿ Tuvo usted dificultad en detener la orina cuando era niña? ☐

12. ¿ Cuando niña, mojaba usted la cama?

13. ¿ Si contesta sí, a qué edad se le quitó el problema de mojar la cama? _____ años

14. ¿ Moja usted la cama ahora? ☐

15. ¿ Que es la cantidad de orina que usted pasa usualmente? (Por favor marque) mucho ☐, regular ☐, poco ☐, muy poquito ☐

16. ¿ Nota usted un goteo de orina al levantarse después de haber orinado? ☐

17. ¿ Pierde usted orina repentinamente al toser fuerte ☐, estornudar ☐, vomitar ☐?

18. ¿ Si lo anterior sucede, en que posición o posiciones occure? (Favor de marcar donde corresponda) de pie ☐, sentada ☐, acostada ☐.

19. ¿ Pierde usted orina sin toser ☐, estornudar ☐, o vomitar ☐? (Favor de marcar donde corresponda).

20. ¿ Si indique que sí cuando occure? Andando ☐, corriendo ☐, haciendo fuerza ☐, acostada ☐, en cambio de posición ☐, despues de relaciones sexuales ☐, durante el acto sexual ☐.

21. ¿ Cuando esta usted orinando generalmente puede contenerse y dejar de orinar? ☐

22. ¿ Cuando empezó su problema de las vías urinarias? durante el embarzo ☐, después del nacimiento de su nene ☐?

23. ¿ Empezo su problema después de una operación? ☐

24. ¿ Si contesta sí, que operación fue:
☐ Historectomía(extirpacion de la matríz) operación abdomina (Radical ☐)
☐ Historectomía (extirpación de la matríz) operación vaginal
☐ Extirpación de un tumor, operación abdominal
☐ Operación de reparación vaginal
☐ Suspensión del útero o la vejiga
☐ Cesarea
Otro operación (Describa) _____
_____

25. ¿ Empezo su problema después del tratamiento de radiología? ☐

26. ¿ Si ya no menstrua usted, la menopausia ha empeorado su padecimiento? ☐

27. ¿ Pierde usted control de la orina cuando tose ☐, estornuda ☐, ríe ☐, levanta algo ☐, hace algun esfuerzo o vomita ☐, después de relaciones sexuales ☐, durante el acto sexual ☐?

28. ¿ Tiene usted dificultad deteniendo la orina si usted de repente se levanta después de haber estado sentada o acostada? ☐

29. ¿ Tiene usted que usar algo de protección porque se moja siempre con la orina que pierde? ☐

30. ¿ Si usa proteción a que edad empezó usted a usarlo? _____

31. ¿ Cuando usa usted proteción? (Favor de marcar donde corresponda). Algunas veces ☐, Siempre ☐, Durante el día ☐, Durante la noche ☐.

32. ¿ Es su problema de las vías urinarias lo suficientemente serio que usted desea recurrir a la cirugia para corregirlo? ☐

33. ¿ Favor de hacer una lista de las medicinas que usted esta tomando ahora?(incluyendo pastillas anticonceptivas).

Coda	Medicina	Tiempo del uso

34. ¿ Cuando pierde usted la orina accidentalmente, se da usted cuenta de que esta orinando? ☐

© 1978 DONALD R. OSTERGARD, MD

Form 1B, Page 1. History (Spanish).

DATOS BASICOS DEL SISTEMA
GINECO-UROLOGICO
HISTORIA GINECOUROLOGICA

DONALD R. OSTERGARD, M.D.
WOMEN'S HOSPITAL
MEMORIAL HOSPITAL MEDICAL CENTER
UNIVERSITY OF CALIFORNIA IRVINE
2801 ATLANTIC AVENUE, P.O. BOX 1428
LONG BEACH, CA 90801 (213) 595-3824

Form 1B
Pagina 2

FECHA_____
CHART NO. _____
PATIENT NO._____

NOMBRE_____ , _____
ULTIMO   PRIMERO

INSTRUCCIONES A LA PACIENTE: Favor de chequear (marcar) el cuadro si contesta sí.

35. ¿ Tiene usted siempre un deseo incontrolable de orinar antes de vaciar la vejiga? ☐

36. ¿ Pierde usted orina antes de

37. ¿ Si contesta sí, esta pérdida de la orina le causa dolor? ☐

38. ¿ Tiene usted que apurarse para llegar al baño ☐ o puede usted demorarse ☐ (favor de marcar donde corresponda).

39. ¿ Puede usted sobreponerse el deseo incontrolable y fuerte de orinar? Usualmente ☐, Algunas veces ☐, Rara vez ☐. (Favor de marcar donde corresponda).

40. ¿ Tiene usted una necesidad poderosa e incomoda de orinar con la vejiga llena? ☐

41. ¿ Tiene usted necesidad poderosa e incomoda de orinar con la vejiga vacia? ☐

42. ¿ Cuantas veces se levanta usted de la cama en la noche para orinar? _____ veces.

43. ¿ Cuantas veces orina usted durante la primera hora después de acostarse? _____ veces.

44. ¿ Siente usted un deseo de orinar tan fuerte e incomodo que la despierta? ☐

45. ¿ Esta usted generalmente despierta y solo orina cuando esta levantada? ☐

46. ¿ Después de orinar puede usted generalmente volverse a dormir? ☐

47. ¿ Que cantidad de líquido toma usted generalmente antes de acostarse? _____ tazas.

48. ¿ Tiene usted algun malestar en el área arriba o al lado de la vejiga? ☐

49. ¿ Tiene usted dolor al orinar? ☐

50. ¿ Tiene usted dolor durante todo el tiempo en que esta orinado? ☐

51. ¿ Siente usted dolor solamente al terminar de orinar? ☐

52. ¿ Siempre se siente que su vejiga esta vacia después de haber pasado la orina? ☐

53. ¿ Tiene usted dolor al orinar después de haber tenido relaciones íntimas? ☐

54. ¿ Siente usted la necesidad de orinar mas frecuentemente después de tener relaciones íntimas? ☐

55. ¿ La incomodidad que siente usted desaparece completamente de la vejiga después de orinar? ☐

56. ¿ Cuántas veces orina usted durante el día? cada _____ horas.

57. ¿ Es necessario para usted orinar frecuentemente? ☐

58. ¿ Cuando usted ve, oye o toca agua corriendo, ésto le causa perder la orina? ☐

59. ¿ Siente usted deseos de orinar mas frecuentemente cuando viaja en automovil? ☐

60. ¿ Esta su ropa humeda ☐, mojada ☐, empapada ☐, o deja usted charcos en el suelo ☐? (Favor de marcar donde corresponda).

61. ¿ La pérdida de orina que usted tiene consiste en un goteo constante que la mantiene mojada? ☐

62. ¿ Esta usted alguna vez sin darse cuenta de que esta a punto de perder orina o de perder el control sobre la facultad de orinar?

63. ¿ Con que frecuencia ocurre lo anterior? _____ / día _____ / semana.

64. ¿ Tiene usted generalmente dificultad en comenzar a orinar? ☐

65. ¿ Con frecuencia necesita usted que le saquen la orina por medio de un tubo debido a que no puede orinar? ☐

HISTORIA UROLOGICA DE LA FAMILIA

¿ Tienen (o tenían) su madre natural, su hermana, su tía o su abuela problemas con la pérdida de la orina cuando era nina o adulta?
(Si contesta sí, favor de contestar lo siguiente.)

	MADRE	HERMANA	TIA	ABUELA
¿ Le operaron para corregir el problema?	☐	☐	☐	☐
¿ Usaba toalla sanitaria para protejerse de la pérdida de la orina?	☐	☐	☐	☐
¿ A que edad empezó su problema de la orina?	___	___	___	___
¿ Cuantos años tuvo ud. cuando ella empezó su problema?	___	___	___	___
¿ Mojaba la cama cuando era niña?	☐	☐	☐	☐
¿ A que edad dejó de mojar la cama?	___	___	___	___

RESUMEN

En el espacio abajo, por favor describa en pocas palabras su problema de la orina. _____
_____
_____
_____
_____
_____

© 1978 DONALD R. OSTERGARD, MD

A9

Form 1B, Page 2.   History (Spanish).

URG-DATA BASE SYSTEM
URODYNAMICS AND GYNECOLOGIC UROLOGY
INITIAL HISTORY AND PHYSICAL EXAMINATION

DONALD R. OSTERGARD, M.D.
WOMEN'S HOSPITAL
MEMORIAL HOSPITAL MEDICAL CENTER
UNIVERSITY OF CALIFORNIA IRVINE
2801 ATLANTIC AVENUE, P.O. BOX 1428
LONG BEACH, CA 90801 (213) 595-3824

Form 2

Name: _____ _____
          LAST   FIRST

DATE: _____
CHART NO. _____
PATIENT NO. _____

CHECKED BOXES INDICATE APPLICABLE OR POSITVE RESPONSE.

I HISTORY

Age _____ LMP _____ Weight _____
Gravida _____ Para _____ Abortions _____
Age of Menarche _____ Age of Menopause _____
Menopausal Status: Pre ☐   Peri ☐   Post ☐
Other Positive History: _____
_____

II PHYSICAL EXAMINATION   Normal ☐

	Mild	Moderate	Severe
Cystocele	☐	☐	☐
Rectocele	☐	☐	☐
Urethral Displacement	☐	☐	☐
Enterocele	☐	☐	☐

Caruncle ☐   Fistula ☐ Type:
Other Positive Findings: _____

III NEUROLOGICAL EVALUATION   Normal ☐

Rectal Evaluation   (check if abnormal)
 Contractions-Voluntary ☐   with Cough ☐   With hold ☐
 Tone: Normal ☐   Abnormal ☐
Reflexes (check if abnormal)
 Bulbocavernosus ☐   Anal ☐: Right ☐   Left ☐
 Babinski Present ☐
 DTR's: Patellar ☐   Ankle ☐
Proprioception ☐
Sensory: L5☐ S1☐ S2☐ S3☐ S4☐   Abnormal on
Motor: L5☐ S1☐ S2☐ S3☐ S4☐   Right ☐ Left ☐
Other:

IV UROFLOWMETRY   †SPONT   †INST

	†SPONT	†INST
Voiding Mechanism — Vesical Contraction		☐
Voiding Mechanism — Urethra		*R☐ C☐ NC☐
Voiding Mechanism — Voluntary Strain		☐
Flow Rate (cc/sec) Maximum/Mean	/	/
Urine Volume (cc) In/Voided	/	/
Flowtime (sec)		
Time to Maximum Flow (sec)		
Residual Urine (cc)		
Maximum Intravesical Pressure (cm/H₂0)		
Resistance = P/F^2		
Time: UP↓ to VP↑ (sec)	+☐ -☐	
Normal voiding for patient?	YES☐ NO☐	YES☐ NO☐
Interpretation	N☐ Ab☐	N☐ Ab☐

V UROLOG SUMMARY (units = minutes/ozs)

		daytime	nighttime
Frequency	Average	q	q
	Minimum/Maximum	/	/
Voided Amount	Average		
	Minimum/Maximum	/	/

VI MISCELLANEOUS TESTS

Residual Urine _____ cc Urethral Anatomical Length _____ cm
"Q" Tip Test (Measure from Horizontal) Change: _____
   Resting Angle + ☐ – ☐ _____°
   Straining Angle + ☐ – ☐ _____°
   Rotation: _____° Direction: Right☐ Left☐

VII URETHROSCOPY   Anesthesia: Topical ☐ Local ☐

Urethro - Vesical Junction	Closes	No Change	Opens
Response to Hold	☐	☐	☐
Response to Cough	☐	☐	☐
Response to Valsalva	☐	☐	☐

Mobility: Fixed☐   Minimal☐   Moderate☐   Extreme☐
Palpation of Urethra with Scope in Place: Diverticula ☐

Description	Bladder Trigone	UV Junction	URETHRA Proximal	URETHRA Mid	URETHRA Distal
Red	☐	☐	☐	☐	☐
Granular	☐	☐	☐	☐	☐
Shaggy	☐	☐	☐	☐	☐
Polyps	☐	☐	☐	☐	☐
Cysts	☐	☐	☐	☐	☐
Exudate	☐	☐	☐	☐	☐
Diverticulum	☐	☐	☐	☐	☐
Other	☐	☐	☐	☐	☐

Photo: Frame _____
   ☐ Roll No. _____ Camera _____
Video ☐   Tape No. _____   Frames _____

VIII MEDICATIONS   None ☐

Code	Drug	Dose	Freq.	Dur/Treatment	Rx'd
	Macrodantin	50 mg.	tid	5 days	
	Vaginal Estrogen	—			
	Pyridium	100 mg	tid	3 days	

IX TREATMENT PROCEDURES   None ☐

Anesthesia: Local ☐   Topical ☐   Calibration To _____ F
Dilatation to _____ F   Bleeding ☐   Pain ☐

X SUMMARY OF MEDICAL HISTORY and SELF EVALUATION

☐ Dysuria _____ + ☐ Freq. q. _____ hrs. ☐ Urgency _____ +
☐ Nocturia ✕ _____   Incontinence: ☐ Stress _____ +
☐ Post Void Fullness _____ +   ☐ Urge _____ +

LAB ORDERED: Urine C&S ☐   Negative ☐ Positive ☐   ON _____
OTHER ☐
RETURN APPOINTMENT:

© 1978 DONALD R. OSTERGARD MD
*R=RELAXES   C=CONTRACTS NC=NO CHANGE † =SPONTANEOUS/INSTRUMENTED _____ MD.   A10

Form 2.   Initial history and physical exam.

URG-DATA BASE SYSTEM
URODYNAMICS AND GYNECOLOGIC UROLOGY
URODYNAMICS VISIT SUMMARY

DONALD R. OSTERGARD, M.D.
WOMEN'S HOSPITAL
MEMORIAL HOSPITAL MEDICAL CENTER
UNIVERSITY OF CALIFORNIA IRVINE
2801 ATLANTIC AVENUE, P.O. BOX 1428
LONG BEACH, CA 90801 (213) 595-3824

FORM 3
PAGE 1

New ☐
Returning ☐
Postpartum _____ Weeks
DATE _____
CHART NO. _____
PATIENT NO. _____

NAME _____ _____
LAST   FIRST

CHECKED BOXES INDICATE APPLICABLE OR POSITIVE RESPONSE

I. CURRENT MEDICATIONS   None ☐

CODE	DRUG*	DOSE	FREQ.	DUR. OF USE	SUBJECTIVE RESPONSE**
					1—5—10
					1—5—10
					1—5—10

*includes contraceptives
** <5 = worse, 5 = no response, >5 = better, 10 = cured

II. SUBJECTIVE RESPONSES TO PREVIOUS TREATMENTS   NONE ☐

TREATMENT	RESPONSE	COMMENTS
Dilatation	1____ 5____ 10	
Cryosurgery	1____ 5____ 10	
	1____ 5____ 10	
	1____ 5____ 10	
	1____ 5____ 10	

III. INTERVAL HISTORY   LMP _____   CYCLE DAY NO. _____

Dysuria: ☐ _____ + Freq ☐ q _____ hrs. Urgency ☐ _____ +
Nocturia: ☐ × _____ Incontinence: Stress ☐ _____
Post Void Fullness ☐ _____ + Urge ☐ _____ +

IV. CYSTOMETRICS and EMG

		H_2O	CO_2
VOLUME	FIRST SENSATION	_____ cc	_____ cc
	FULLNESS	_____ cc	
	MAXIMUM	_____ cc	_____ cc

VOUNTARY TERMINAL CONTRACTION   None ☐

	Inhibited	☐	☐
	Uninhibited	☐	☐
Urethral Sphincter Response	Relaxes	†P☐ †E☐	P☐ E☐
	Contracts	P☐ E☐	P☐ E☐
	No Change	P☐ E☐	P☐ E☐
Pressure Change (cmH_2O)		+ ☐	+ ☐
Anal Sphincter Response	Relaxes	E☐	E☐
	Contracts	E☐	E☐
	No Change	E☐	E☐

VESICAL CONTRACTIONS   None ☐

	Inhibited	☐	☐
	Uninhibited	☐	☐
Spontaneous		☐	☐
Induced by:	Jolt	☐	☐
	Cough	☐	☐
	Filling	☐	☐
Bladder Volume		_____ cc	_____ cc
Urethral Sphincter Response	Relaxes	P☐ E☐	P☐ E☐
	Contracts	P☐ E☐	P☐ E☐
	No Change	P☐ E☐	P☐ E☐
Pressure Change (cmH_2O)		+ ☐	+ ☐
Anal Sphincter Response	Relaxes	E☐	E☐
	Contracts	E☐	E☐
	No Change	E☐	E☐

†P = Pressure Response   E = EMG Response

V. URETHRAL PRESSURE and EMG

		Sitting		Standing		Units
		Bladder Filling				
		Empty	Full	Empty	Full	
PROFILE: Area						Cm²
LENGTH	Functional					Cm
	Total					Cm
PRESSURE	Closing					CmH_2O
	Maximum					CmH_2O
DISTANCE: Bladder → Max						Cm
Max → Zero						Cm

URETHRAL SPHINCTER RESPONSE   (@Maximum Urethral Pressure)

	Sitting Empty	Sitting Full	Standing Empty	Standing Full	
Relaxes	P☐ E☐	P☐ E☐	P☐ E☐	P☐ E☐	
Contracts	P☐ E☐	P☐ E☐	P☐ E☐	P☐ E☐	
No Change	P☐ E☐	P☐ E☐	P☐ E☐	P☐ E☐	
Urethral Pressure Change	+ / −	+ / −	+ / −	+ / −	CmH_2O
Vesical Pressure Change	+ / −	+ / −	+ / −	+ / −	CmH_2O
Actual Urethral Pressure Change	+ / −	+ / −	+ / −	+ / −	CmH_2O
TRUE INTRA-VESICAL PRESSURE					CmH_2O

CLOSING PRESSURE						
	Strain	+ −	+ −	+ −	+ −	CmH_2O
	Cough	+ −	+ −	+ −	+ −	
	Jolt	+ −	+ −	+ −	+ −	
PRESSURE EQUALIZATION		+ −	+ −	+ −	+ −	
COUGH UCPP		+ −	+ −	+ −	+ −	

VI. URETHROSCOPY: ANESTHESIA: Topical ☐   Local ☐

URETHRO-VESICAL JUNCTION	Closes	No Change	Opens
Response to Hold	☐	☐	☐
Response to Cough	☐	☐	☐
Response to Valsalva	☐	☐	☐

Mobility: Fixed ☐ Minimal ☐ Moderate ☐ Extreme ☐
Palpation of Urethra with Scope in Place: Diverticula ☐

DESCRIPTION	Bladder Trigone	UV Junction	URETHRA Proximal	URETHRA Mid	URETHRA Distal
Red	☐	☐	☐	☐	☐
Granular	☐	☐	☐	☐	☐
Shaggy	☐	☐	☐	☐	☐
Polyps	☐	☐	☐	☐	☐
Cysts	☐	☐	☐	☐	☐
Exudate	☐	☐	☐	☐	☐
Diverticulum	☐	☐	☐	☐	☐
Other					

Photo: Frames ☐   Roll No. _____ Camera _____
Video _____ Tape No. _____ Frames _____

© 1978 Donald R. Ostergard, M.D.   A11

Form 3, Page 1. Visit summary (urodynamics).

URG DATA BASE SYSTEM
URODYNAMICS AND GYNECOLOGIC UROLOGY
URODYNAMICS VISIT SUMMARY

DONALD R. OSTERGARD, M.D.
WOMEN'S HOSPITAL
MEMORIAL HOSPITAL MEDICAL CENTER
UNIVERSITY OF CALIFORNIA IRVINE
2801 ATLANTIC AVENUE, P.O. BOX 1428
LONG BEACH, CA 90801 (213) 595-3824

FORM 3
PAGE 2

DATE _____
CHART NO. _____
PATIENT NO. _____

NAME _____
        Last   First

CHECKED BOXES INDICATE APPLICABLE OR POSITIVE RESPONSE

VII. MISCELLANEOUS UROLOGICAL

Urolog Summary (units = minutes/ozs)

Frequency:		Daytime	Nighttime
Average		q	q
Minimum / Maximum		/	/
Voided Amount: Average		ozs	ozs
Minimum / Maximum		/	/

VIII. ELECTROMYOGRAPHIC STIMULATION

Anal Sphincter response to urethral stimulation:
Normal ☐ Abnormal ☐ Latency _____ Msec

Perineal Relaxation:
No Effect ☐   Response: Abolished ☐ Decreased ☐

Interpretation: Normal ☐ Abnormal ☐

IX. UROFLOWMETRY   † SPONT.   † INST.

Voiding Mechanism	Vesical Contractions	☐	☐
	Urethra	* R☐ C☐ NC☐	* R☐ C☐ NC☐
	Voluntary Strain	☐	☐
Flow Rate (cc/sec) Max/Mean		/	/
Urine Volume (cc) In/Voided		/	/
Flowtime (sec)			
Time to Max. Flow (sec)			
Residual Urine (cc)			
Max. Intravesical Press. (cm/H_2O)			
Resistance = P/F^2			
Time: UP to VP (sec)		☐☐ ___	☐☐ ___
Normal Voiding for patient?		yes☐ no☐	yes☐ no☐
Interpretation		N☐ Ab☐	N☐ Ab☐

X. MEDICATIONS   None☐

Code	Drug	Dose	Freq.	Duration/Treatment	Rx'd
	Macrodantin	50 mg		3 days	
	Vaginal Estrogen				
	Pyridium	100 mg		5days	

XI. TREATMENT PROCEDURES   None ☐

Anesthesia: Local ☐ Topical ☐

Dilation ☐ To _____F   Bleeding ☐

Calibration   To _____I   Pain ☐

Distention ☐:   Diverticula ☐   Other ☐

Cryosurgery ☐ (See Form 5) Polyps ☐   Caruncled ☐

Surgery: Suspension ☐ Anterior Repair ☐ Sling ☐
Diverticulectomy ☐ Repeat ☐ Other ☐ Spence ☐
Urethrotomy ☐ Dilation ☐ To _____F

XII. LABORATORY

Urine C&S ordered ☐:
  Neg ☐ Pos ☐ on _____ (date)

XIII. XRAYS   VCUG ☐   TRATNER ☐   IVP ☐

XIV. CONSULTATIONS REQUESTED   CYSTOSCOPY ☐

Psychiatry ☐ Urology ☐ Neurology ☐ EMG ☐ Other ☐

XV. DIAGNOSIS codes: No Change ☐

1._____
   _____ Code: _____

2._____
   _____ Code: _____

3._____
   _____ Code: _____

4._____
   _____ Code: _____

COMMENTS/INTERVAL HISTORY AND SELF EVALUATION SUMMARY

† SPONTANEOUS \ INSTRUMENTED   * R=RELAXES   C=CONTRACTS   NC=NO CHANGE

©1978 DONALD R. OSTERGARD, MD

RETURN APPOINTMENT DATE _____   _____ MD   A12

Form 3, Page 2.   Visit summary (urodynamics).

URG-DATA BASE SYSTEM
URODYNAMICS AND GYNECOLOGIC UROLOGY
ROUTINE VISIT SUMMARY

DONALD R. OSTERGARD, M.D.
WOMEN'S HOSPITAL
MEMORIAL HOSPITAL MEDICAL CENTER
UNIVERSITY OF CALIFORNIA IRVINE
2801 ATLANTIC AVENUE, P.O. BOX 1428
LONG BEACH, CA 90801 (213) 595-3824

New ☐   FORM 4
Returning ☐
Postpartum _____ Weeks
DATE: _____
CHART NO. _____
PATIENT NO. _____

NAME _____ _____
                Last   First
CHECKED BOXES INDICATE APPLICABLE OR POSITIVE RESPONSES

I. CURRENT MEDICATIONS   None ☐

CODE	DRUG*	DOSE	FREQ.	DUR. OF USE	SUBJECTIVE RESPONSE**
					1__5__10
					1__5__10
					1__5__10

* includes contraceptives
** < 5 = worse 5 = no response > 5 = improved 10 = no symptoms

II. SUBJECTIVE RESPONSES TO PREVIOUS TREATMENTS   None ☐

TREATMENT	RESPONSE	COMMENTS
Dilatation	1___5___10	
Cryosurgery	1___5___10	
	1___5___10	
	1___5___10	
	1___5___10	

III. INTERVAL HISTORY LMP_____ CYCLE DAY NO._____

Dysuria: ☐____ + Freq ☐ q____hrs. Urgency ☐ _____+
Nocturia: ☐ × _____   Incontinence: Stress ☐ _____+
Post Void Fullness ☐_____+   Urge ☐ _____+

IV. URETHROSCOPY: Anesthesia: Topical ☐ Local ☐

Urethro - Vesical Junction	Closes	No Change	Opens
Response to Hold	☐	☐	☐
Response to Cough	☐	☐	☐
Response to Valsalva	☐	☐	☐

Mobility: Fixed ☐   Minimal ☐   Moderate ☐   Extreme ☐
Palpation of Urethra with Scope in Place: Diverticula ☐

Description	Bladder Trigone	UV Junction	URETHRA Proximal	Mid	Distal
Red	☐	☐	☐	☐	☐
Granular	☐	☐	☐	☐	☐
Shaggy	☐	☐	☐	☐	☐
Polyps	☐	☐	☐	☐	☐
Cysts	☐	☐	☐	☐	☐
Exudate	☐	☐	☐	☐	☐
Diverticulum	☐	☐	☐	☐	☐
Other					

Photo: Frame _____
☐ Roll No.   Camera _____
Video ☐   Tape No. _____   Frames _____

V. MISCELLANEOUS UROLOGICAL

Urolog Summary (units = minutes/ozs)

		daytime	nighttime
Frequency	Average	q	q
	Minimum/Maximum	/	/
Voided Amount	Average		
	Minimum/Maximum	/	/

VI. UROFLOWMETRY   SPONT.   INST.

			SPONT.	INST.
Voiding Mechanism		Vesical Contraction		☐
		Urethra		+R☐ C☐ NC☐
		Voluntary Strain		☐
	Flow Rate(cc/sec) Maximum/Mean		/	/
	Urine Volume (cc) In/Voided		/	/
	Flowtime (sec)			
	Time to Maximum Flow (sec)			
	Residual Urine (cc)			
Maximum Intravesical Pressure(cm/H$_2$0)				
Resistance = P/F2				
Time: UP↓ to VP↑ (sec)				☐ ☐
Normal Voiding for patient?			YES☐ NO☐	YES☐ NO☐
Interpretation			N☐ Ab☐	N☐ Ab☐

VII. TREATMENT PROCEDURES   None ☐

Anesthesia: Local ☐   General ☐   Topical ☐
Dilation ☐ To _____ F   Bleeding ☐
Calibration To _____ F   Pain ☐
Cryosurgery ☐   (See Form 5)
Surgery: Suspension ☐ Anterior Repair ☐ Sling ☐
Diverticulectomy ☐ Repeat ☐ Other ☐ Spence ☐
Urethrotomy ☐   Dilation ☐ To_____F

VIII. MEDICATIONS   None ☐

Code	Drug	Dose	Freq.	Dur/Treatment	Rx'd
	Macro-dantin	50 mg.	tid	5 days	
	Vaginal Estrogen				
	Pyridium	100 mg	tid	3 days	

IX. LABORATORY

Urine C&S ordered ☐:
Negative ☐ Positive ☐ on_____(date)

X. XRAYS   VCUG ☐   TRATNER ☐   IVP ☐

XI. CONSULTATIONS REQUESTED: CYSTOSCOPY ☐

Psychiatry ☐ Urology ☐ Neurology ☐ EMG ☐ Other ☐

XII. DIAGNOSIS codes: No Change ☐

1. _____
   _____ Code: _____
2. _____
   _____ Code: _____

COMMENTS:

© 1978 DONALD R. OSTERGARD, MD

+ R = RELAXES   C = CONTRACTS   NC = NO CHANGE   RETURN APPOINTMENT DATE _____ _____MD.   A13
† = SPONTANEOUS/INSTRUMENTED

Form 4.   Visit summary (routine).

URG-DATA BASE SYSTEM
URODYNAMICS AND GYNECOLOGIC UROLOGY
MISCELLANEOUS SPECIAL EVALUATIONS

DONALD R. OSTERGARD, M.D.
WOMEN'S HOSPITAL
MEMORIAL HOSPITAL MEDICAL CENTER
UNIVERSITY OF CALIFORNIA IRVINE
2801 ATLANTIC AVENUE, P.O. BOX 1428
LONG BEACH, CA 90801 (213) 595-3824

FORM 5

NAME _____ , _____
Last   First

DATE: _____
CHART NO. _____
PATIENT NO. _____

CHECKED BOXES INDICATE APPLICABLE OR POSITIVE RESPONSE

I. SPECIAL EVALUATIONS

☐ Ice Water Test
_____ cc Introduced into Bladder
Time to Expulsion _____ sec. ____ No Expulsion ☐
Maximum Bladder Pressure _____ cm H_2O
Subjective Sensation:
None ☐ Mild ☐ Moderate ☐ Severe ☐
Interpretation: Normal ☐ Abnormal ☐

CRYOSURGERY

	Bladder Trigone	UV Junction	URETHRA Proximal	URETHRA Mid	URETHRA Distal
Temp. °C	____ °C	____ °C	____ °C	____ °C	____ °C
TIME	____ sec	____ sec	____ sec	____ sec	____ sec
	____ sec	____ sec	____ sec	____ sec	____ sec
	____ sec	____ sec	____ sec	____ sec	____ sec

☐ Propantheline Test ☐ Bethanechol Test
☐ Phentolamine Test (minutes after injection: _____)
☐ Pudendal Block (minutes after injection: _____)
☐ Alpha Stimulation Test _____

NOTES

		Baseline	15 min	30 min	Units
Pulse/BP		/	/	/	
UCPP (Empty)	Max. Pressure				cmH₂O
	Closing Pressure				cmH₂O
	Functional Length				cm
UCPP (Full)	Max. Pressure				cmH₂O
	Closing Pressure				cmH₂O
	Functional Length				cm
Cystometry	1st Desire Vol				cc
CO₂ ☐	Fullness Volume				cc
H₂O ☐	Capacity				cc
	Uninhibited Contr.	YES☐ NO ☐	YES☐ NO ☐	YES☐ NO ☐	
Uroflow	Voiding pressure				cmH₂O
	Maximum Flow				cc/sec
	Voided Volume				cc
	Resistance				

Therapeutic Benefit Anticipated   yes ☐   no ☐

COMMENTS:

A14

Form 5.   Miscellaneous special evaluations.

URG-DATA BASE SYSTEM
URODYNAMICS AND GYNECOLOGIC UROLOGY
PATIENT'S RESPONSE CHART

DONALD R. OSTERGARD, M.D.
WOMEN'S HOSPITAL
MEMORIAL HOSPITAL MEDICAL CENTER
UNIVERSITY OF CALIFORNIA IRVINE
2801 ATLANTIC AVENUE, P.O. BOX 1428
LONG BEACH, CA 90801 (213) 595-3824

Form 6A

DATE _____
CHART NO. _____
PATIENT NO. _____

NAME _____ , _____
　　　　　　　Last　　　　　　　　　　　First

INSTRUCTIONS

You are under treatment for your urinary complaints. We are anxious to learn more from you regarding your urinary problem and any change which may occur. We are also interested in any other symptom that is currently present or may develop in your general condition. The accurate completion of this form will enable us to help you in the best way possible. Below is a list of symptoms. Each is followed by 4 columns with dates marked at the top. On the date indicated, please circle the correct choice for each item.

THE NUMBERS REFER TO THESE PHRASES:

0 - NONE
1 - A LITTLE
2 - SOME
3 - QUITE A BIT
4 - UNBEARABLE

Reporting Date	——	——	——	——
Number of capsules this date	——	——	——	——
1) Nausea	0 1 2 3 4	0 1 2 3 4	0 1 2 3 4	0 1 2 3 4
2) Vomiting	0 1 2 3 4	0 1 2 3 4	0 1 2 3 4	0 1 2 3 4
3) Diarrhea	0 1 2 3 4	0 1 2 3 4	0 1 2 3 4	0 1 2 3 4
4) Loss of appetite	0 1 2 3 4	0 1 2 3 4	0 1 2 3 4	0 1 2 3 4
5) Dryness of mouth	0 1 2 3 4	0 1 2 3 4	0 1 2 3 4	0 1 2 3 4
6) Dizziness	0 1 2 3 4	0 1 2 3 4	0 1 2 3 4	0 1 2 3 4
7) Weakness	0 1 2 3 4	0 1 2 3 4	0 1 2 3 4	0 1 2 3 4
8) Change of vision	0 1 2 3 4	0 1 2 3 4	0 1 2 3 4	0 1 2 3 4
9) Sleeplessness	0 1 2 3 4	0 1 2 3 4	0 1 2 3 4	0 1 2 3 4
10) Sleepiness	0 1 2 3 4	0 1 2 3 4	0 1 2 3 4	0 1 2 3 4
11) Palpitations	0 1 2 3 4	0 1 2 3 4	0 1 2 3 4	0 1 2 3 4
12) Trembling	0 1 2 3 4	0 1 2 3 4	0 1 2 3 4	0 1 2 3 4
13) Nervousness	0 1 2 3 4	0 1 2 3 4	0 1 2 3 4	0 1 2 3 4
14) Tension	0 1 2 3 4	0 1 2 3 4	0 1 2 3 4	0 1 2 3 4
15) Depression	0 1 2 3 4	0 1 2 3 4	0 1 2 3 4	0 1 2 3 4
16) Uncomfortably strong need to pass urine	0 1 2 3 4	0 1 2 3 4	0 1 2 3 4	0 1 2 3 4
17) Burning when passing urine	0 1 2 3 4	0 1 2 3 4	0 1 2 3 4	0 1 2 3 4
18) Sensation of continued need to pass urine after emptying bladder	0 1 2 3 4	0 1 2 3 4	0 1 2 3 4	0 1 2 3 4
19) Loss of urine with coughing or straining	0 1 2 3 4	0 1 2 3 4	0 1 2 3 4	0 1 2 3 4
20) Loss of urine before reaching toilet	0 1 2 3 4	0 1 2 3 4	0 1 2 3 4	0 1 2 3 4
21) Lower abdominal pressure	0 1 2 3 4	0 1 2 3 4	0 1 2 3 4	0 1 2 3 4
22) Lower abdominal pain	0 1 2 3 4	0 1 2 3 4	0 1 2 3 4	0 1 2 3 4
25) Backache	0 1 2 3 4	0 1 2 3 4	0 1 2 3 4	0 1 2 3 4
24) Painful intercourse	0 1 2 3 4	0 1 2 3 4	0 1 2 3 4	0 1 2 3 4
25) Indicate number of headaches in last 24 hours.	——	——	——	——
26) Indicate number of hours between times you pass urine.	——	——	——	——
27) Indicate number of times you pass urine at night.	——	——	——	——
28) Indicate number of times you pass urine during first hour after going to bed.	——	——	——	——
PHYSICIAN USE ONLY:				
LMP _____ Cycle Day	——	——	——	——

A15

Form 6A. Patient's response chart (English).

DATOS BASICOS DEL SISTEMA GINECO –
UROLOGICO
HOJA DE REPUESTAS DE LA PACIENTE

DONALD R. OSTERGARD, M.D.
WOMEN'S HOSPITAL
MEMORIAL HOSPITAL MEDICAL CENTER
UNIVERSITY OF CALIFORNIA IRVINE
2801 ATLANTIC AVENUE, P.O. BOX 1428
LONG BEACH, CA 90801 (213) 595-3824

Form 6B

FECHA: _____
CHART NO. _____
PATIENT NO. _____

Nombre _____

INSTRUCCIONES

Usted esta bajo tratamiento para su padecimiento de las vías urinarias. Estamos deseosos de conocer más a fondo los detalles de su problema de las vías urinarias y estar al tanto de cualquier cambio que pueda ocurrir. Estamos tambien interesados en cualquier otro síntoma que esta presente en estos momentos o puede desarrollarse en su estado general. El llenar esta forma con exactitud nos ayudará a atender a usted en la mejor forma posible. Cada uno de estos, tiene 4 columnas con fechas marcadas arriba. En la fecha indicada, por favor haga un circulo en la contestación correcta para cada síntoma.

LOS NUMEROS SE REFIEREN
A ESTAS FASES:

0 - NINGUNA
1 - UN POCO
2 - ALGO
3 - BASTANTE
4 - INAGUANTABLE

1) Nausea	0 1 2 3 4	0 1 2 3 4	0 1 2 3 4	0 1 2 3 4
2) Vómito	0 1 2 3 4	0 1 2 3 4	0 1 2 3 4	0 1 2 3 4
3) Diarrea	0 1 2 3 4	0 1 2 3 4	0 1 2 3 4	0 1 2 3 4
4) Pérdida de apetito	0 1 2 3 4	0 1 2 3 4	0 1 2 3 4	0 1 2 3 4
5) Boca seca	0 1 2 3 4	0 1 2 3 4	0 1 2 3 4	0 1 2 3 4
6) Mareos	0 1 2 3 4	0 1 2 3 4	0 1 2 3 4	0 1 2 3 4
7) Debilidad	0 1 2 3 4	0 1 2 3 4	0 1 2 3 4	0 1 2 3 4
8) Problemas de la vista	0 1 2 3 4	0 1 2 3 4	0 1 2 3 4	0 1 2 3 4
9) Falta de sueño	0 1 2 3 4	0 1 2 3 4	0 1 2 3 4	0 1 2 3 4
10) Exceso de sueño	0 1 2 3 4	0 1 2 3 4	0 1 2 3 4	0 1 2 3 4
11) Palpitaciones	0 1 2 3 4	0 1 2 3 4	0 1 2 3 4	0 1 2 3 4
12) Temblor	0 1 2 3 4	0 1 2 3 4	0 1 2 3 4	0 1 2 3 4
13) Nerviosidad	0 1 2 3 4	0 1 2 3 4	0 1 2 3 4	0 1 2 3 4
14) Tensión	0 1 2 3 4	0 1 2 3 4	0 1 2 3 4	0 1 2 3 4
15) Depresión	0 1 2 3 4	0 1 2 3 4	0 1 2 3 4	0 1 2 3 4
16) Deseo incontrolable de orinar	0 1 2 3 4	0 1 2 3 4	0 1 2 3 4	0 1 2 3 4
17) Ardor al orinar	0 1 2 3 4	0 1 2 3 4	0 1 2 3 4	0 1 2 3 4
18) Sensación de necesidad de seguir orinando aun después de haber vaciado la vejiga	0 1 2 3 4	0 1 2 3 4	0 1 2 3 4	0 1 2 3 4
19) Perdida de orina al toser	0 1 2 3 4	0 1 2 3 4	0 1 2 3 4	0 1 2 3 4
20) Pérdida de orina antes de llegar al baño	0 1 2 3 4	0 1 2 3 4	0 1 2 3 4	0 1 2 3 4
21) Presión en la región púbica	0 1 2 3 4	0 1 2 3 4	0 1 2 3 4	0 1 2 3 4
22) Dolor en la parte inferior del abdomen	0 1 2 3 4	0 1 2 3 4	0 1 2 3 4	0 1 2 3 4
23) Dolor de espalda	0 1 2 3 4	0 1 2 3 4	0 1 2 3 4	0 1 2 3 4
24) Dolor al tener relaciones intimas	0 1 2 3 4	0 1 2 3 4	0 1 2 3 4	0 1 2 3 4
25) Indique cuantos dolores de cabeza en las últimas 24 horas	_____	_____	_____	_____
26) Indique cada cuantas horas tiene que orinar	_____	_____	_____	_____
27) Cuantas veces orina en la noche?	_____	_____	_____	_____
28) Indique el número de veces que orina durante la primera hora despés de que va a la cama	_____	_____	_____	_____
Para el Medico Solamente: LMP _____ Cycle Day _____	_____	_____	_____	_____

A16

Form 6B. Patient's response chart (Spanish).

URG - DATA BASE SYSTEM
URODYNAMICS AND GYNECOLOGIC UROLOGY
RADIOLOGIC PROCEDURES

DONALD R. OSTERGARD, M.D.
WOMEN'S HOSPITAL
MEMORIAL HOSPITAL MEDICAL CENTER
UNIVERSITY OF CALIFORNIA IRVINE
2801 ATLANTIC AVENUE, P.O. BOX 1428
LONG BEACH, CA 90801 (213) 595-3824

NAME _____ , _____

First   Last

DATE _____
CHART NO. _____
PATIENT NO. _____

DYNAMIC CYSTOURETHROGAPHY

Volume of contrast used: _____ cc.

Supine or scout films: Reflux ☐

Diverticula ☐
Bladder ☐
Urethra ☐

VIEW	NON-STRAIN	STRAIN
AP (Erect with catheter)	Cystocele ☐ Funneling ☐ Vesical Neck Displacement _____ cm Other: _____ _____ _____ _____	Cystocle ☐ Funneling ☐ Vesical Neck Displacement _____ cm Other: _____ _____ _____ _____

Lateral (erect with catheter)	Describe:
	    Urethral
	        Displacement ☐
	       Cystocele ☐
	       Funneling ☐
	Other: _____
	_____
	_____
		UV angle: no change ☐
		           flattens ☐
		Vesical neck Displacement: _____ cm
		Urethral Displacement ☐
		Cystocele ☐
		Other: _____
		_____
		_____

Oblique (erect without catheter)	Describe: _____ _____ _____ _____ _____ _____ _____	Response to cough: True SI ☐ Delayed urine loss ☐ Other: _____ _____ _____ _____ _____

VOIDING CYSTOURETHROUGRAPHY	URETHROGRAM

Urethral Appearance
  Normal   ☐
  Abnormal ☐
Obstruction
  Yes ☐
  No ☐
	Normal ☐
	Diverticula ☐ Number _____
	Location: Normal ☐
	             Distal ☐
	             Proximal ☐

Diagnosis: _____
_____
_____
_____
_____
_____

Comments: _____
_____
_____
_____
_____
_____
_____

Code _____ _____ _____

_____ M.D.

A17

Form 7. Radiologic procedures.

URG-DATA BASE SYSTEM
URODYNAMICS AND GYNECOLOGIC UROLOGY
UROLOG

DONALD R. OSTERGARD, M.D.
WOMEN'S HOSPITAL
MEMORIAL HOSPITAL MEDICAL CENTER
UNIVERSITY OF CALIFORNIA IRVINE
2801 ATLANTIC AVENUE, P.O. BOX 1428
LONG BEACH, CA 90801 (213) 595-3824

FORM 8

DATE _____
CHART NO. _____
PATIENT NO. _____

NAME: _____ , _____
　　　　　　　　Last　　　　　　　　　First

INSTRUCTIONS : EACH TIME YOU PASS URINE, WRITE DOWN THE TIME AND THE AMOUNT OF URINE WHICH YOU PASS.

TIME	AMOUNT	TIME	AMOUNT

© 1978 DONALD R. OSTERGARD, MD

A18

Form 8. Urolog.

**URG-DATA BASE SYSTEM
URODYNAMICS AND GYNECOLOGIC
UROLOGY PATIENT SUMMARY**

DONALD R. OSTERGARD, M.D.
WOMEN'S HOSPITAL
MEMORIAL HOSPITAL MEDICAL CENTER
UNIVERSITY OF CALIFORNIA IRVINE
2801 ATLANTIC AVENUE, P.O. BOX 1428
LONG BEACH, CA 90801 (213) 595-3824

Form 9

DATE _____
CHARTNO. _____
PATIENT NO. _____

NAME _____ / _____
　　　　Last　　　　　　　First

I. PATIENT DATA

Address _____　　Tel. No. ( ) _____
Birthdate _____　Marital Status: M☐ S☐ D☐ P☐ W☐　Race: W☐ N☐ S☐ O☐ AI☐
Also Known as _____　　Soc. Sec. No. _____
Spouse: Name _____ Address _____
　　　　　　　　　　　　　　　Tel. No. ( ) _____

Person who will always be aware of patient's whereabouts—Relationship: _____
　　Name _____ Address _____
　　　　　　　　　　　　　　　Tel. No. ( ) _____

Referred by Physician
　　Name _____ Address _____
　　　　　　　　　　　　　　　Tel. No. ( ) _____

VISIT SUMMARY (One line per visit)　　　　　**INITIALS**

Urine C&S☐

SPECIAL NOTES:　　　　　　　　　　　　A19

© 1978 DONALD R. OSTERGARD, MD

Form 9. Patient summary.

Index

Index